Controversies in Clear Aligner Therapy

Anderson T. Huang • Darren Huang

Controversies in Clear Aligner Therapy

Contemporary Perspectives, Limitations, and Solutions

Springer

Anderson T. Huang
Department of Orthodontics
New York University, College of Dentistry
New York, NY, USA

Darren Huang
Department of Orthodontics
New York University, College of Dentistry
New York, NY, USA

ISBN 978-3-030-92809-4 ISBN 978-3-030-92810-0 (eBook)
https://doi.org/10.1007/978-3-030-92810-0

This Springer imprint is published by the registered company Springer Nature Switzerland AG
The registered company address is: Gewerbestrasse 11, 6330 Cham, Switzerland

For Johnny

Foreword

Authoring an orthodontic textbook to address controversies is refreshing, ambitious, and evidence of self-reflection by the authors who have gained a good amount of experience with clear aligners. In the age of evidence-based practice in health care, this was a much-needed effort to examine critically, 22 years after the launch of *Invisalign*, the current knowledge regarding the treatment of malocclusions with clear aligners.

As Chair of the Department at New York University where Drs. Anderson and Darren Huang teach orthodontics, I am honored to write the Foreword to their book, **Controversies in Clear Aligner Therapy: Contemporary Perspectives, Limitations, and Solutions**. They are both graduates of the College of Dentistry and of the Advanced Education programs. Dr. Anderson Huang's long interest in clear aligner therapy has been well known in the Department of Orthodontics for many years. He is joined by his son Darren, a more recent graduate, who shares the same clinical interest and educational perspectives. As orthodontists, neither one is inclined to settle for less than excellence.

One of my goals as Chair of the Department of Orthodontics is to educate students to consider the best interest of the patients they care for, and therefore to adopt a best-practice approach to treatment planning. With this in mind, there is a dearth of books devoted to clear aligners other than those which explain how to use the appliances and how to plan and sequence tooth movements with the aligners. As a practitioner, I find such information much needed, and I believe that sharing one's experience on any treatment modality with one's orthodontist peers is valuable and respectable. Like many, I was at first a dubious user of clear aligners for orthodontic treatment. Some movements, such as extrusion or rotations, were difficult to accomplish and frequently required fixed appliances to achieve treatment goals to satisfaction.

It is undeniable that 20 years later, orthodontic treatment with clear aligners has become more sophisticated; for example, the software platforms have made communication with technicians easier. With software improvements, practitioners have learned to plan tooth movement better, and this brought their treatment goals and planning to higher grounds. However, despite these improvements, there are still many global questions practitioners have regarding this treatment modality no matter the type of aligner one may prefer or select.

What sets this work apart is the authors' reflections and their acknowledgement that there are debate and disagreements on the effectiveness of clear aligners. To name a few: their use during interceptive treatment, as substitute to functional appliances, the predictability of root movements, is there too much interproximal enamel reduction being used, or excessive expansion prescribed. Additionally, how effectively can one correct an open bite with clear aligners, when many have been humbled by attempting bite closure with mere fixed appliances.

Such reflective work is welcome by all orthodontists interested in using clear aligners on a routine basis. After all, it took many years of practice and learning from mistakes to master the use of fixed appliances whether on the labial or lingual side of the dental arches. For those who first thought that clear aligners would be the panacea of orthodontic treatment, one just needs to recall the enthusiasm generated by the wide accessibility to straight-wire appliances and the belief that orthodontic treatment could be rendered by any practitioner no matter their degree of knowledge or experience.

I think you will find this book very useful and refreshing to read; you are not the only one to have questions, strong convictions, and doubts, and yet wish to better yourself in treating patients with clear aligners because you understand that they are here to stay.

I applaud Drs. Anderson and Darren Huang for researching and writing this book, for being thorough in their thinking, and for demonstrating critical judgment on the efficacy of treatment with clear aligners. With these efforts, we are all going to improve our treatment of patients with clear aligners.

Olivier Nicolay
Chair, Department of Orthodontics
New York University
New York, NY, USA
August 30, 2021

Preface

Since the introduction of the Invisalign appliance in 1999, clear aligner therapy has gradually become a significant modality of orthodontic treatment for the modern orthodontist and an area of intensive scientific research in the orthodontic field. The first clear aligners were limited to the treatment of mild malocclusions in adult patients. In the last 20 years, technological developments in clear aligner software, improvements in aligner materials and their functionality, and innovations in treatment methods have expanded the capabilities of clear aligner therapy for the treatment of complex malocclusions in children, adolescents, and adults. Clear aligner therapy is rapidly evolving and represents one of the next frontiers for orthodontic treatment.

Despite these advances, clear aligner therapy remains limited by significant deficiencies resulting in clinical dilemmas for the practitioner, from the use of clear aligners for interceptive treatment, complex movements, Class II therapy, overcorrection, to the treatment of vertical problems. With the rapid growth of clear aligner therapy within the field, there has arisen a dense forest of contradictory and controversial opinions and methodologies for treatment. Our own experience with clear aligner therapy has been a humbling but enlightening process, one in which we have had to negotiate the appliance's limitations over the course of its evolution. Additionally, aside from a limited number of systematic reviews and meta-analyses, there are few texts that deeply engage with the limitations of clear aligner therapy and their implications. Therefore, there exists a need for a critical appraisal of the current body of knowledge to determine viable treatment approaches in addressing these dilemmas.

To address this need, we do not intend this book to be an exhaustive survey of clear aligner therapy or a stepwise guide with generalized formulas for the management of malocclusions with clear aligners. Instead, our aim is to provide rigorous, scientific evidence-based evaluations of the current status of knowledge regarding controversial dilemmas within clear aligner therapy, while mapping out solutions for their management. Each chapter will focus on a dilemma, which we have frequently encountered in clinical practice and the scientific literature. We will comprehensively analyze each dilemma with a discussion of the current state of affairs in the context of the latest research, its clinical implications including the limitations the dilemma bears on the treatment of specific malocclusions, and our strategies for solutions. As learning tools, we have included numerous cases for study with their virtual setups. Additionally, we have incorporated a series of prototypes, figures illustrating suggested technological modifications, and future clinical applications with clear aligners.

Because we aim to be as impartial and comprehensive as possible in our evaluations of these dilemmas, we have included discussions of clear aligner systems alternative to Invisalign. However, this is not always possible because certain aspects of clear aligner therapy with the Invisalign system are currently significantly advanced and not yet available in the alternative systems, such as a developed bite jump function or optimized attachments. Nevertheless, we believe these alternative systems, in addition to clinician-printed aligners (via in-office 3D printers), will become increasingly viable for the treatment of both simple and complex malocclusions.

This book seeks to address the ambiguity and confusion surrounding the most pressing and troubling clinical dilemmas in clear aligner therapy. It intends to provide the clinician greater clarity and understanding on these dilemmas, as well as paradigms for their resolution. We hope this book can serve as a valuable contribution to the discussion surrounding these topics and that it will assist readers in making more informed and effective clinical decisions in their delivery of clear aligner treatments.

New York, NY Anderson Huang
New York, NY Darren Huang

Acknowledgments

We are deeply grateful to Dr. Olivier Nicolay, Dr. Jae Hyun Park, and Dr. George Anastassov, who believed in this project from the very start and offered their early support and invaluable guidance. We sincerely thank Springer Nature and our generous and perceptive editors, Alison Wolf, Priyadarshini Vasudevan, and Shilpa Sheetal, for graciously offering us the opportunity to realize our project and patiently directing us from proposal to publication.

We thank the New York University College of Dentistry Department of Orthodontics for their commitment to an evidence-based best-practice approach to orthodontic practice, their continued innovations in clear aligner research and therapy, and for creating space for us to nurture our ideas for optimal patient care.

We thank Dr. Mitchell J. Lipp for his insight, friendship, and support.

We would like to express our love and gratitude for our family, Jennifer and Madeline, for their patience, enthusiasm, and support, throughout this entire project.

Contents

Abbreviations

AAO	American Association of Orthodontists
ANB	A-point-nasion-B-point angle
BSSO	Bilateral sagittal split osteotomy
CBCT	Cone-beam computed tomography
IHA	In-house aligner
IMPA	Incisor mandibular plane angle
IPR	Interproximal reduction
MA	Mandibular advancement
PDL	Periodontal ligament
RME	Rapid maxillary expansion
RPFM	Reverse pull face mask
SNA	Sella-nasion-A-point angle
SNB	Sella-nasion-B-point angle
TAD	Temporary anchorage device
U1-SN	Upper incisor-sella-nasion angle
VCC	Virtual C-chain
VGB	Virtual gable bend

Optimizing Diagnosis and Treatment Planning with Clear Aligner Software

1

Contents

Clear Aligner Software: A Brief History

In orthodontic therapy with clear aligners, the judicious manipulation of the software constitutes a significant aspect of treatment planning and is critical for successful outcomes. The first software for clear aligner therapy was introduced by the founders of Align Technology and the inventors of the Invisalign appliance to the American Congress of Orthodontists in 1999 [1]. The technology adopted computer-aided design/computer-aided manufacturing (CAD/CAM) techniques to fabricate a series of aligners that gradually moved teeth into their desired positions. The first generation of the Invisalign software, known as the Clincheck, was primarily designed for the resolution of simple malocclusions, such as mild and moderate crowding, minor space closure, and minor root movements [2]. Subsequent generations of the Invisalign clear aligner appliance improved both the aligner material and its capabilities as well as the functionality of the software. Typically, software innovations allowed for finer control during the virtual setup through the addition of more features for tooth positioning, the addition of auxiliaries, and treatment planning. The technological development of Invisalign's clear aligner appliance has expanded its range to the potential treatment of more complex malocclusions. However, many of Invisalign's claims regarding the efficacy of its appliance, such as the resolution of significant rotations, extrusions and intrusions of 2.5 mm in anterior teeth, and root movements of up to 4 mm in posterior teeth, have not been properly substantiated [2].

Importantly, in 2015, Invisalign introduced a number of innovations, including the Clincheck Pro, alongside alterations in aligner material and

A. T. Huang, D. Huang, *Controversies in Clear Aligner Therapy*,
https://doi.org/10.1007/978-3-030-92810-0_1

the addition of a number of features for the management of cases involving first premolar extractions [3]. At the time of writing, the current version of the Clincheck software is the Clincheck Pro 5.0, which is essentially the original Clincheck Pro with a number of modifications. Since its first iteration, Clincheck has not been web-based but needs to be downloaded as an application. As a result, it remains prone to discontinuities from server disruptions. The Clincheck Pro 5.0 remained unavailable as web-based software. Notably, the 2015 update incorporated into the software the 3D toolbar, which allows for the positioning of individual teeth in all dimensions, updated its SmartTrack polymer aligner material, increased functionality for the placement, orientation, and sizing of attachments and cuts, widened capabilities for expansion and contraction of either the maxillary or the mandibular arch, and allowed the addition and removal of sites of interproximal reduction for space management [3, 4]. The update also added a number of features to assist in treatment planning, including an automatic Bolton analysis, the visualization of occlusal contacts, and a "dual view," which compares the clinician's modifications to Invisalign's initial setup.

In recent years, a variety of dental suppliers have created competing clear aligner appliances along with their respective software. In 2018, 3M launched its Clarity clear aligner system and its web-based software for treatment planning. Also in 2018, Dentsply Sirona introduced its Suresmile aligners and Elemetrix software as another clear aligner alternative. Both 3M and Dentsply Sirona's software differ significantly from that of Clincheck and offer distinct advantages for the clinician.

Despite Invisalign's continued innovations, its Clincheck Pro software remains limited by a number of deficiencies, which potentially compromise ideal treatment outcomes. These limitations range from lack of optimization for single tooth movement to a failure in correcting skeletal discrepancies to unrealistic modeling of soft tissue changes. For instance, the Clincheck software currently lacks proper integration of soft and hard tissues. As a result, the treatment simulation fails to realistically model soft tissue changes produced by orthodontic movements. It is important that the clinician is mindful of these deficiencies so that they can anticipate the effects of their mechanotherapy and minimize any unfavorable outcomes.

In the following chapter, we discuss the major limitations of Invisalign's Clincheck software, which range from a lack of functionality for optimizing single tooth movement to improper modeling of soft tissues. In our discussion of single tooth movement, we will focus on the judicious manipulation of attachments. When viable, we will propose solutions for overcoming these limitations in the software. Thereafter, we will survey the lesser-known alternative software and discuss how their differing features might be used to the clinician's advantage for delivering successful orthodontic treatment.

Major Deficiencies in the Invisalign Clincheck Software

Single Tooth Movement: Incompatibilities in Attachment Design

Studies have shown that the addition of attachments onto teeth improves the accuracy of specific types of orthodontic tooth movements [5]. Simon et al. reported the best accuracy in the bodily distalization of upper molars of at least 1.5 mm when movements were supported by attachments on the tooth surfaces [6]. Clinically, we have observed that the use of attachments prevents excessive tipping of molars during distalization. However, we note that though the difference in accuracy for distalization between teeth with attachments was greater than that of teeth without attachments, it was not by a statistically significant margin [6].

Studies have also investigated the effects of attachment use on the efficacy of other types of movements. A clinical trial in 2005 supported the use of attachments to improve the accuracy of rotational movements [7]. Simon et al. observed that in premolar rotations of >10°, the use of attachments and the degree of movement per aligner both had a great impact on predictability [6]. A systematic review in 2015 also recommended the use of attachments to improve the predictability of rotational movements [5]. Nevertheless, other studies have shown conflicting results and claimed that the use of attachments does not aid in stimulating derotation for canines [8]. A 2019 systematic review also concluded there is a lack of evidence to support the use of attachments for derotation [2]. Despite the lack of consensus in the current evidence, it is still recommended to place attachments on teeth for derotation, especially exceeding 15°, for treatment predictability [5].

There is a greater consensus for the use of attachments in improving the predictability of extrusive movements. The treatment of vertical problems, especially deep overbite, is especially challenging for clear aligners. In a clinical trial, extrusion was found to be the least accurate tooth movement [9]. Therefore, it is recommended that attachments be placed on teeth requiring extrusion for predictability [2].

It is evident that the use of attachments is able to stimulate certain orthodontic movements [10]. In its most recent generations, Invisalign's Clincheck Pro has incorporated a number of features that expanded the clinician's control over attachments as well as their capabilities for controlling tooth movement. Specifically, when the clinician decides to place an attachment, they are able to choose its shape, whether an ellipsoid, mesial or distally beveled vertical attachment, or a gingival or incisally beveled horizontal attachment (Fig. 1.1). Secondly, the clinician is also able to determine the size of the attachment—3, 4, or 5 mm in length (Fig. 1.2). Thirdly, the clinician is able to position the attachment both in terms of its location on the tooth surface and the orientation of its bevel (Fig. 1.3).

Despite these capabilities, there remain shortcomings in the Clincheck software's attachment design that compromise treatment predictability. Notably, because of the limited configurations available, the attachment cannot properly adapt to the full range of tooth surfaces. For instance, the software limits the minimum size of attachments so that they cannot be incorporated onto tooth surfaces that are deficient in crown length. This situation arises when attachments are required for distalizing maxillary molars with short clinical crowns (Fig. 1.4). In such cases, the vertical beveled attachment would most ideally support the distalizing movements. However, because of the short clinical crowns in the maxillary molars, the Clincheck software will automatically trigger the placement of horizontal beveled attachments instead of the desired vertical beveled attachments (Fig. 1.5). As a result, the predictability of the distalizing movement is

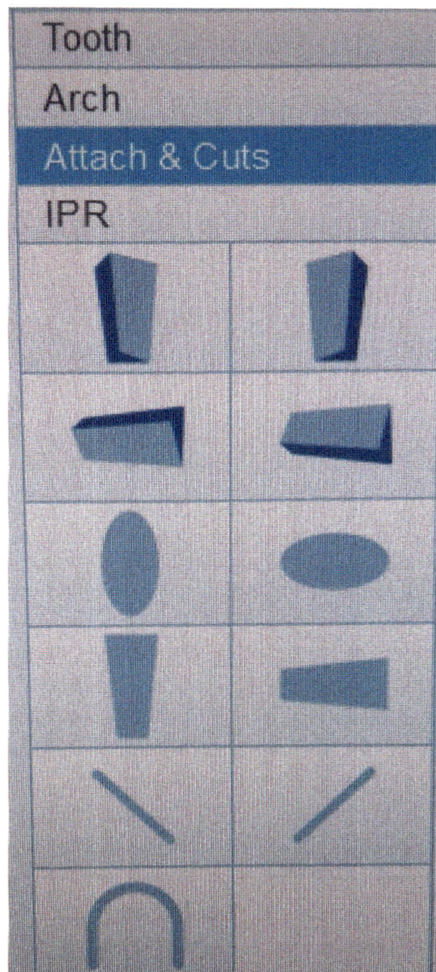

Fig. 1.1 Invisalign allows for a wide range of attachments, including the horizontal bevel, vertical bevel, and ellipsoid

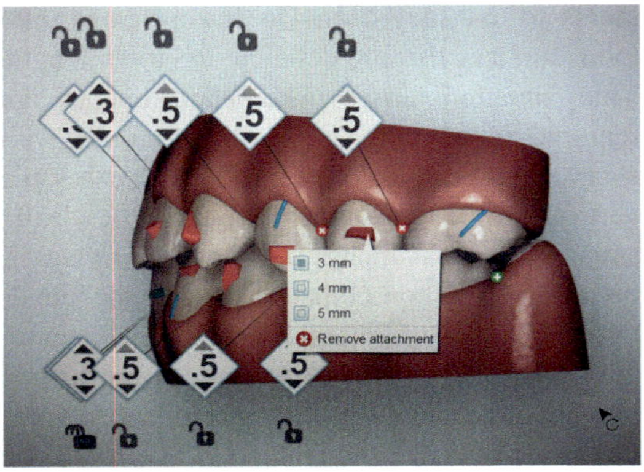

Fig. 1.2 Invisalign Clincheck allows for the clinician to adjust the length of the adjustment from 3 to 5 mm. However, at present, the adjustment of other dimensions (height and depth) remains limited

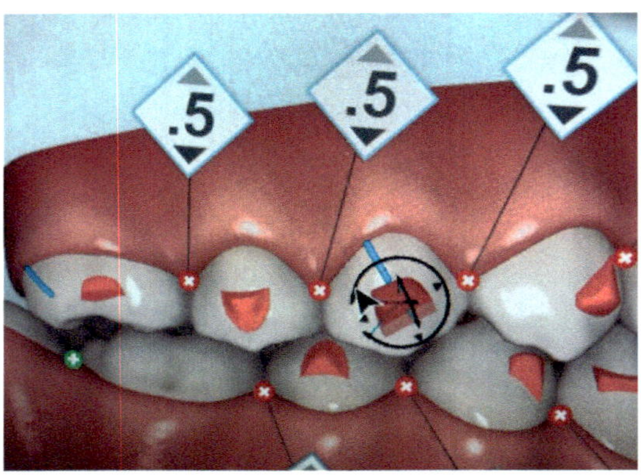

Fig. 1.3 Invisalign Clincheck permits the clinician to rotate the attachment in all dimensions. This allows the clinician the freedom to position the active surface of the attachment to optimize desired tooth movements

limited by the use of a nonideally configured attachment. The solution for this incompatibility between attachment size and tooth morphology would be for the software to allow for attachments with lengths smaller than 3 mm. Though this option does not yet exist for the most recent generation of Clincheck software, it has already been made available by alternative software, such as 3M Clarity (which we will discuss later in this chapter).

During the initial setup of a Clincheck for a particular case, the Invisalign technician will often incorporate specialized attachments known as optimized attachments (Fig. 1.6). The latter is

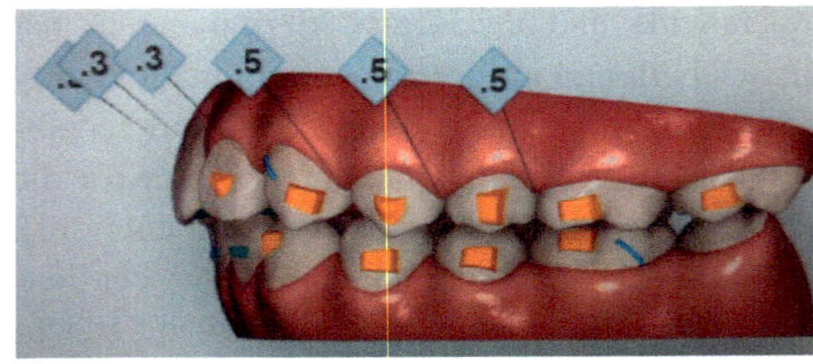

Fig. 1.4 Horizontal beveled attachments were placed on molars requiring distalization, whereas the more optimally designed attachments would have been vertical beveled. However, Invisalign's dimensional limitations prohibit the placement of vertical beveled attachments due to the molars' short clinical crowns

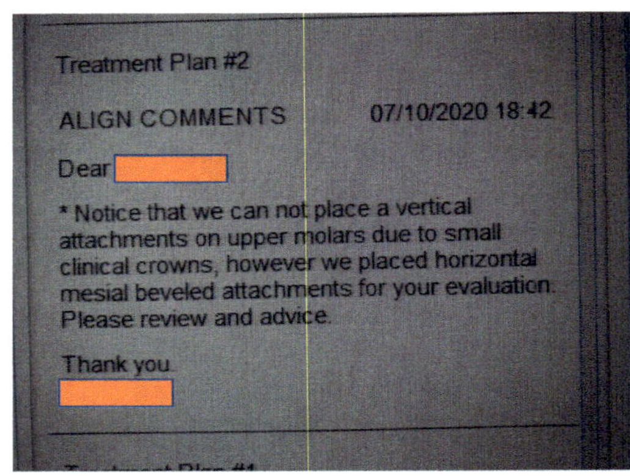
Treatment Plan #2

ALIGN COMMENTS 07/10/2020 18:42

Dear [redacted]

* Notice that we can not place a vertical attachments on upper molars due to small clinical crowns, however we placed horizontal mesial beveled attachments for your evaluation. Please review and advice.

Thank you
[redacted]

Fig. 1.5 An Invisalign error message flags the necessary substitution of horizontal for vertical beveled attachments due to short clinical crowns

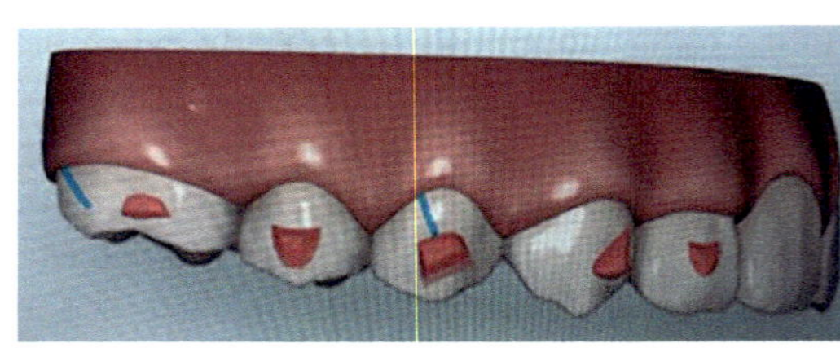

Fig. 1.6 Invisalign optimized attachments have been placed on the right maxillary lateral incisor, the right maxillary canine, right maxillary second premolar, and the right maxillary first molar

configured in such a way to enhance specific movements, including extrusion, root movement, and rotation. A recent clinical trial showed that optimized attachments allowed for less difference between predicted and achieved tooth movement when compared to differences with non-optimized (conventional) attachments [11]. Ironically, the manner in which these optimized attachments are applied actually becomes a limitation in optimizing treatment outcomes. Namely, once the Invisalign technician places these optimized attachments onto tooth surfaces, they cannot be modified by the clinician except for their elimination. The clinician is not able to reposition or reorient the optimized attachment on the tooth surface. At present, if the clinician desires the reconfiguration of the attachment, they have to resort to placing a conventional attachment, which may be less ideal for enhancing the specific type of tooth movement. The most ideal solution would be for the software to allow the clinician greater control over the configuration of the optimized attachments.

Therefore, the current generation of Clincheck Pro, despite its advances, restricts attachment design through firstly, size limitations and secondly, the default placement of optimized attachments. As a result, the clinician must negotiate these limitations by resorting to the use of nonideal configurations or forgoing the placement of attachments altogether. Because attachments are often required to improve root control and to facilitate a variety of movements such as rotation, extrusion, and distalization, limitations in their design adversely affect treatment predictability [6].

Single Tooth Movement: Limitations in Torque Application

Historically, torque control has been problematic for clear aligners. Studies have shown clear aligner therapy is not as effective in controlling torque as fixed appliances [12]. A clinical trial reported an average accuracy of 50.3% for anterior torque movements as compared to 39.95% for premolar rotation and 87.65% for molar distalization [6]. Invisalign, along with dental suppliers, such as 3M, have incorporated a variety of features, including the alteration of aligner geometry, for the generation of adequate force systems and the enhancement of torque control on specific teeth. Simon et al. has concluded that either the alteration of aligner geometry (the power ridge in the Invisalign appliance) or the use of attachments is practicable for increasing the predictability of torquing movements [6]. The same study also found that there was no significant difference in the predictability of maxillary incisor torque whether the movement was supplemented by an ellipsoid attachment or a power ridge [6]. Another study found that minor activation through the modification of aligner material near the gingival margin or the use of properly configured attachments could improve root control during torquing movements of a maxillary central incisor [13]. Though few studies on the topic have been performed, the current scientific evidence supports the alteration of aligner geometry to enhance torquing movements with clear aligners.

Currently, Invisalign alters aligner geometry for torque control through the addition of power ridges, which are lines of pressure close to the gingival margins of particular teeth (we more comprehensively discuss their application and efficacy in Chap. 8). There are also points of pressure that are applied at the incisal region on the opposite surface of the tooth. For instance, lingual root torque for a maxillary incisor is created through a coupling effect: a larger force is applied at the gingival margin, while a smaller force in the opposing direction is applied at the linguoincisal region (Fig. 1.7). The additive effect of the two forces creates a moment for lingual root torque. The Clincheck Pro software severely limits the clinician in their ability to incorporate and manipulate power ridges for root control. Firstly, the power ridges can only be applied to the maxillary and mandibular incisors; canines and posterior teeth cannot be equipped with power ridges so any torquing movements for these teeth cannot be enhanced with auxiliary alterations in aligner geometry. Secondly, the power ridges can only be applied on the labial surfaces of the incisors for lingual root torque. At present, power ridges cannot be placed on any lingual surfaces for the enhancement of labial root torque.

Thirdly, the clinician can adjust neither the placement of the power ridge nor that of the pressure point. Ideally, the Clincheck software would

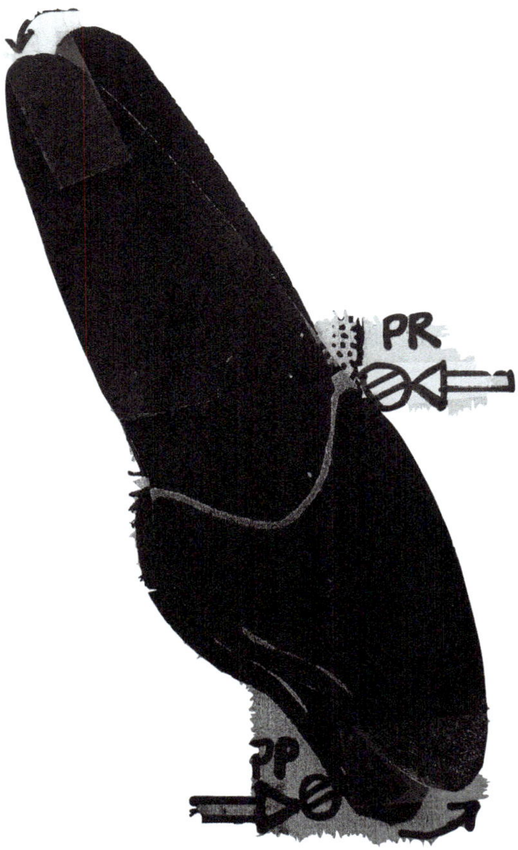

Fig. 1.7 A coupling effect is created by a labial force from a power ridge and a lingual force from a pressure point to generate lingual root torque. *PR* power ridge; *PP* pressure point.

allow the clinician the capability to position both the power ridge and the pressure point. The control over both auxiliaries would allow the clinician greater ability to control crown and root movements in the buccolingual dimension. For example, there are instances during orthodontic treatment when the clinician desires a lingual movement of the root while preventing excessive labial movement of the crown (Fig. 1.8a,b). This scenario is common during the late stages of cases involving the extractions of the four first premolars. In fixed appliances, for the mandibular incisors, the clinician can achieve the desired crown and root movements by placing lingual root torque in a rectangular wire in addition to applying a distalizing force at the crown level through a strong cinch-back, a power-chain, or some other means. At present, such simultaneous crown and root movements cannot be effectively programmed by the Clincheck software (Fig. 1.9a,b). If the clinician requests a power ridge on the mandibular incisors, then the power ridge would stimulate the root to travel lingually. However, the crown would also be stimulated to travel labially. With the addition of the power ridge on the labiogingival area of the tooth, it would be difficult to program a simultaneous lingual force to the crown surface. If the clinician were able to program a pressure point on the middle third of the crown surface, they would be able to apply the necessary distalizing force to prevent excessive labial tipping of the crown.

Fourthly, when power ridges are applied to maxillary or mandibular incisors, they are placed for a specific number of aligners or stages. For instance, in a treatment that requires 20 active aligners, power ridges may only be applied in 10, 15, or all 20 aligners to the designated teeth. One of the most critical issues with the application of power ridges through the Clincheck software is that the power ridge is not precisely calibrated for a particular amount of lingual root torque movement. That is, the clinician cannot know the degrees of lingual root torque applied to the tooth per each stage of power ridges.

One of the current solutions for these limitations in power ridge and pressure point placement and configuration within the Clincheck software is to apply these auxiliaries with hand instruments during the course of treatment (we will further discuss the use of hand instruments in Chap. 11). For instance, if during treatment, a maxillary canine crown requires additional lingual root torque, one can apply with a horizontal dimple plier a power ridge on the labiogingival surface of the canine crown in addition to a pressure point on the linguoincisal region with a dimple plier.

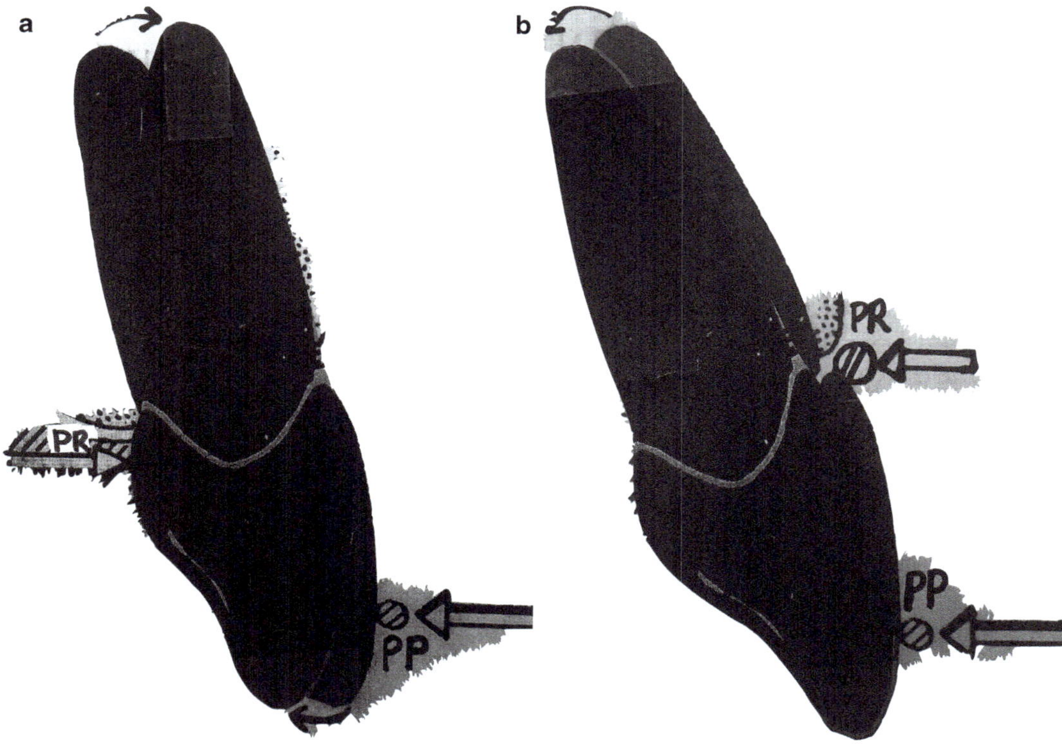

Fig. 1.8 (**a**) Buccal root torque applied with both a power ridge at the lingual surface and a pressure point from the labial. *PR* power ridge; *PP* pressure point. (**b**) Lingual root torque with controlled root tipping applied with a power ridge at the cervical area of the labial surface and a pressure point applied at the labial surface near the incisal edge. *PR* power ridge; *PP* pressure point

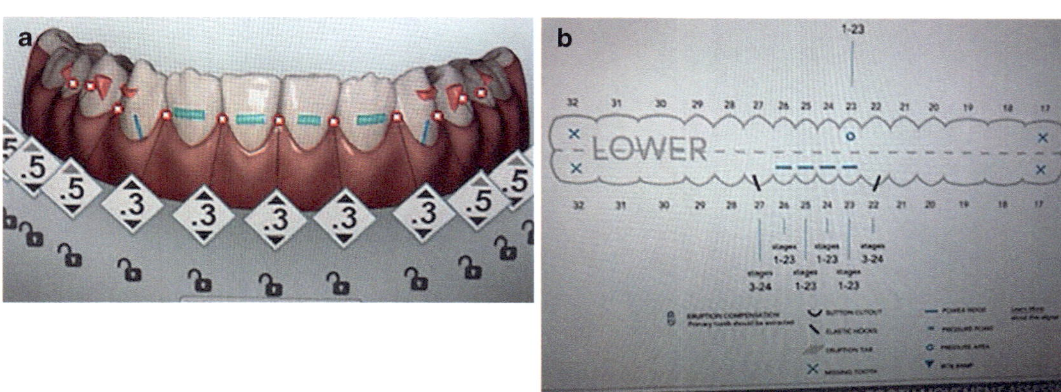

Fig. 1.9 (**a**) Power ridges can be applied to the cervical area of the labial surfaces of maxillary and mandibular incisors. However, they cannot be applied in any other region, such as any lingual surface or on the posterior teeth. (**b**) A pressure area has been placed on the lingual region of tooth #23. At present, pressure areas cannot be determined by the clinician and are placed at default by the software

Single Tooth Movement: Limitations during Extraction Therapy

Extraction therapy remains challenging for clear aligners (we discuss in detail the efficacy and overcoming limitations of clear aligner extraction therapy in Chap. 9). Studies have shown that despite advances, they still cannot treat complex cases, including extraction cases, as successfully as fixed appliances [14]. Notably, a clinical trial analyzed the differences between actual and predicted tooth movements in cases involving the extractions of two maxillary first premolars [15]. The study found that following treatment, the molars tipped mesially more than predicted in addition to other discrepancies between predicted and actual movements in incisor torque and vertical position [15]. In 2015, Invisalign introduced the G6 protocol for improving the effectiveness of extraction therapy with clear aligners [3]. Specifically, for cases involving premolar extractions, Invisalign programs an optimized retraction attachment, optimized anchorage attachments for the premolars and molars, and the incorporation of a virtual gable bend, which creates moments on the anterior and posterior segments to counteract unwanted crown tipping.

The use of the G6 protocol has been shown to slightly improve control of first molar movement as compared to the use of conventional attachments in cases involving two first premolar extractions [15]. The G6 protocol automatically incorporates a virtual gable bend but it remains unclear the amount of counteracting force the bend provides to the anterior and posterior segments adjacent to the extraction space. One of the weaknesses of the Clincheck software is that it fails to visualize the movements provided by the virtual gable bend. When the clinician requests the virtual gable bend, the software will show counteracting forces applied to the designated teeth but neither the amount of degrees produced nor the specific number of stages (Fig. 1.10). The lack of visualization deprives the clinician of a means to control the extent of crown tipping in the adjacent teeth during extraction space closure. As we will discuss in Chap. 9, crown tipping during extraction space closure remains one of the foremost challenges to extraction therapy with clear aligners.

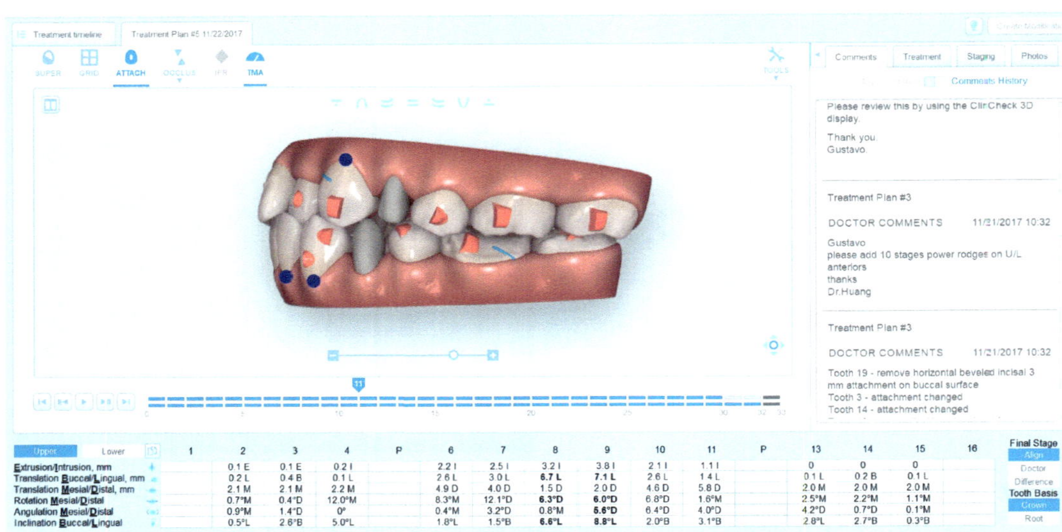

Fig. 1.10 Though a virtual gable bend (VGB) has been requested and forces have been applied to the teeth adjacent to the extraction space to prevent unwanted tipping, it cannot be determined the amount of degrees of counteracting force applied by the VGB per aligner

Deficiencies in Hard and Soft Tissue Modeling

Studies have shown that three-dimensional soft tissue modeling is a useful modality for optimizing esthetics during treatment planning [16]. A modern form of diagnosis and treatment planning seems to require the integration of facial modeling for the prediction of soft tissue changes as a result of treatment, especially in extraction cases and cases involving orthognathic surgery, which are often characterized by extensive facial changes [17].

At present, the Clincheck software does allow for partial integration of soft tissue during the simulation of the patient's malocclusion. In the treatment plan simulation, the clinician can observe the movements of both the marginal and attached gingiva along with the simulated movement of the teeth. However, the current software fails to accurately predict the movements of both marginal and attached gingival tissue. For instance, in cases involving the extraction of a mandibular incisor, the clinician can anticipate the development of a black triangle between the incisors adjacent to the extraction space, especially in older patients. The Clincheck simulation of the teeth and soft tissue movements will not express the development of black triangles and instead models the marginal gingiva so that it unrealistically fills in the interproximal embrasure between the incisors adjacent to the extraction space. The poor accuracy of the Invisalign software's soft tissue modeling remains a deficiency for the clinician who seeks to predict soft tissue changes as a result of treatment.

The Clincheck software also lacks any sort of facial modeling. At present, there is no integration of the facial soft tissues, including upper and lower lips, nose, or chin, with hard tissues. Presently, the clinician cannot model alterations in the facial soft tissues on the Clincheck software. It would be more ideal for diagnosis and treatment planning if there were functional integration of the hard and soft tissues so that facial features could be modeled along with the teeth. Studies have created 3D simulations of soft tissue norms for forecasting facial outcomes as a result of orthodontic treatment [18]. Ideally, the Clincheck software could model facial soft tissue changes by calibrating them to hard tissue changes in accordance with demographic norms, such as ethnicity, gender, age, and skeletal class. Alternative software, like that of Dentsply Sirona, have begun an integration between hard and facial soft tissues, through features such as the "lip trace," which superimposes teeth movements from the frontal view with the patient's actual lip contours.

Similarly, the Clincheck software is limited by liabilities in its visualization of hard tissues. Most notably, though the amount and degree of root movement for all teeth are displayed in the software's assessment table, the roots themselves cannot be visualized in three dimensions because they remain concealed by the gingival tissues. As a result, it is difficult for the clinician to assess the precise orientation of any root at a particular stage during treatment. This unpredictability is especially disadvantageous for the treatment of complex cases that involve significant root movement, such as those involving extractions or significant retraction of the maxillary and mandibular incisors. As we will discuss later in this chapter, the 3M software allows for the option of viewing teeth movement without any soft tissues so that the roots can be more precisely visualized at any point in time during the simulated treatment plan.

Limitations in the Correction of Skeletal Discrepancies

Studies have shown that clear aligners are limited in their capabilities to resolve large anteroposterior discrepancies [10]. In late 2018, Invisalign introduced the mandibular advancement feature for the correction of Class II skeletal discrepancies (we discuss the efficacy of the mandibular advancement feature in Chap. 3). Prior to this feature, the Clincheck software resorted to a "bite jump," a significant interarch simulated movement whether in the anteroposterior, transverse, or vertical dimension, as a means of correcting large skeletal discrepancies in the simulated treatment plan.

As we will further discuss in Chap. 10, the bite jump is frequently mis-prescribed by both clinicians and the Clincheck software. Clincheck currently offers a tooth movement assessment, which expresses the difficulty of individual tooth movements (Fig. 1.11). However, the software fails to recognize and indicate the difficulty of interarch movements, most notably the bite jump. As a result, Clincheck allows clinicians to freely prescribe bite jumps in unrealistic scenarios—such as a bite jump paired with Class II or Class III elastics for the correction of a large anteroposterior skeletal discrepancy or the incorporation of an anteroposterior bite jump in a nongrowing patient (Fig. 1.12). In these cases, the Clincheck software allows or automatically prescribes a bite jump in a situation where such an extensive skeletal correction could not feasibly occur. The unrealistic bite jump would produce an overestimation of the amount of skeletal correction. Ideally, the Clincheck software would allow for the incorporation of bite jumps only when indicated. The realistic simulation of bite jumps is significant for achieving successful outcomes with the correction of skeletal discrepancies with clear aligners.

Limitations in Diagnostic Tools

The Invisalign software provides a number of diagnostic tools for the clinician during the design of the treatment plan, most notably the Bolton analysis for the mandibular anterior teeth relative to the maxillary anterior teeth as well as the mandibular posterior teeth relative to the maxillary posterior teeth, the tooth movement assessment for difficult movements, and the tooth movement table, which records the total amount of movement in all three orders. Though the software allows for the uploading of the cephalometric radiograph for reference, one of its deficiencies is its lack of integration of cephalometric values, such as SNA, SNB, ANB, U1-SN, IMPA, Sn-GoGn, and other measurements important for the development of the patient's treatment plan. Cephalometric analyses, though there remains a lack of consensus regarding which measurements are the most essential, remain the gold standard for orthodontic clinical routine and the diagnosis of growth and developmental abnormalities [19, 20]. Dentsply Sirona has started to functionally integrate the cephalometric radiograph into treatment planning by allowing the clinician the ability to superimpose the simulated teeth

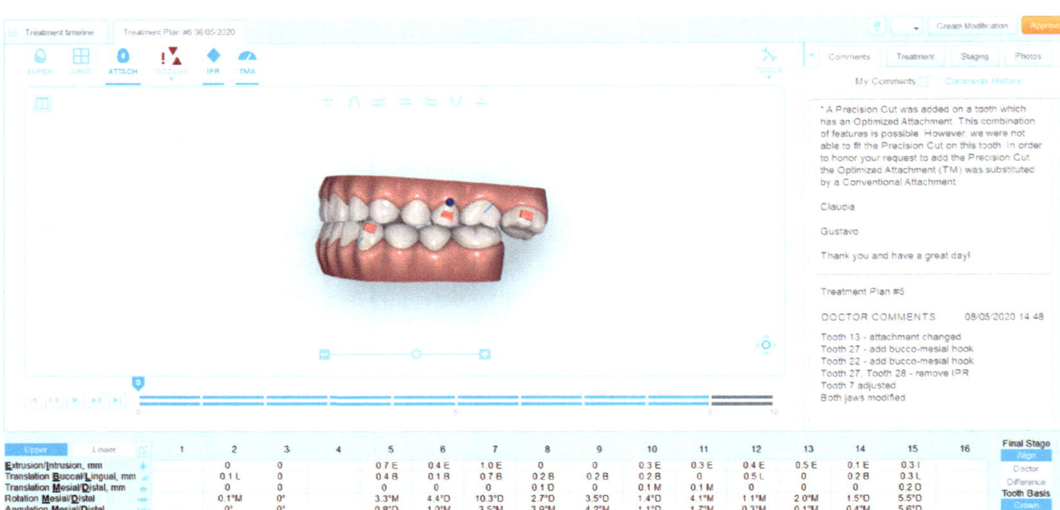

Fig. 1.11 The tooth movement assessment table is displayed at the bottom of the virtual setup in the Invisalign Clincheck. The blue dot on the simulation indicates a difficult movement

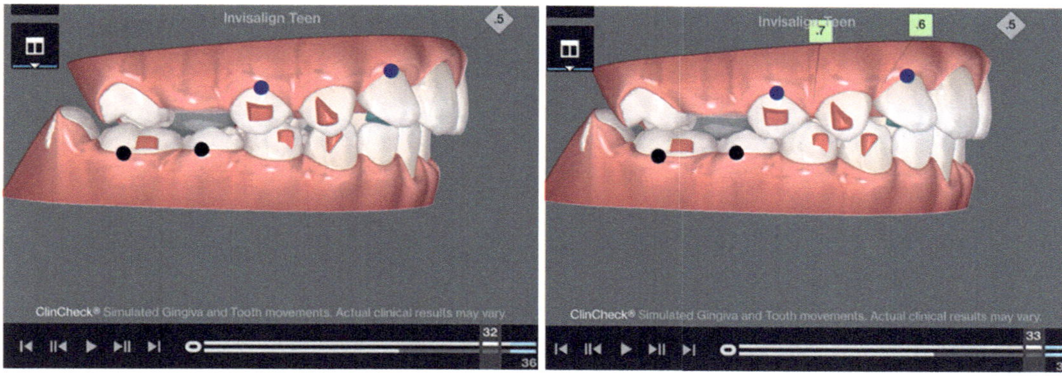

Fig. 1.12 A bite jump is depicted in aligner stage 33. The software simulates the forward advancement of the mandible from the use of Class II elastics. However, this bite jump is unrealistic due to the absence of significant growth forecasted for the patient or Class II mechanotherapy that could feasibly produce such a change in the position of the mandible, such as the use of the MA appliance or a Class II orthopedic appliance, like the cervical-pull headgear

movements over the radiograph. However, like Invisalign, it has not been able to incorporate cephalometric analyses into the software.

The 3M Software

In 2018, 3M introduced its Clarity aligners along with their software for diagnosis and treatment planning [21]. Because of their recent development, limited research has been performed on the efficacy of the aligners as compared to either fixed appliances or Invisalign clear aligners. The 3M software is deficient in a number of aspects, particularly in its ability to plan the treatment of complex cases, such as those involving extractions and the correction of severe skeletal discrepancies. Nevertheless, the software has incorporated a number of unique features, which offer distinct capabilities for the clinician during diagnosis and treatment planning.

Optimizing Single Tooth Movement: Capabilities and Limitations of Attachment Design

Studies have shown the significance of attachment design for the optimization of tooth movement [10]. One of the capabilities of the 3M software is its free manipulation of attachments during the treatment planning stage. We have discussed the importance of attachment shape and size for the placement of attachments on the crowns of teeth with abnormal morphology, such as those with small crown height or diminutive cusps. The 3M software allows for the manipulation of the attachment in all three dimensions—length, width, and depth (Fig. 1.13). Notably, each dimension can be reduced to a minimal size—2 mm in length, 1 mm in width, and 0.5 mm in depth for the bar attachment (Fig. 1.14). Therefore, unlike the attachments of the Invisalign software, the small volume of 3M's attachments can be adapted to even abnormally small clinical crowns.

Despite the software's capability for adjusting attachment size, it remains limited in regards to shape. At present, the only shapes available are the bar and bevel. There are also no optimized default attachments automatically incorporated by the software. Recent clinical trials have suggested that optimized attachments play a role in improving the accuracy of movements, particularly extrusion and rotation [22]. The 3M software's limited range in attachment shape adversely affects the predictability of traditionally difficult tooth movements for clear aligners.

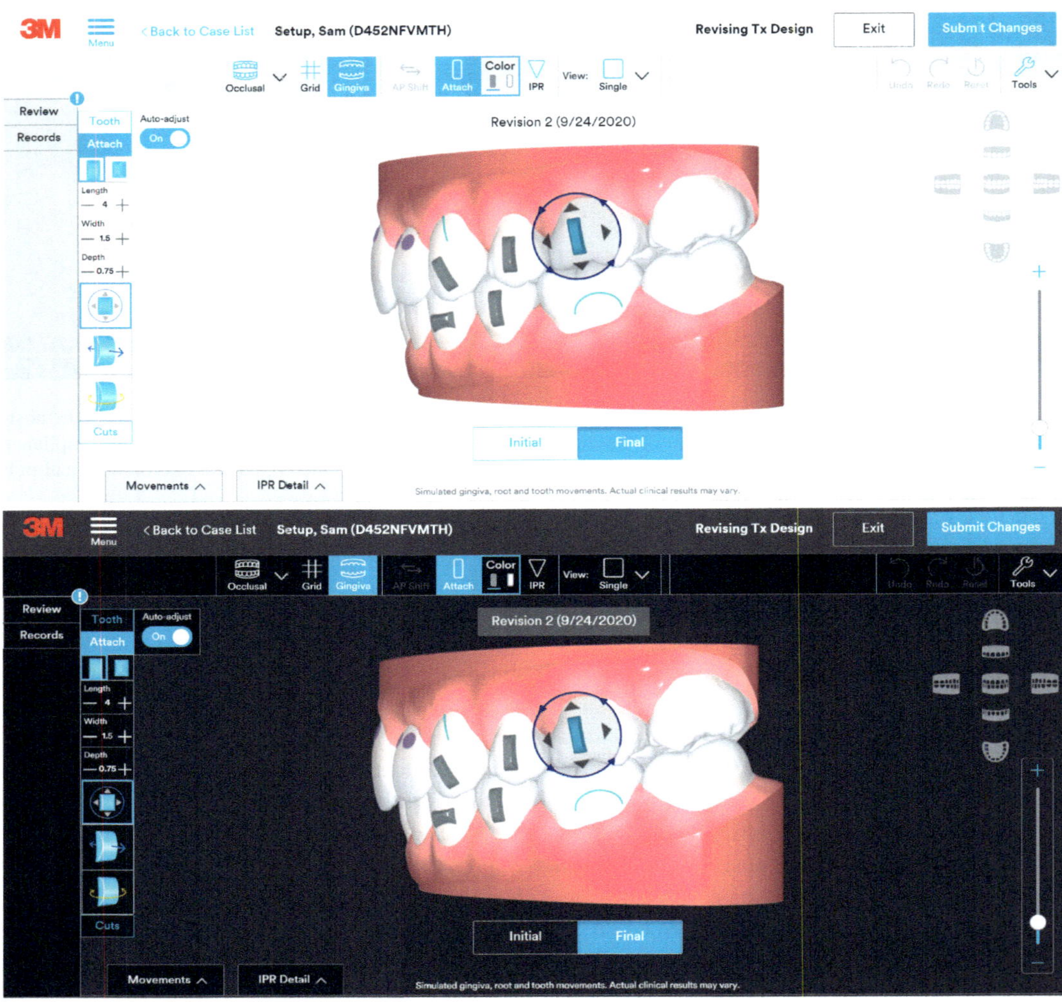

Fig. 1.13 The attachments in the 3M™ Oral Care Portal software can be customized in all three dimensions: length, width, and height. They can also be minimized to small volumes to accommodate teeth with small clinical crowns or abnormal morphology

Optimizing Single Tooth Movement: Torque Application and Bite Opening

Like Invisalign, 3M employs alterations of aligner geometry for the enhancement of root torquing movements. Instead of power ridges, 3M uses individual points of pressure, known as "torque points" (Fig. 1.15). The 3M software also limits the placement of their torque points on the maxillary and mandibular incisors so that they cannot be placed on the canines or the posterior teeth. Similar to the power ridges of Invisalign Clincheck, the torque points can only be placed on the labial surfaces of crowns so they cannot enhance buccal root torque. Therefore, the accuracy of buccal-lingual torquing movements can be compromised, especially on teeth which typically struggle with lingual root torque, such as the second molars [22].

For bite opening of deep bite cases, 3M also allows for bite ramps on the lingual surfaces of the maxillary anterior teeth. These are slight enlargements on the lingual surfaces that prematurely occlude with the mandibular anterior teeth

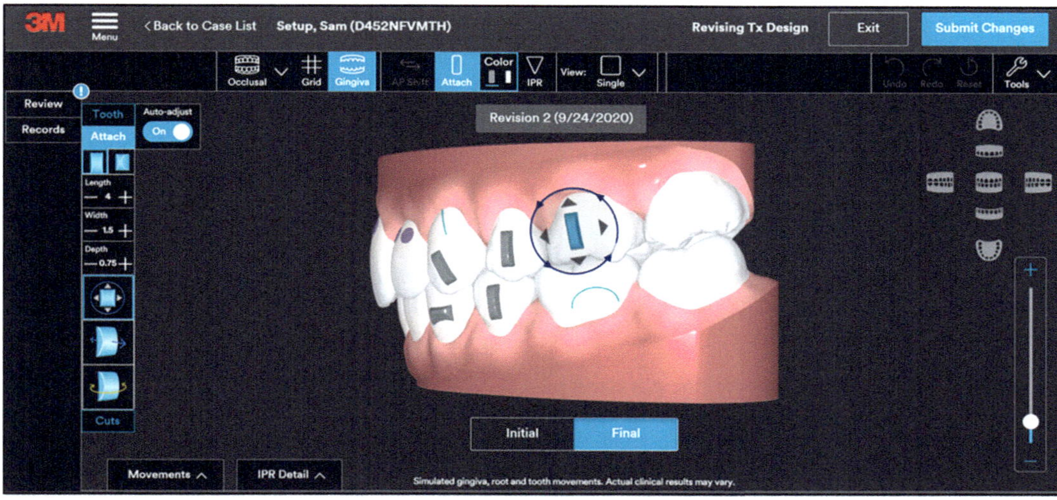

*	Height	Width	Length
Bar	.5, .75, 1mm	1, 1.5, 2 mm	2, 3, 4 mm
Beveled	.5, .75. 1mm	1.5, 2, 2.5 mm	2, 3, 4, 5, 6 mm

*This chart indicates the parameters of height, width, and length for attachments that the 3M Treatment Design Team works within. The clinician still has the option to modify within these parameters.

Fig. 1.14 The 3M™ Oral Care Portal software allows for an attachment's minimum size to be 2 mm in length, 1 mm in width, and 0.5 mm in depth for bar attachments. For beveled attachments, the minimum size parameter is 2 mm in length, 1.5 mm in width, and 0.5 mm in depth

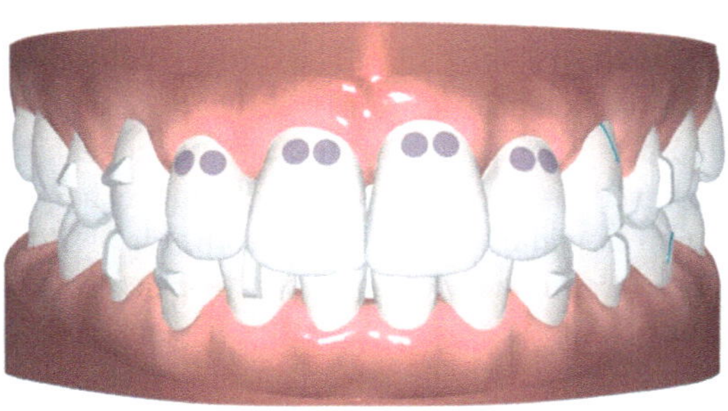

Fig. 1.15 The 3M software employs torque points for lingual root torque, available only on the labial surfaces of maxillary and mandibular incisors

for posterior disocclusion and additional intrusive forces on the maxillary anterior teeth (Fig. 1.16). The software automatically installs the bite ramps on the lingual surfaces of the maxillary anterior teeth when it detects the presence of a deep overbite. Bite opening remains one of the most challenging movements for clear aligner therapy [23]. One of the weaknesses of the 3M software (and the Invisalign software) in regards to application of the bite ramps is the fact that neither the position nor the size of the bite ramps can be adjusted by the clinician. In certain cases, like a Class II patient with both a deep overbite and large overjet, the default bite ramps are not adequately gingival to occlude with the mandibular anterior teeth. As a result, the efficacy of bite opening can be compromised due to the lack of disocclusion of the posterior teeth.

Hard and Soft Tissue Modeling

One of the unique features of the 3M software is its detailing of the gingival soft tissues (Fig. 1.17). The software allows for the evaluation of soft tissue responses to treatment, such as the development of black triangles. In 3M's view of the teeth and gingival movements, the background can also be dimmed to better visualize soft tissue changes. Nevertheless, the software has neither been able to incorporate any simulation of facial

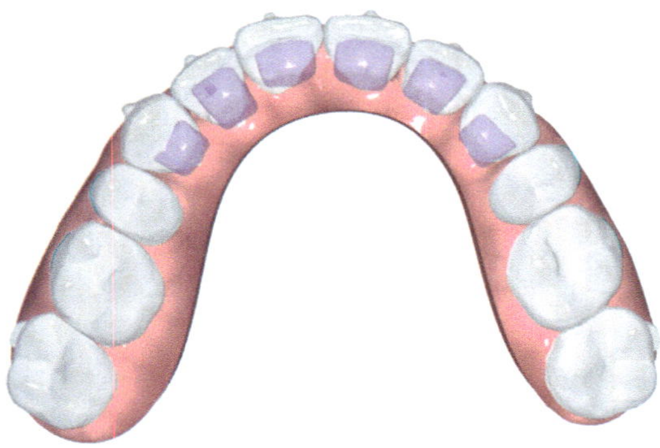

Fig. 1.16 The 3M software allows for the placement of bite ramps on the lingual surfaces of the maxillary anterior teeth for disocclusion of the posterior teeth during deep bite opening

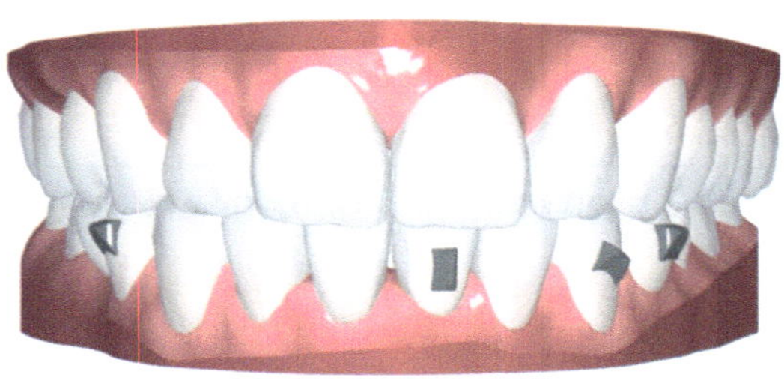

Fig. 1.17 The gingival architecture in the 3M™ Oral Care Portal software is highly realistic and can be simulated to show its responses to teeth movement

changes as a response to treatment nor has it been able to integrate cephalometric analyses.

Limitations in the Treatment of Complex Malocclusions

The 3M software, most likely because of its recent development, has not yet incorporated specific features for the treatment of complex malocclusions. Most notably, it lacks a bite jump option so it cannot accurately model cases involving extensive interarch changes, such as mandibular autorotation as a result of maxillary molar intrusion, mandibular growth in a growing patient, and orthognathic surgical corrections. At present, the software seems less capable than Invisalign in the treatment of skeletal discrepancies and remains most adequate for malocclusions of mild to moderate severity.

Dentsply Sirona Suresmile Software

Like 3M, Dentsply Sirona introduced its Suresmile clear aligner product and the respective software in 2018 [24]. The supplier's model was unique in that it allowed clinicians an option of greater control over tooth movements so that they could treatment plan teeth movements stage-by-stage without a technician's initial setup. The latter option also allows clinicians in-house aligner (IHA) fabrication.[1] Clinicians are able to use the Suresmile software for in-office 3D printing of aligners at fairly reasonable service fees. The software remains early in its development and lacks functions such as optimized attachments and the bite jump for the treatment of complex malocclusions. However, it is unique among the current forms of software in its advanced integration of radiographic data.

Optimizing Single Tooth Movement: Attachment Design

Presently, the Suresmile software offers only three types of attachments—ellipsoid, horizontal, and vertical (Fig. 1.18a). The software allows for modification in attachment size, but only in depth and not in length or width. Attachments can be designed for a minimal volume of 5 mm in height, 2 mm in width, and 1 mm in depth (Fig. 1.18b). These requirements in size limit the placement of attachments onto abnormally shaped crowns. Likewise, the minimal range of attachment shapes also limits the enhancement of complex tooth movements, such as root control.

[1] Suresmile refers to this option as do-it-yourself (DIY) fabrication of aligners. However, because of the controversial associations of DIY aligners with direct-to-consumer products, which completely omit a medical professional from treatment, we elect to use the alternative term, in-house aligner (IHA), for the rest of the book.

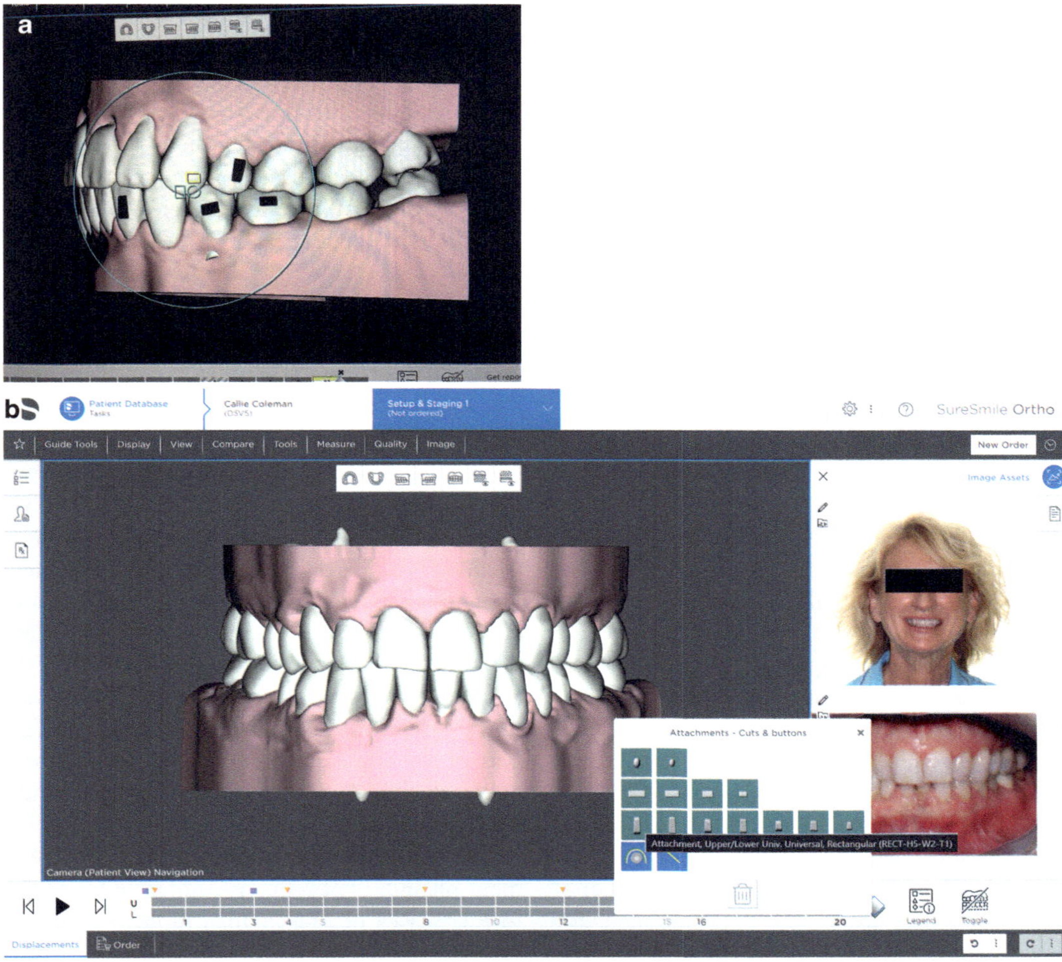

Fig. 1.18 (**a**) The Suresmile software allows only horizontal, vertical, and ellipsoid attachments. At present, no optimized attachments are available. (**b**) In the Dentsply Suresmile software, attachment volume can be minimized to 5 mm in height, 2 mm in width, and 1 mm in depth

Optimizing Single Tooth Movement: Torque Application and Bite Ramps

The Suresmile software remains undeveloped in its features for the enhancement of torquing movements. We have discussed how the modification of aligner geometry can enhance torquing movements, which can be difficult for aligners due to the nature of the material [13]. Suresmile currently lacks any modifications of aligner material for the purpose of torque in the manner of power ridges or torquing points.

Similarly, the Suresmile software lacks the capability to add bite ramps in deep bite cases, whether automatically or manually requested by the clinician. As a result, there are currently no means for Suresmile to disocclude posterior teeth in deep bite cases.

Hard and Soft Tissue Modeling

The Suresmile software is advanced in its integration of hard and soft tissue for treatment planning. Specifically, it allows for the "lip trace" option, which superimposes the patient's photographed lips from the frontal smile photo onto the simulated tooth movements (Fig. 1.19). The feature

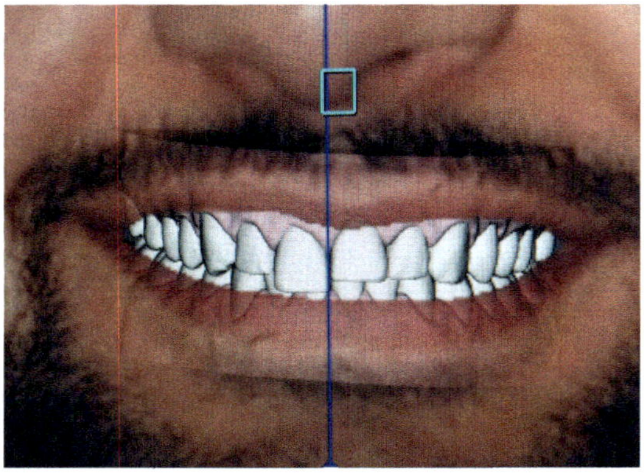

Fig. 1.19 The Suresmile software is unique in that it allows the superimposition of the patient's lips from their smile photo onto the simulated teeth movements

can be useful for planning the extent of intrusion of the maxillary incisors, as well as the amount of expansion in the maxillary posterior segments. The software has also incorporated realistic modeling of the patient gingiva in response to tooth movements. It offers a "comparison gingiva" option, which juxtaposes the initial and final gingival architecture. These features for soft tissue modeling facilitate treatment planning but the real-time simulation of other soft tissues, such as lips in profile, have not yet been introduced.

The software has also assimilated a number of hard tissue diagnostic tools. For instance, the cephalometric radiograph can be superimposed over the simulated teeth movements so they can be assessed with more certainty. Secondly, the software is capable of linking CBCT imaging so that both root movements and the bony housing can be visualized (Fig. 1.20). Studies have shown that the use of 3D imaging can allow for more accurate predictions of orthodontic tooth movement [25]. The CBCT integration would allow for such applications as eruption compensation for permanent teeth, whether impacted or otherwise, planning for the degree of expansion or proclination, and the planning of root movements.

Treatment of Complex Malocclusions

The Suresmile software currently lacks specific features for the treatment of complex malocclusions, such as a bite jump function, a mandibular advancement feature for the treatment of growing individuals, optimized attachments, and a virtual gable bend for extraction situations. The clinician should take caution in using the product and the software in treating cases of complexity, such as those involving extractions, skeletal discrepancies, and orthognathic surgery.

uLab Software

The uLab software is unique among the various software in that it gives the clinician the freedom to create the initial setup and plan all tooth movements during the treatment planning stage. This more independent type of treatment planning seems to represent the future form of clear aligner therapy. There is an option for a software-coordinated tooth setup either for the maxillary and mandibular anterior teeth or both of the entire arches, but it remains rudimentary and always requires additional modification on the part of the clinician to achieve ideal alignment and occlusion. The current software is characterized by versatility in attachment design and the enhancement of tooth movements during treatment planning but remains limited in its ability to treat cases of greater than mild to moderate severity.

Optimizing Single Tooth Movement: Attachment Design

The uLab software allows for adjustment of attachments in all three dimensions—length, width, and depth. It has also incorporated a "copy-paste" function so that clinicians can save a specific attachment design to a library for reuse on another tooth in the future (Fig. 1.21). The attachments have been designed for a wide range of sizes and shapes and can be adapted for small clinical crowns and teeth with abnormal morphology. Nevertheless, at present, the software has not yet incorporated default or optimized attachments for complex tooth movements, though an update is planned for fall 2020.

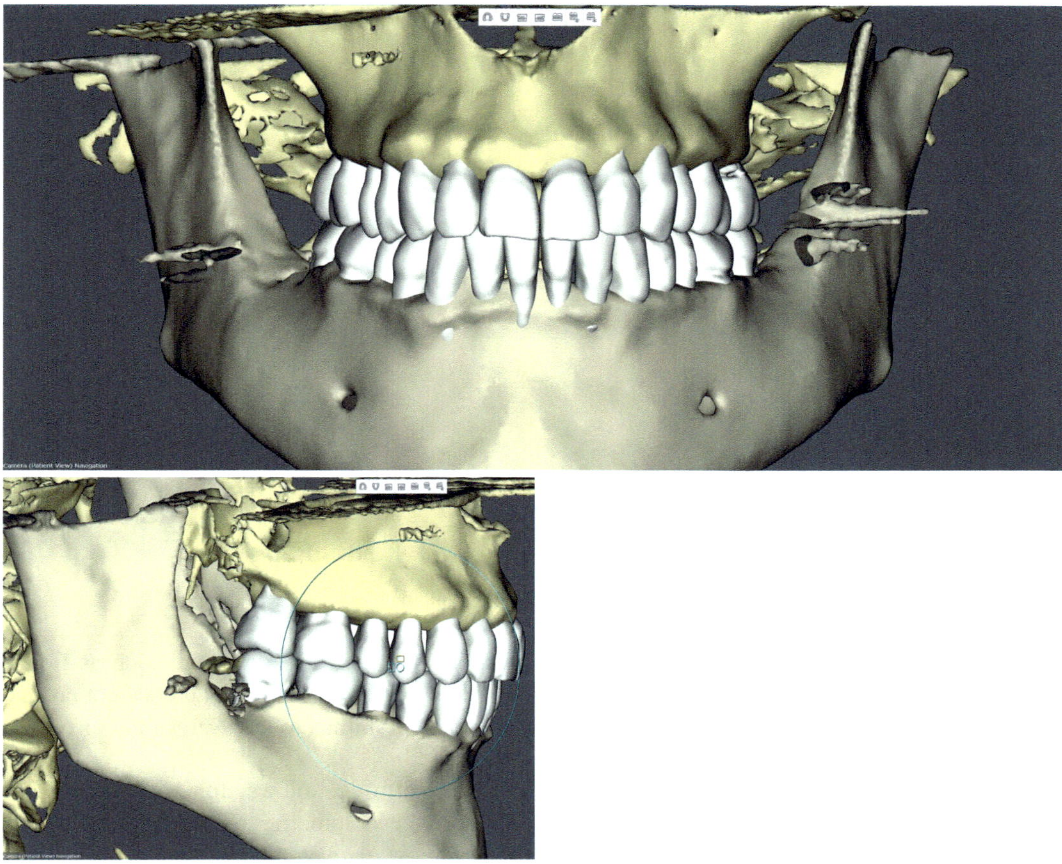

Fig. 1.20 The Suresmile software allows for integration of CBCT imaging and the cephalometric radiograph with the simulated tooth movements

Fig. 1.21 The uLab software allows for a wide variety of attachments and pressure points

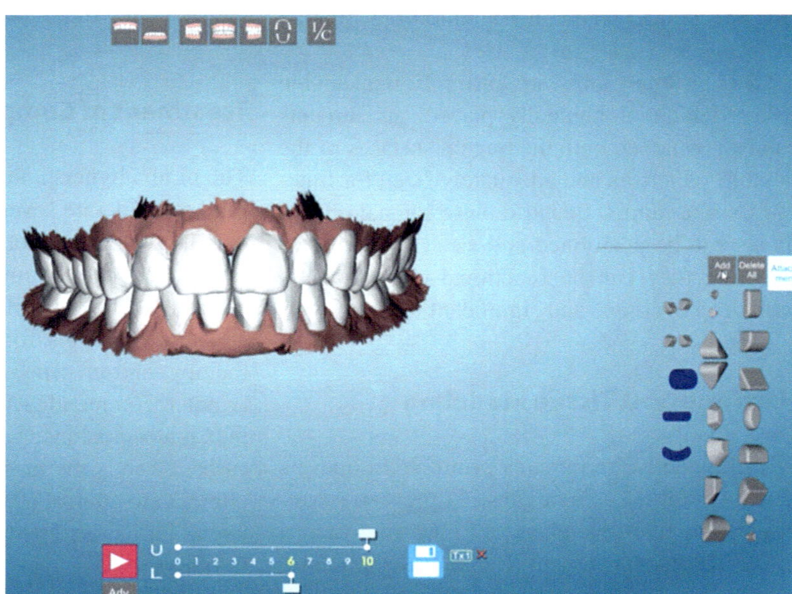

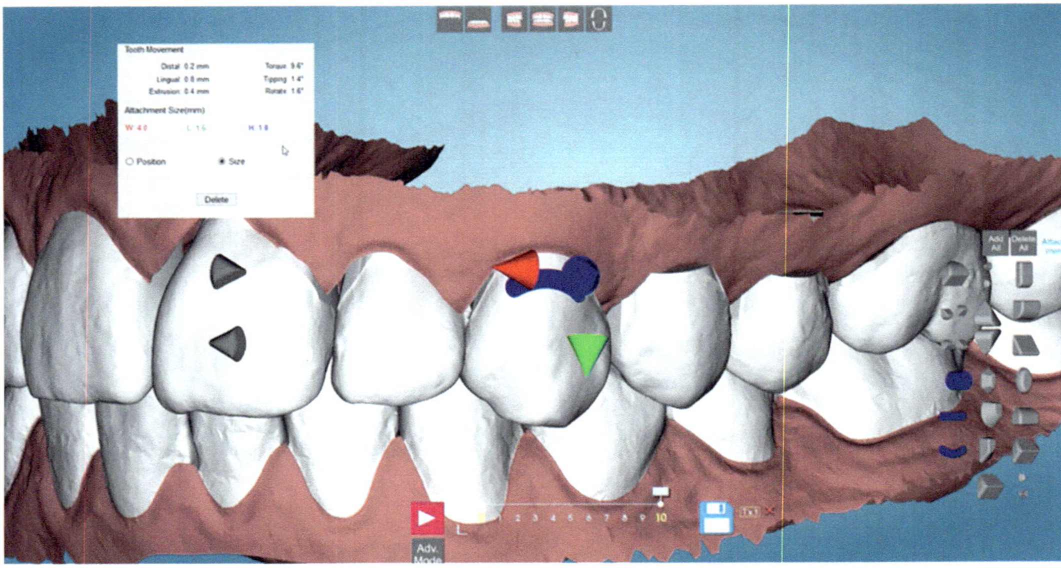

Fig. 1.22 Pressure points can be placed on all surfaces and fully manipulated in the uLab software

Optimizing Single Tooth Movement: Torque Application and Bite Ramps

Like 3M software, uLab employs pressure points for the application of either buccal or lingual root torque. The uLab software permits the placement of the pressure points anywhere on the crown of both anterior and posterior teeth so that lingual root torque can be enhanced by applying a pressure point on the gingival third of the labial surface and another on the incisal third of the lingual surface (Fig. 1.22) [13].

Though bite ramps are currently unavailable either default or manually placed, attachments can be positioned onto the lingual surfaces of the maxillary incisors and adequately sized for function as bite ramps. Because these lingual attachments can be positioned and sized with relative freedom, they can be functional even in cases with deep overbites and significant overjet.

Hard and Soft Tissue Modeling

The uLab software remains primitive in both its hard and soft tissue modeling. At present, it cannot display real-time changes to the gingiva as a result of teeth movement. It also lacks any integration of the facial soft tissue, such as lips in frontal view, lips in profile, and does not possess any feature similar to the Suresmile software's "lip trace."

The software allows for viewing of the untraced cephalometric radiograph but cannot superimpose it over the simulated teeth movements. It has not been developed for integration of CBCT imaging and therefore cannot visualize root movements or the bony housing along with the simulated tooth movements.

Treatment of Complex Malocclusions

The uLab aligners and software are adequate for mild to moderate severity malocclusions but are unequipped for severe malocclusions. It currently lacks a bite jump feature for skeletal discrepancies, any form of mandibular advancement, and any protocols for bite opening, extraction therapy, and growing individuals. The clinician is not recommended to employ uLab for complex malocclusions. Nevertheless, for less severe cases, uLab is the most suited for IHAs, for the clinician to control all stages of tooth movement from initial setup to 3D printing aligners in-house.

The Ideal Clear Aligner Software

In light of the numerous deficiencies that mark the current forms of software, we conclude this chapter by proposing the characteristics that comprise an ideal clear aligner software (Table 1.1) Recent editorials have also advocated the creation of an AAO-based staging software for doctor control over data, workflow, and the delivery of treatment, as opposed to partnering with an external corporation [26]. A software controlled by the orthodontic specialty organization would create a more flexible treatment option for patients. Also, the collection and analysis of data would allow for improved efficacy of evidence-based clear aligner treatments. In light of these recommendations, the following represents a paradigm for a software that can optimize the accuracy of tooth movement, incorporate modern and comprehensive diagnostic and treatment planning tools involving both hard and soft tissue modeling, and realistically plan for the treatment of complex malocclusions (Table 1.2).

Optimizing Tooth Movement: Attachment Design

The ideal software should allow for the clinician to freely customize attachments in all three dimensions—length, width, and depth. The minimal dimensions should be small enough to

Table 1.1 Comparison between major types of clear aligner software

Type of software	Invisalign Clincheck	3M software	Suresmile	uLab
Attachment design	Wide range of shapes. Optimized and default available. Limitations on minimal size.	Limited shapes. No optimized or default. Small volume available for teeth with abnormal morphology.	Limited shapes. No optimized or default. Limitations on minimal size.	Wide range of shapes. No optimized or default. Copy and paste function. Small volume available for teeth with abnormal morphology.
Torque application and bite opening	Power ridges for torque application: limited to labial surfaces and incisors. No clinician adjustment. Bite ramps on lingual surfaces of U3-3. No clinician adjustment.	Pressure points for torque application: limited to labial surfaces and incisors. No clinician adjustment. Bite ramps on lingual surfaces of U3-3. No clinician adjustment.	No alterations in aligner geometry for torque application. No bite ramps available for bite opening.	Pressure points can be applied in any area. Fully adjustable by clinician. Lingual attachments can be employed as bite ramps on any surface. Fully adjustable.
Hard and soft tissue modeling	Limited; primitive gingiva modeling, no facial soft tissue modeling. No integration of cephalometric and CBCT radiographs.	Real-time gingiva modeling, no facial soft tissue modeling. No integration of cephalometric and CBCT radiographs.	Real-time gingiva modeling. Lip trace option available. Integration of CBCT, cephalometric radiograph superimposition available.	Limited; primitive gingiva modeling, no facial soft tissue modeling. No integration of cephalometric and CBCT radiographs.
Treatment of complex malocclusions	Bite jump, mandibular advancement, extraction protocols available. Able to treat complex malocclusions.	No bite jump or mandibular advancement. Virtual gable bend available for extraction cases. Mild-moderate severity malocclusions.	No bite jump or mandibular advancement. No extraction protocols. Mild-moderate severity malocclusions.	No bite jump or mandibular advancement. No extraction protocols. Mild-moderate severity malocclusions.
In-house aligner fabrication	Not compatible.	Not compatible.	Option available.	Compatible.

Table 1.2 Characteristics of an ideal aligner software

Parameter	Characteristics
Attachment design	Freely customizable attachments in all three dimensions and sizes.
Torque application	Free placement of pressure points and lines.
Hard and soft tissue modeling	Integration of soft tissue and CBCT modeling.
Treatment of complex malocclusions	• Realistic bite jump • Surgical planning • Standardization of extensive movements • Realistic growth modeling
In-house aligner fabrication	Compatible.

adapt to small clinical crowns, such as small vertical attachments on diminutive maxillary molars for distalization. Attachment shapes should also be available in a wide array to enhance complex tooth movements, such as coupled, tear-drop shaped attachments, in the fashion of Invisalign's optimized root control attachments, which can be placed facing opposite directions on a tooth crown to enhance root control.

Optimizing Tooth Movement: Torque Application

The ideal software would provide the clinician with fine control of tooth movements in the third order. The uLab software currently permits the greatest freedom for the manipulation of the third order. Similarly, the ideal software would allow for the placement of multiple pressure points on either labial or lingual surfaces and in both anterior and posterior teeth. The accuracy of torquing movements has been shown to be problematic. Studies on the efficacy of tooth movement in nonextraction Invisalign cases have shown statistically significant differences between predicted and actual facial crown torque in the mandibular first and second molars as well as the maxillary first and second molars [27]. The application of pressure points in these problematic areas would allow for greater predictability in torque control [6].

Hard and Soft Tissue Modeling

Real-time hard and soft tissue responses to orthodontic treatment would be fully integrated into an ideal software. The software would allow for the superimposition of the cephalometric radiograph with the simulated teeth movements along with the initial and predicted final measurements. The software would also incorporate soft tissue modeling, including the responses of the gingival tissues, lips, and soft tissue chin to tooth movement. The integration of CBCT imaging would allow for visualization of root movements and the bony housing.

Treatment of Complex Malocclusions

The ideal software would develop realistic and comprehensive features for the treatment of complex malocclusions. The bite jump, which we previously discussed is often overused or unrealistically applied in treatment plans involving skeletal discrepancies, could be monitored by the software so that alerts or warnings could be flagged for movements that are either unpredictable or unfeasible. In other words, the tooth movement assessment tool, which flags difficult tooth movements, would also monitor for difficult interarch movements.

The ideal software would also incorporate more realistic surgical planning so that surgical movements would not only be simulated by bite jumps but also in the manner of virtual model surgery, which is the most commonly accepted method of planning for orthognathic surgery [28]. For instance, in a two-jaw surgery to correct a Class III skeletal patient, the software would be able to precisely simulate the movements of a mandibular setback in addition to a maxillary impaction and advancement rather than resort to a simple bite jump, which would only approximate the surgery by displaying a mandibular setback. Ideally, the software would also simulate surgeries for TMJ disorders such as osteotomies and distraction osteogenesis in the treatment of TMJ ankylosis. Such simulations would be similar to those modeled by imaging software, such as Dolphin, which have been shown to facilitate virtual surgical planning in surgeries for the treatment of TMJ disorders [29].

It would also be important for the ideal software to standardize extensive movements, such as the virtual gable bend, the virtual C-chain, and the bite jump. That is, the software would calibrate a stage of a virtual gable bend to a certain degree of root tipping for each of the teeth adjacent to the extraction space. Similarly, the software would calibrate a single stage of a virtual C-chain to a specific percentage of shrinkage, while a single bite jump would correspond to a certain amount of millimeters of both maxillary and mandibular movement. Such standardization would allow for increased predictability during extraction space closure, finishing, and the correction of skeletal discrepancies.

Lastly, the ideal software would be able to model treatment in growing individuals so that the treatment simulation would include the effects on the jaws due to growth. For instance, in the treatment of children in mixed dentition, forward and downward movement of the maxilla and mandible could be incorporated into the treatment simulation in accordance with craniofacial growth norms [30]. The addition of increments in maxillary and mandibular growth would be particularly useful in treatment planning clear aligner cases involving growing patients who require mandibular advancement or Phase I treatment.

3D Printer Compatibility

As previously mentioned, the future of clear aligner therapy seems to lie in IHA fabrication, in which the clinician sets the majority, if not all, of tooth and interarch movements and 3D prints each aligner in-office. Therefore, it would be important for the ideal software to allow the option for the clinician to control tooth movements from initial setup as well as offer high compatibility with the major brands of 3D printers.

References

1. Bouchez R. Clinical success in Invisalign orthodontic treatment. Paris: Quintessence International; 2010.
2. Galan-Lopez L, Barcia-Gonzalez J, Plasencia E. A systematic review of the accuracy and efficiency of dental movements with Invisalign®. Korean J Orthod. 2019;49(3):140–9.
3. Align Technology. Invisalign for adults and teens. www.invisalign.com/braces-for-adults-and-teens (2020). Accessed 19 Jul 2020.
4. Align Technology. Align Technology receive US patents for Smarttrack Invisalign aligner material. Align Tech (2017). http://investor.aligntech.com/news-releases/news-release-details/align-technology-receives-us-patents-smarttrackr-invisalignr. Accessed 22 Jul 2020.
5. Rossini G, Parrini S, Castroflorio T, Deregibus A, Debernardi CL. Efficacy of clear aligners in controlling orthodontic tooth movement: a systematic review. Angle Orthod. 2015;85(5):881–9.
6. Simon M, Keilig L, Schwarze J, Jung BA, Bourauel C. Treatment outcome and efficacy of an aligner technique—regarding incisor torque, premolar derotation and molar distalization. BMC Oral Health. 2014;14:68.
7. Djeu G, Shelton C, Maganzini A. Outcome assessments of Invisalign and traditional orthodontic treatment compared with the American Board of Orthodontics objective grading system. Am J Orthod Dentofac Orthop. 2005;128:292–8.
8. Kravitz ND, Kusnoto B, Agran B, Viana G. Influence of attachments and interproximal reduction on the accuracy of canine rotation with Invisalign. A prospective clinical study. Angle Orthod. 2008;78:682–7.
9. Kravitz ND, Kusnoto B, BeGole E, Obrez A, Agran B. How well does Invisalign work? A prospective clinical study evaluating the efficacy of tooth movement with Invisalign. Am J Orthod Dentofac Orthop. 2009;135:27–35.
10. Papadimitriou A, Mousoulea S, Gkantidis N, Kloukos D. Clinical effectiveness of Invisalign® orthodontic treatment: a systematic review. Prog Orthod. 2018;19(1):37.
11. Dai F-F, Xu T-M, Shu G. Comparison of achieved and predicted tooth movement of maxillary first molars and central incisors: first premolar extraction treatment with Invisalign. Angle Orthod. 2019;89(5):679–87.
12. Ke Y, Zhu Y, Zhu M. A comparison of treatment effectiveness between clear aligner and fixed appliance therapies. BMC Oral Health. 2019;19(1):24.
13. Hahn W, Zapf A, Dathe H, et al. Torquing an upper central incisor with aligners—acting forces and biomechanical principles. Eur J Orthod. 2010;32(6):607–13.
14. Gu J, Tang JS, Skulski B, Fields HW Jr, Beck FM, Firestone AR, et al. Evaluation of Invisalign treatment effectiveness and efficiency compared with conventional fixed appliances using the peer assessment

rating index. Am J Orthod Dentofac Orthop. 2017;151(2):259–66.
15. Dai F-F, Tian-Min X, Shu G. Comparison of achieved and predicted tooth movement of maxillary first molars and central incisors: first premolar extraction treatment with Invisalign. Angle Orthod. 2019;89(5):679–87.
16. Holberg C, Heine A, Geis P, et al. Three-dimensional soft tissue prediction using finite elements. J Orofac Orthop. 2005;66:122–34.
17. Noguchi N, Tsuji M, Shigematsu M, Goto M. An orthognathic simulation system integrating teeth, jaw, and face data using 3D cephalometry. Int J Oral Maxillofac Surg. 2007;36:640–5.
18. Nanda V, Gutman B, Bar E, et al. Quantitative analysis of 3-dimensional facial soft tissue photographic images: technical methods and clinical application. Prog Orthod. 2015; https://doi.org/10.1186/s40510-015-0082-0.
19. Heil A, Lazo Gonzalez E, Hilgenfeld T, et al. Lateral cephalometric analysis for treatment planning in orthodontics based on MRI compared with radiographs: a feasibility study in children and adolescents. PLoS One. 2017;12(3):e0174524.
20. American Association of Orthodontists. Clinical Practice Guidelines for Orthodontics and Dentofacial Orthopedics. 2014. https://www.aaoinfo.org/system/files/media/documents/2014Cllinical Practice Guidelines.pdf. Accessed 21 Jul 2020.
21. 3M. Clear Aligners. Types of Braces and Treatment. 3M. 2020. https://www.3m.com/3M/en_US/types-of-braces-and-treatment-us/clear-aligners/. Accessed 22 Jul 2020.
22. Haouili N, Kravitz ND, Vaid NR, Ferguson DJ, Makki L. Has Invisalign improved? A prospective follow-up study on the efficacy of tooth movement with Invisalign. Am J Orthod Denofac Orthop. 2020;158(3):420–5.
23. Khosravi R, Cohanim B, Hujoel P, Daher S, Neal M, Liu W, et al. Management of overbite with the Invisalign appliance. Am J Orthod Dentofac Orthop. 2017;151:691–9.
24. Suresmile Aligners. Suresmile. https://www.suresmile.com/device-fabrication/suresmile-aligners/ (2019). Accessed 23 Jul 2020.
25. Maki K, Inou N, Takanishi A, Miller AJ. Computer-assisted simulations in orthodontic diagnosis and the application of a new cone beam X-ray computed tomography. Orthod Craniofacial Res. 2003;6(1):95–101.
26. Riolo C, Vaden J. Taking control of our workflow and data. Am J Orthod Dentofac Orthop. 2021;160:331–4.
27. Grünheid T, Loh C, Larson BE. How accurate is Invisalign in nonextraction cases? Are predicted tooth positions achieved? Angle Orthod. 2017;87(6):809–15.
28. Hammoudeh JA, Howell LK, Boutros S, Scott MA, Urata MM. Current status of surgical planning for orthognathic surgery: traditional methods versus 3D surgical planning. Plast Reconstr Surg Glob Open. 2015;3(2):e307.
29. Chen K, Xiao D, Abotaleb B, Chen H, Li Y, Zhu S. Accuracy of virtual surgical planning in treatment of temporomandibular joint ankylosis using distraction osteogenesis: comparison of planned and actual results. J Oral Maxillofac Surg. 2018;76(11):2422.e1–2422.e20.
30. Buschang PH, Roldan S, Tadlock L. Guidelines for assessing the growth and development of orthodontic patients. Semin Orthod. 2017;23(4):321–35.

Adapting Clear Aligner Therapy to Interceptive Treatment for Early Mixed Dentitions: Are They the Same as Late Teen or Adult Treatment?

2

Contents

Clear Aligner Therapy for Interceptive Treatment: Challenges and Considerations

Historically, clear aligner therapy was originally designed for the treatment of mild malocclusions in adults. However, in 2019, Invisalign adapted their clear aligners for interceptive treatment (Phase I treatment) of children in the early mixed dentition with the introduction of a group of features collectively known as Invisalign First treatment [1]. The updates included optimized support attachments and force systems for increased predictability of dental expansion, optimized retention attachments for improved adherence to teeth with short clinical crowns, eruption compensation for erupting incisors, canines, and premolars, and treatment planning modalities for movements of primary teeth [1]. Because of their recent development, the efficacy of these updates has not been rigorously tested in the scientific literature. However, early clinical trials and clinical application suggest a number of deficiencies in Invisalign First that limit both treatment predictability and efficacy. Phase I therapy poses unique challenges for clear aligner therapy. Though Invisalign First features can replace certain modalities in Phase I treatment with conventional fixed appliances, they often require supplementation or significant modification to achieve the effects necessary for the treatment of the full range of malocclusions in the early mixed dentition.

One of the most critical components of conventional Phase I therapy is growth modification in growing individuals for the correction of Class II and Class III skeletal discrepancies. The precise timing of intervention for Class II discrepancies remains controversial, though studies have shown that significant long-term improvement of

A. T. Huang, D. Huang, *Controversies in Clear Aligner Therapy*,
https://doi.org/10.1007/978-3-030-92810-0_2

Class II skeletal relationships occurs when treatment is started at the outset of puberty [2]. Nevertheless, there is an increased acceptance that though early intervention in Class II malocclusions may not be more effective long-term, it is more efficient than later treatment [3]. However, there is a greater consensus that early intervention is most optimal for the correction of Class III skeletal discrepancies. It has been shown that maxillary protraction (traditionally with rapid maxillary expansion and reverse-pull facemask) is most successful when performed in the early mixed dentition [4]. Importantly, conventional Phase I therapy also typically includes rapid maxillary expansion (RME), involving the widening of the maxillary basal bone prior to the fusion of the maxillary sutures at 14–15 in females and 15–16 in males [5]. Early expansion is often used for the purposes of the correction of transverse discrepancies, increased effectiveness of maxillary protraction, elimination of functional shift, and the resolution of arch length deficiency. Baccetti et al. observed that RME treatment in the pre-peak period of puberty resulted in greater transverse skeletal changes than those when RME treatment was initiated in the post-peak period [6]. Therefore, it is essential that an adaptation of clear aligner therapy for interceptive treatment allows for the incorporation of growth modification and orthopedic treatment effects.

One of the challenges of Phase I therapy is that significant dental changes occur over a short time frame. For instance, an effective appliance for the interceptive treatment of patients in the early mixed dentition needs to accommodate the exfoliation of primary teeth and the eruption of succedaneous teeth. This can be problematic for an appliance like clear aligners, which cannot be readily modified during a course of aligners.

Phase I therapy also requires the management of children, who are generally not as compliant or as motivated as the adult or late teenager population [7]. Clear aligner therapy may require certain modifications to address hyperactive or noncompliant children, especially because aligners are more susceptible to wear and breakage than traditional Phase I fixed appliances, i.e., rapid palatal expander, mandibular lingual arches, transpalatal arches, and transpalatal-Nance arches.

In this chapter, we discuss the effectiveness of clear aligners in their application to Phase I therapy. We describe the major features of the most current form of clear aligners for Phase I therapy, its applications for treatment, its deficiencies, and propose current and future solutions to maximize its effectiveness.

Major Features of Clear Aligner Interceptive Treatment

Expansion

For interceptive treatment, Invisalign clear aligners rely heavily on expansion for arch length development. The treatment effects of expansion with clear aligners simulate those of traditional Phase I appliances with expansion capabilities, such as the lip bumper, the inner bow of the headgear, RME, mandibular lingual arches, transpalatal arches, transpalatal-Nance arches, and certain functional appliances. At present, Invisalign has incorporated optimized expansion attachments in order to supplement the predictability of expansion movements (Fig. 2.1). There has been a limited number of studies that have assessed the efficacy of expansion with clear aligners in the child or teenage population, but there have been clinical trials investigating its efficacy in adults. It has been observed that maximum expansion with Invisalign should be limited to 2–4 mm [8]. A recent study showed that in adults, Invisalign could achieve 68.31% efficacy of crown expansion movement for maxillary first molars [9]. Another study found a 72.8% efficacy of expansion for the maxilla and 87.7% efficacy of expansion for the mandible [10]. However, it is important to note that most of the crown expansion movement occurred through buccal tipping rather than bodily expansion or skeletal expansion. Houle et al. found that Clincheck's prediction of expansion involved more bodily movement than clinically observed, while more buccal tipping was found than predicted [10]. Therefore, the clinician should be mindful of performing

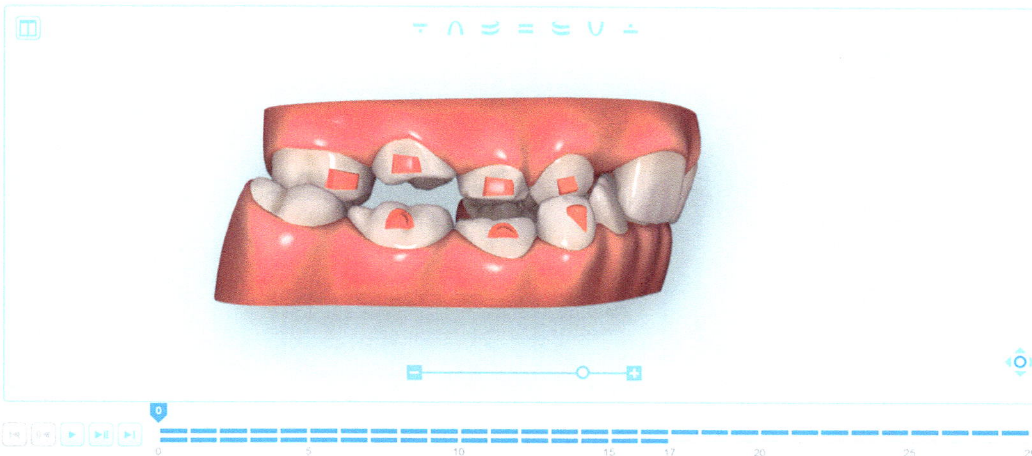

Upper / Lower	30	T	S	R	26	25	24	23	22
Extrusion/Intrusion, mm	0.3 E	1.1 E	1.3 E	0.6 E	0.3 I	0.5 I	1.0 I	0.1 I	0.3 E
Translation Buccal/Lingual, mm	2.6 L	0.2 B	1.7 B	1.2 B	2.5 B	3.3 B	3.9 B	3.9 B	4.6 B
Translation Mesial/Distal, mm	0.3 M	0.1 M	0.3 M	0.2 M	0.5 M	0	0.5 M	1.6 M	0.3 D
Rotation Mesial/Distal	3.6°D	7.0°D	6.4°D	7.8°M	35.6°D	6.7°M	9.3°M	9.1°D	8.1°M
Angulation Mesial/Distal	0.9°M	3.7°M	4.8°M	6.2°M	8.9°M	0.3°D	0°	10.4°M	5.3°M
Inclination Buccal/Lingual	0.4°L	2.0°L	5.7°B	4.0°B	16.2°B	19.7°B	23.1°B	22.7°B	18.3°B

Fig. 2.1 Optimized expansion attachments have been incorporated on the right mandibular first and second primary molars (#S and #T). Both are programmed for buccal translation, as indicated by the tooth movement assessment table

extensive expansion movements, i.e. >4 mm, even in the child population, because the clear aligner appliance primarily relies on buccal tipping for expansion effects. Later in this chapter, we discuss approaches to controlling expansion during interceptive treatment within a safe range.

Eruption Compensation

For the orthodontic treatment of patients in the early mixed dentition, the appliance must accommodate for the frequent exfoliation of primary teeth and the eruption of succedaneous teeth. Invisalign First has incorporated eruption compensation features into its appliance to plan and maintain space for permanent teeth (Fig. 2.2) [1]. Invisalign claims that its eruption compensation algorithm can accurately predict and create the spacing necessary for the maxillary incisors, canines, and premolars [11]. Eruption compensation features have been available for adolescents with Invisalign Teen, which was introduced in 2008. However, research has focused on the effects of the appliance in adults and offers limited evidence regarding the accuracy of the eruption compensation algorithm.

Optimized Attachments

For interceptive treatment, Invisalign has designed specialized optimized attachments for patients in the mixed dentition. As previously mentioned, optimized attachments are automatically placed on both primary and permanent teeth to supplement all types of movements. Like the optimized attachments for permanent teeth, those for the early mixed dentition also enhance a wide range of movements, such as rotation, root tipping, and extrusion (Fig. 2.3). In contrast to both the optimized and nonoptimized attachments for permanent dentition, the Invisalign First optimized attachments are sized for adaptation to the small clinical crowns of primary teeth. However, nonoptimized attachments are still limited in the sense that they cannot be minimized beyond a size of 3 mm.

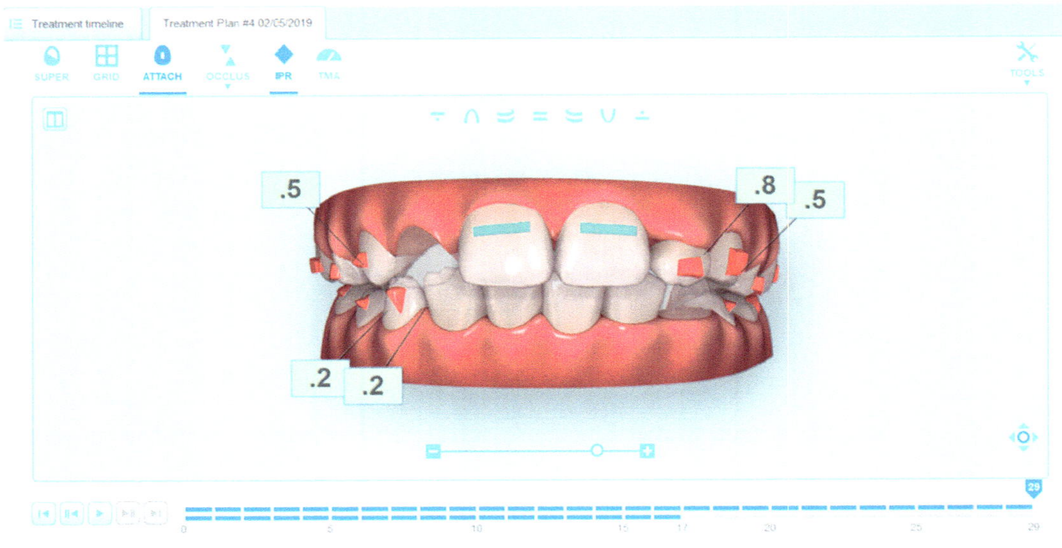

Fig. 2.2 Invisalign First's eruption compensation algorithm has planned for the eruption of the maxillary right lateral incisor and the mandibular left canine

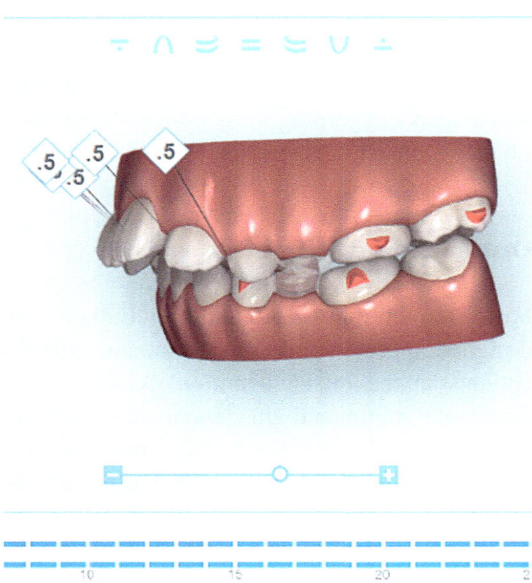

Fig. 2.3 On the left maxillary first molar, the left second maxillary primary molar, and the left second mandibular primary molar, optimized attachments enhance movements such as expansion and derotation

Mandibular Advancement

In 2018, Invisalign introduced its mandibular advancement feature for the correction of skeletal Class II discrepancies. The feature sought to simulate the mandibular repositioning effects of Class II functional appliances, such as the Twin-Block, MARA, Herbst appliance, and other activators. It employs "precision wings," which are extensions from both the maxillary and mandibular aligners that hold the mandible in a forward position (Fig. 2.4). The feature is only available for patients in the mixed dentition, which applies to Invisalign First and Invisalign Teen patients. Only a limited number of pilot studies has investigated the efficacy of the mandibular advancement feature, which we examine further in Chap. 3.

Phase II Treatment

Like more traditional forms of Phase I, interceptive treatment with clear aligners should be completed as efficiently as possible to minimize treatment time [12]. After its completion, patients are typically monitored at 6–12 month intervals until the eruption of the remaining permanent teeth. Because it is common that a significant period of time will elapse before the patient is dentally mature enough for Phase II, the clinician

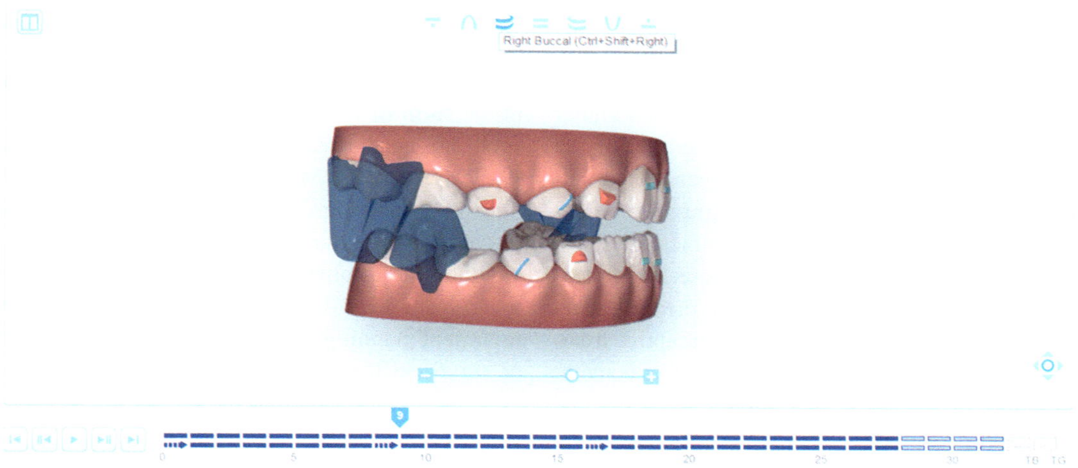

Fig. 2.4 The mandibular advancement feature is simulated in the Clincheck through the extensions from the maxillary and mandibular molars. The simulation demonstrates a 1 mm advancement of the mandible occurring between the eighth and ninth stage. Precision cuts have been designed on the maxillary primary canines and mandibular primary first molars for vertical elastics to maintain a forward repositioned bite

will have to consider retention measures. These may involve more traditional appliances because, at present, Invisalign does not provide retainers that can accommodate the transition of dentition in patients between phase I and II. Interceptive treatment with clear aligners will typically be followed by Phase II treatment in the form of the Invisalign Teen appliance, which shares a number of features with Invisalign First, including the eruption compensation algorithm.

Frequent Midcourse Corrections

During the course of interceptive treatment with clear aligners of patients in the mixed dentition, erupting permanent teeth can often lead to poor tracking, even with the application of the eruption compensation algorithm. In such cases, the clinician must either order a midcourse correction or additional aligners to continue treatment by accommodating for erupting permanent teeth. One of the characteristics of Invisalign First is the greater frequency of midcourse corrections when compared to that of adult or teen Invisalign treatment.

Duration of Aligner Wear

Studies have shown that teenage patients may prefer removable clear aligners to fixed appliances for reasons such as improved esthetics, less hard and soft tissue irritation, no dietary restrictions, and fewer social issues [13]. However, prepubescent children may have more frequent compliance issues with clear aligners than older populations such as chewing or playing with the appliance leading to breakage. In these cases, the duration for each aligner may have to be shortened from the typical 14 days to 5 or 7 days in order to minimize breakage and facilitate treatment.

Treatment Applications

Interceptive treatment with clear aligners can achieve typical Phase I objectives, such as the alleviation of an anterior crossbite, space management for erupting permanent teeth, or correction of anterior crowding, by simulating the dental effects of a maxillary and mandibular 2 × 4 setup in conventional fixed appliances (Fig. 2.5). In the case illustrated in Fig. 2.5, patient V.Z. received a course of conventional Phase I appliances, including treatment with high-pull headgear and lip bumper. The lip bumper expanded the mandibular arch and relieved crowding in the region of the mandibular right canine but the mandibular left canine remain blocked out. A course of clear aligners further expanded the arch to create space for the mandibular left canine. Phase I treatment was followed with Invisalign Teen clear aligners during phase II. In this fashion, interceptive treatment with clear aligners can function like conventional Phase I appliances to relieve crowding and create space for permanent teeth.

However, because clear aligners are not able to produce orthopedic effects, for more severe discrepancies, they may require supplementation in the form of traditional orthopedic appliances, such as headgear, the reverse-pull facemask (RPFM), and the RME. Though Invisalign claims that its mandibular advancement appliance can produce orthopedic effects, it remains uncertain whether the appliance can effectively promote mandibular growth. The clear aligner itself and treatment planning with the software may have to be modified for the incorporation of orthopedic appliances during the course of interceptive treatment.

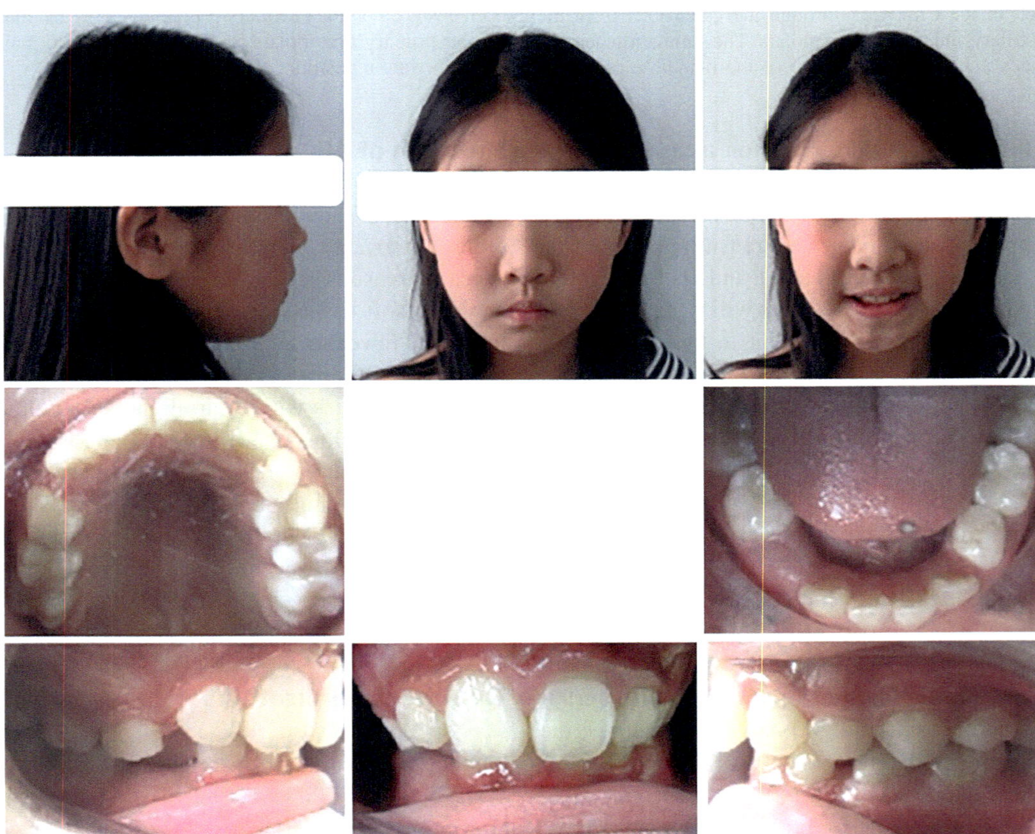

Fig. 2.5 Patient V.Z. received an initial course of treatment with high-pull headgear and lip bumper. Afterward, the mandibular arch was further expanded with a course of Invisalign First clear aligners. Adequate space was created for the left mandibular canine with the course of clear aligners. Phase II treatment involved detailing and finishing, reduction of residual overjet, and correction of canines and molars into Class I relationships

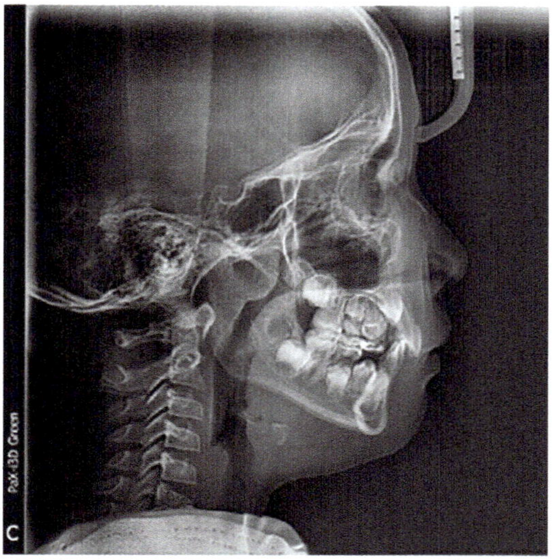

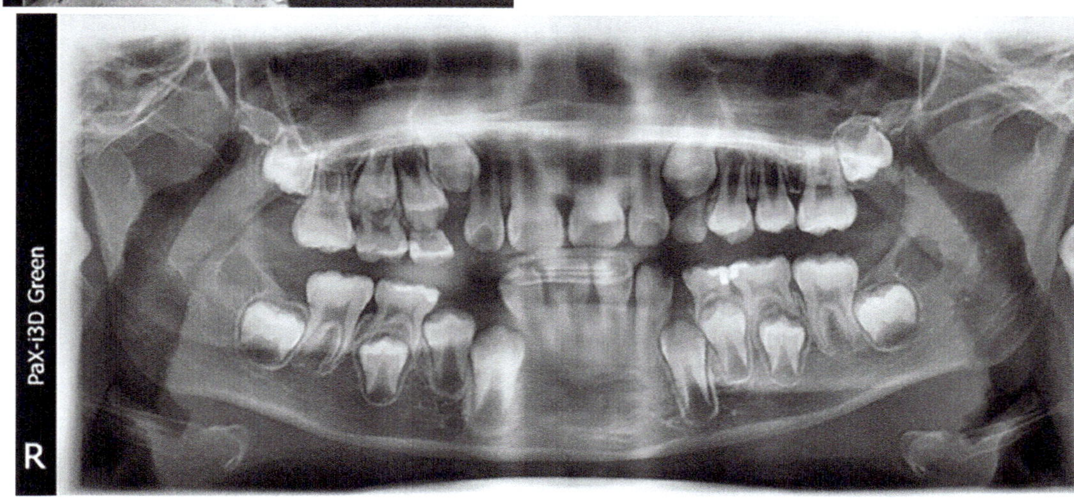

Fig. 2.5 (continued)

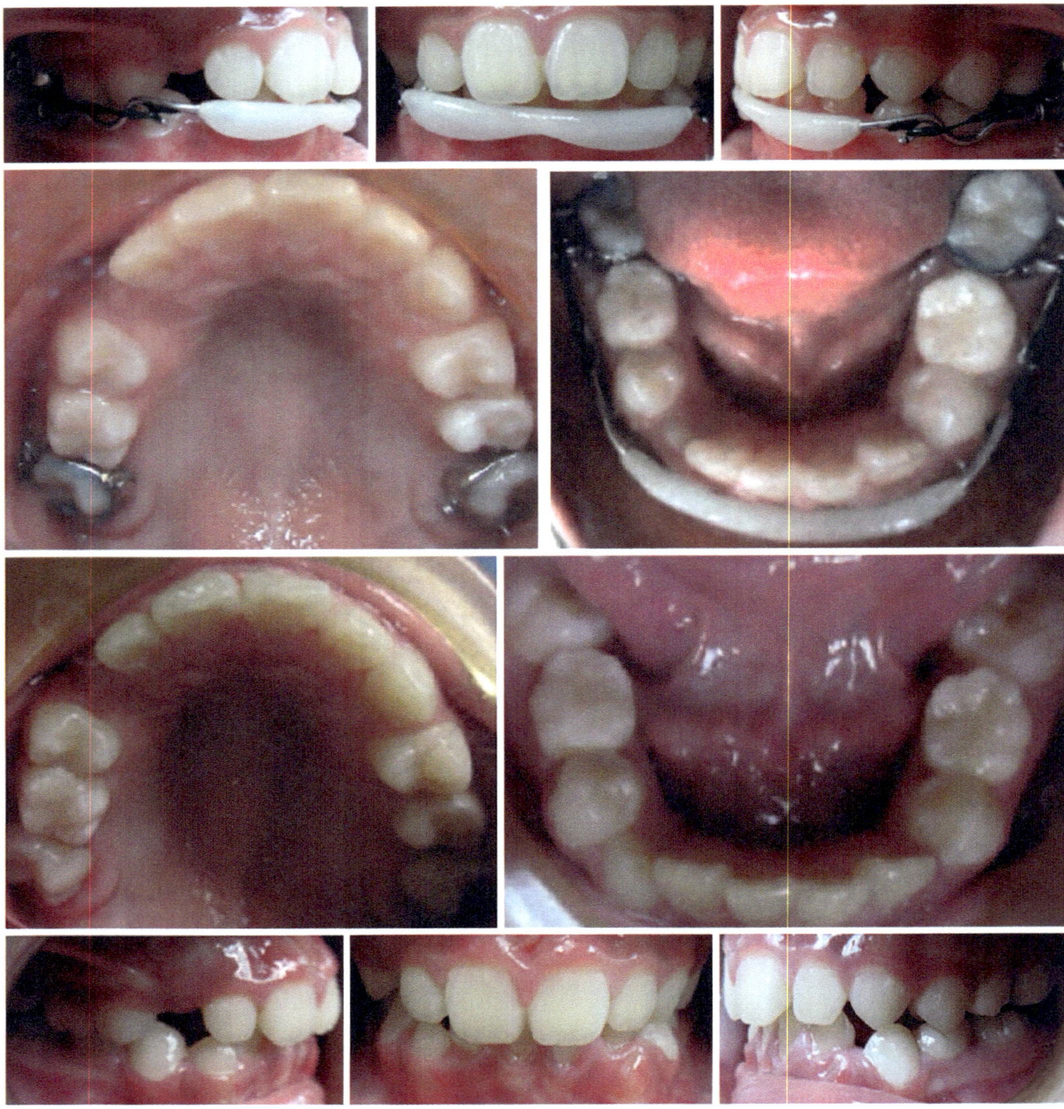

Fig. 2.5 (continued)

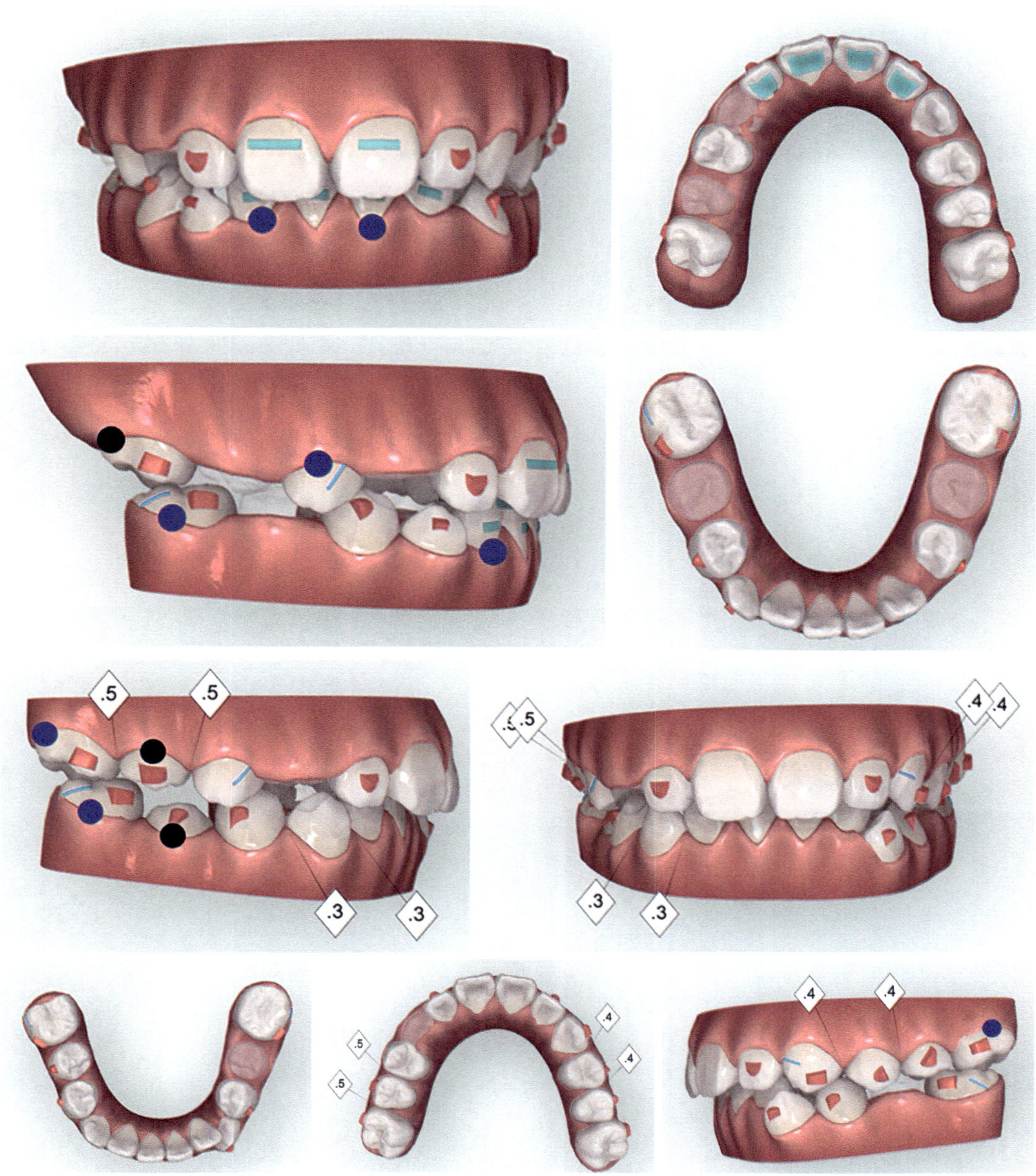

Fig. 2.5 (continued)

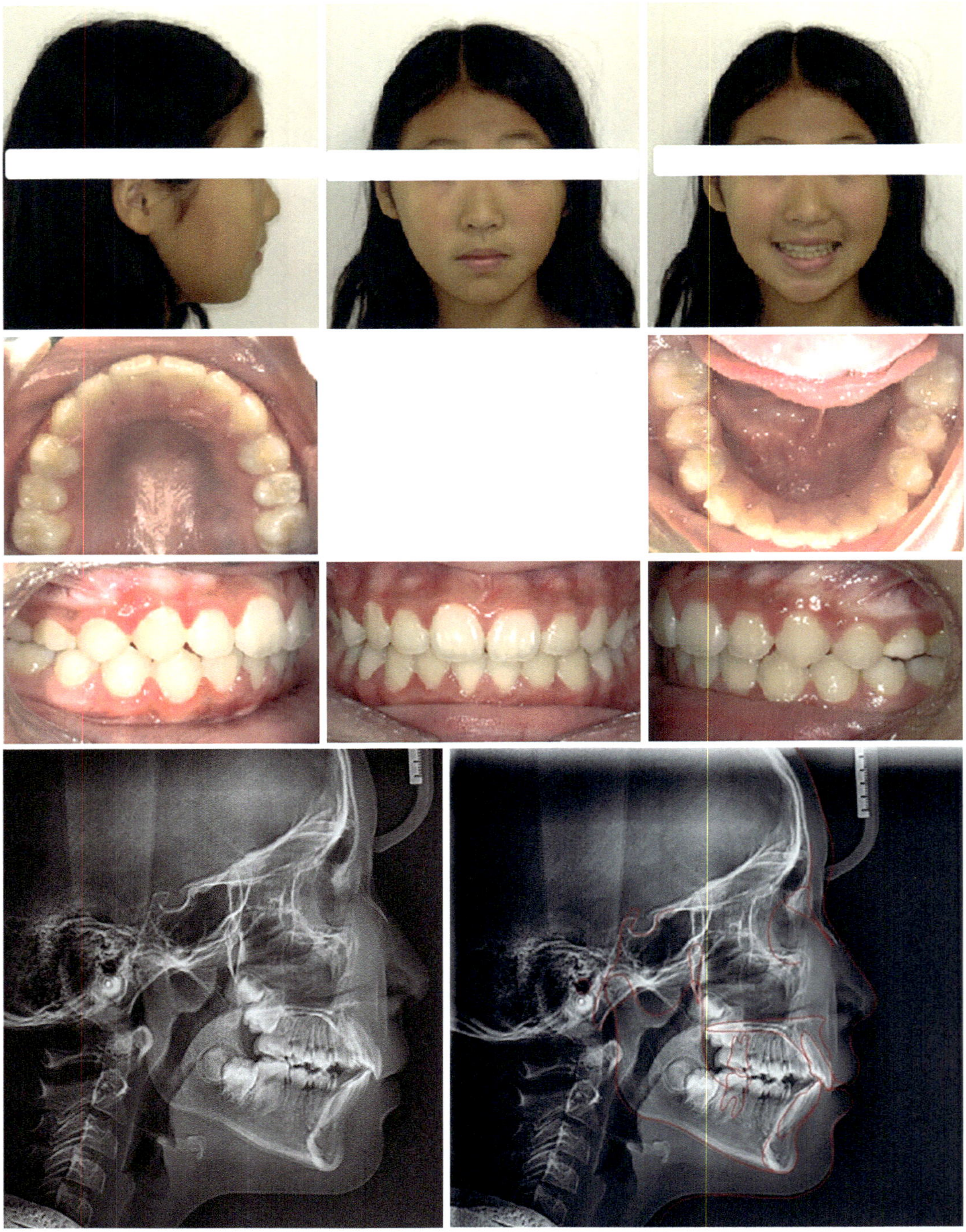

Fig. 2.5 (continued)

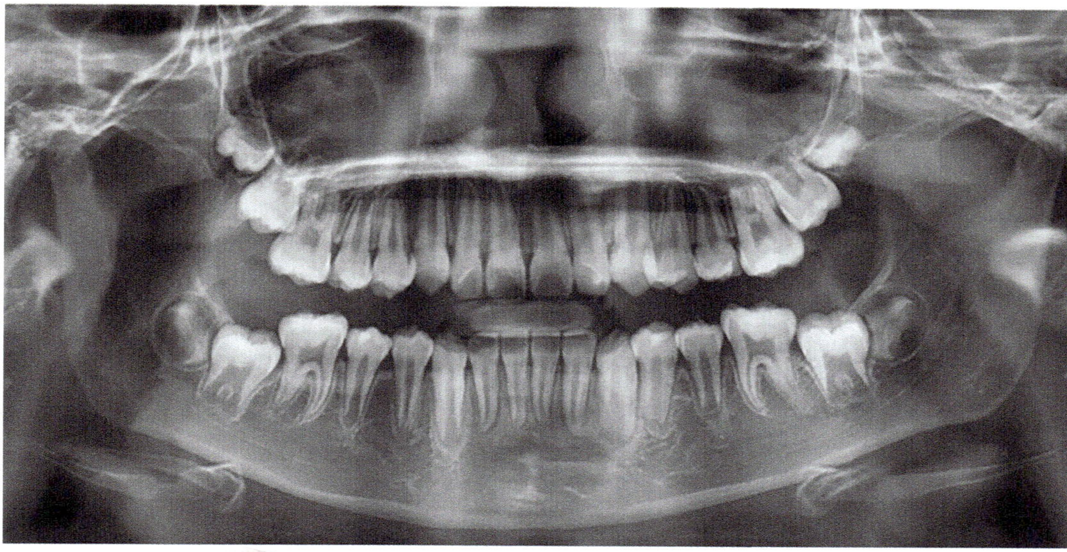

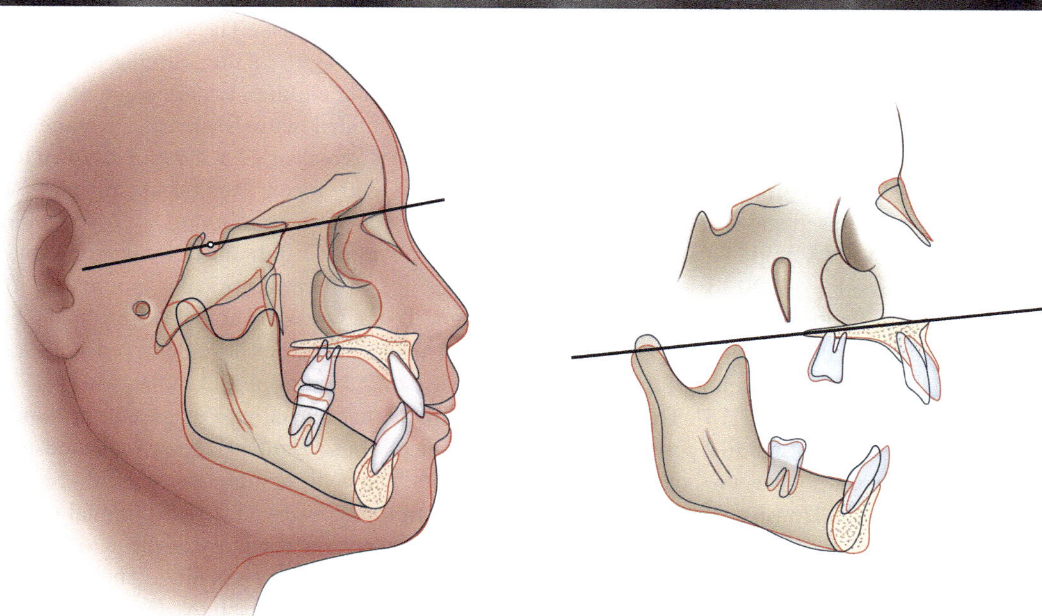

Fig. 2.5 (continued)

The Deficiencies of Interceptive Treatment with Clear Aligners

Limitations in Growth Modification and Prediction

Invisalign has claimed that its mandibular advancement appliance can correct Class II discrepancies by promoting mandibular growth in a "more efficient" manner than conventional functional appliances [14]. These strong claims of greater efficiency have not been supported by any substantial scientific evidence. Like other appliances when first introduced for orthodontic treatment, the mandibular advancement feature requires further research regarding its treatment efficacy.

The Invisalign First appliance is also limited in its compatibility with more conventional orthopedic appliances whose potential treatment effects have been established, most notably the headgear. High-quality studies have noted that headgear treatment can produce skeletal changes in the short term, as demonstrated by a mean annual change in SNA angle (−1.63°/year, 95% Confidence Interval = −2.20 to −1.06°/year) in treated patients compared to untreated patients (though the amount of skeletal change long-term seems to diminish when comparing headgear treated to untreated patients) [15]. The Invisalign First appliance does not readily permit the integration of appliances such as the headgear during a course of aligners. However, for Class III correction, the reverse-pull facemask (RPFM) can be incorporated into aligner wear through precision cuts at the first maxillary molars or alternative means, such as bonding metal buttons onto the first maxillary molars and creating button cutouts in the series of aligners.

In addition to these limitations in the application of orthopedic forces, the Invisalign First appliance also lacks realistic modeling of mandibular growth in prepubertal patients. Presently, the appliance employs the bite jump to simulate mandibular growth during a course of aligners (Fig. 2.6). However, the bite jump is not calibrated to any standard of growth and tends to overestimate the extent of mandibular growth in the prepubescent patient because the software will automatically finish the occlusion as ideally as possible. As a result, the bite jump may produce an unfeasible treatment outcome. The clinician must be cautious that the software does not perform unrealistic movements with bite jumps during treatment planning with Invisalign First.

Range of Expansion

The Invisalign First appliance currently allows the clinician to select among several options for the range of expansion desired for treatment planning a given case. The choices range from <2, 2–4, 4–6, 6–8, to >8 mm. Studies have shown that in growing children (average age of 8 years, 1 month) treated with RME, the average total expansion was measured at the molar crown to be 3.60 mm, with mean skeletal expansion at the molar of 1.60 mm (minimum: 1.12 mm, maximum: 1.97 mm) [16]. In the treatment of growing children with conventional appliances that expand less aggressively, such as the inner bow of the headgear, studies have observed an average increase of 2.31 mm in intermolar width [17]. It is unlikely that Invisalign First, a non-orthopedic appliance whose limit has been indicated to be 2–4 mm, can achieve a greater amount of expansion than those observed in conventional modalities of expansion, particularly the RME, which induces palatal sutural opening. Therefore, it is problematic that Invisalign First allows for choices of expansion that range greater than 4 mm because such expansion movements, when modeled in the treatment simulation, would be unrealistic.

Adaptation to Short Clinical Crowns

As previously discussed, Invisalign First has incorporated optimized retention attachments for increased adherence of its aligners [11]. However, the attachments are often still inadequate to retain the aligner to deciduous teeth with short clinical crowns and to prevent dislodging. These optimized attachments are also not modifiable by the clinician, so their sizes and positions may not be ideal for retention onto the deciduous crown.

Inadequate crown retention can also be problematic for elastics wear in Invisalign First patients. During interceptive treatment with clear aligners, intermaxillary elastics and elastics for RPFM wear are often applied from precision cuts on either or both the maxillary and the mandibular aligners. Even with the addition of retention attachments, the short clinical crowns of deciduous teeth lend themselves to aligner dislodging during elastics wear. An alternative to frequent dislodging can be to bond metal buttons on the teeth for elastics wear. However, the clinician should be mindful that children and prepubescent adolescents are populations that are more prone to the breakage of fixed appliances than adults [18]. The parents of children who elected for Invisalign First over fixed appliances may oppose any fixed appliance because, at the outset, they desired for their children no restrictions in eating and brushing. It is also important to note that the application of force directly onto teeth with metal buttons may result in undesired side effects, such as extrusion of molars during Class II or Class III elastics, or mesialization and rotation of maxillary molars with RPFM wear (Fig. 2.7).

In the case illustrated in Fig. 2.7, the patient I.T. received Phase I treatment with clear aligners supplemented with RPFM. The protraction force was directed to buttons on the maxillary left first premolar because of lack of retention on the short clinical crowns of the first permanent molars. The RPFM allowed for forward advancement of the maxilla but caused the mesialization of the maxillary left first premolar leading to potential impaction of the maxillary left canine. The

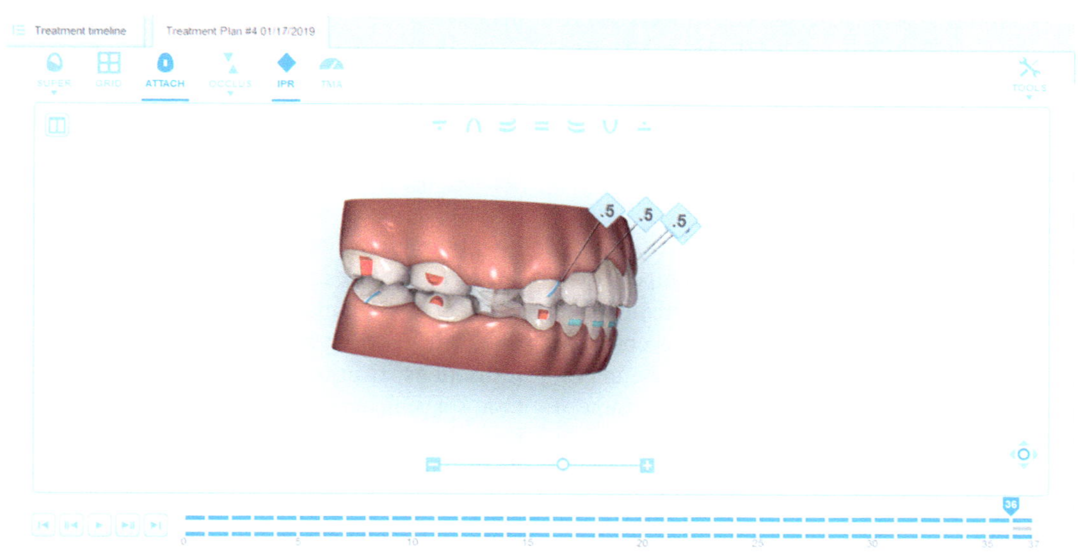

Fig. 2.6 A bite jump was programmed into the Clincheck between stages 36 and 37. It advanced the mandible 3 mm forward.

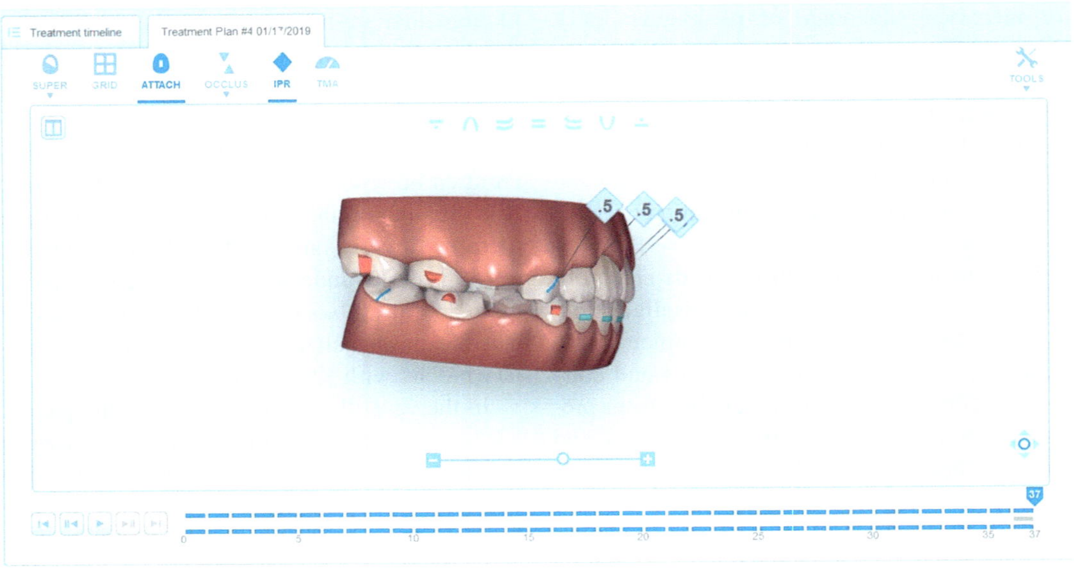

Fig. 2.6 (continued)

patient received a refinement course to distalize the maxillary left first premolar and to ensure adequate space for the eruption of the maxillary left canine. I.T's case evidences the importance of monitoring for adverse side effects when incorporating additional appliances to clear aligners during interceptive treatment.

Software Calibration for Treatment Planning

Invisalign claims that its eruption compensation algorithm for incisors, canines, and premolars is "highly accurate." Clinically, we have observed that the accuracy of the algorithm can be unpredictable. It tends to underestimate the amount of space necessary for the eruption of the permanent tooth, so the clinician must often increase the space originally planned by the software (Fig. 2.8).

Similarly, the software has not calibrated tooth positions and movements to cephalometric data. As a result, the simulated inclinations of the maxillary and mandibular incisors are often not representative of their actual positions as reflected by standardized cephalometric measurements such as IMPA and U1-SN. Therefore, the final incisor positions modeled by the Clincheck do not accurately project what may occur as a result of treatment.

Availability of Clinical Preferences

During the submission of a new patient case prior to the development of the treatment simulation, Invisalign allows the clinician to select certain preferences, including whether to incorporate the mandibular advancement feature, bite opening mechanics, tooth movement restrictions, overjet correction, midline correction, space management, teeth that require eruption compensation, and modalities for decrowding, i.e., anterior interproximal reduction, posterior interproximal reduction, expansion, and proclination. However, these clinical preferences still lack important features for treatment planning, including the placement of precision cuts, timing of attachment placement, and limitations for the expansion of the mandibular intercanine width.

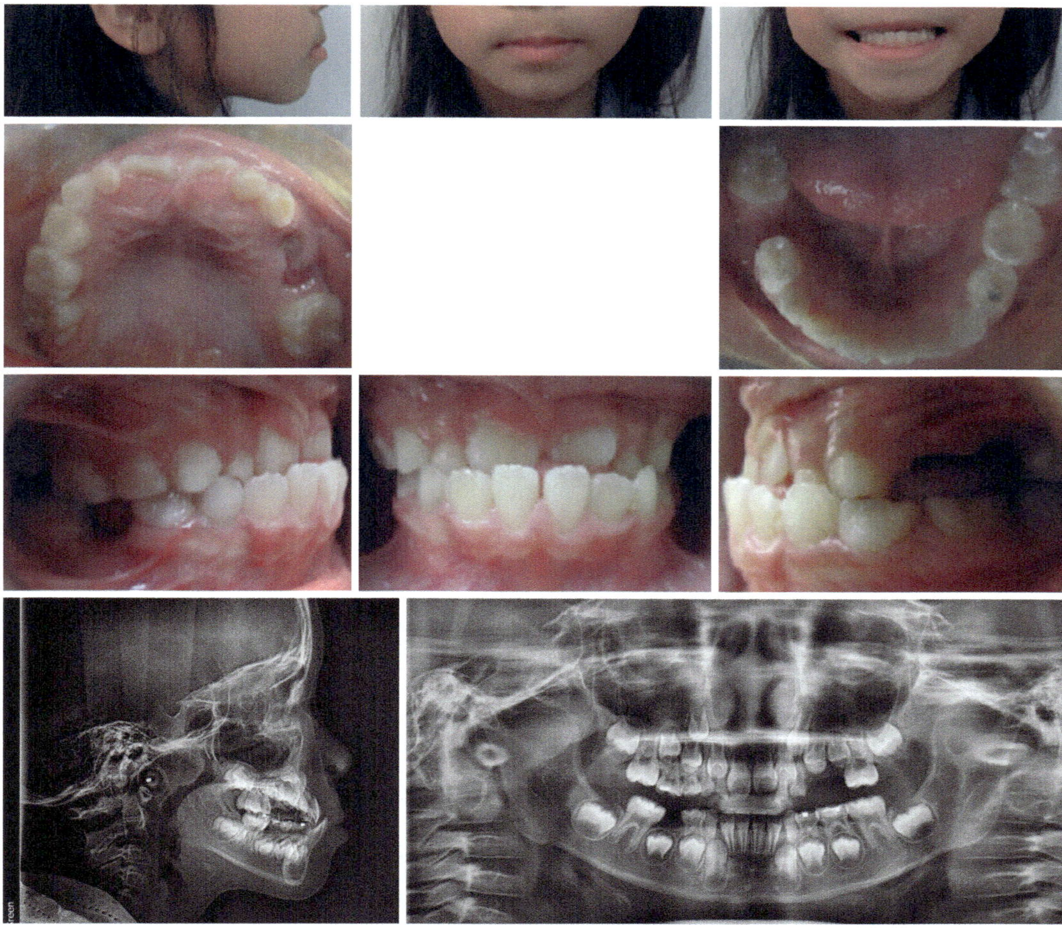

Fig. 2.7 Patient I.T. was treated with RPFM in combination with clear aligners (Invisalign First). The protraction force could not be applied to precision cuts respective to the first maxillary molars due to their short clinical crowns and problems with retention. As a result, the RPFM was applied with elastics to buttons on the left maxillary primary canine and then the left maxillary first premolar after it was erupted. The protraction force assisted in jumping the anterior crossbite and advancing the maxilla. However, it also mesialized the maxillary left first premolar despite encapsulation by the aligner. The undesired movement of the maxillary left first premolar led to possible impaction of the maxillary left canine. Consequently, we incorporated a short refinement course to distalize the left maxillary first premolar to create adequate space for the eruption of the left maxillary canine

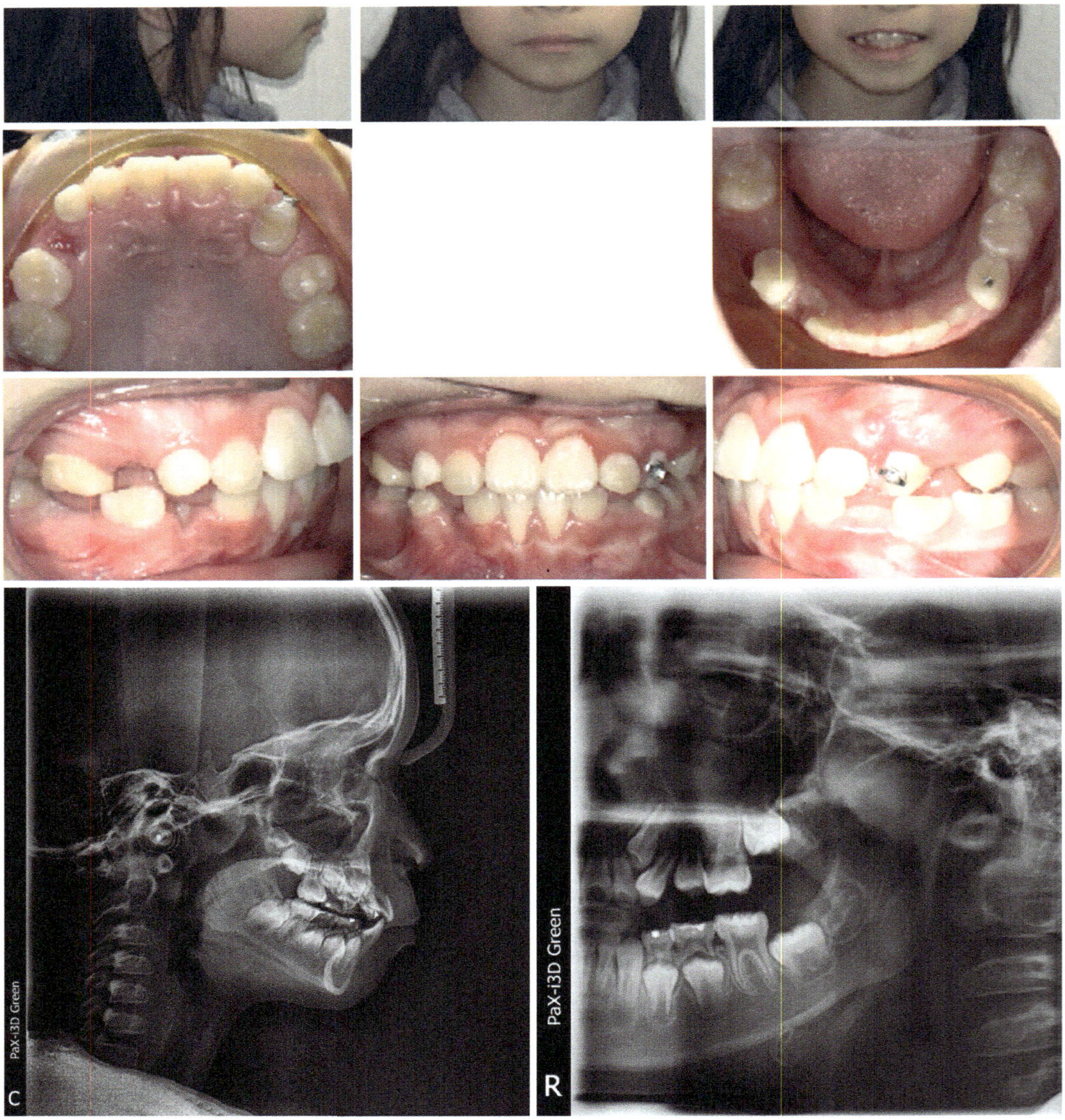

Fig. 2.7 (continued)

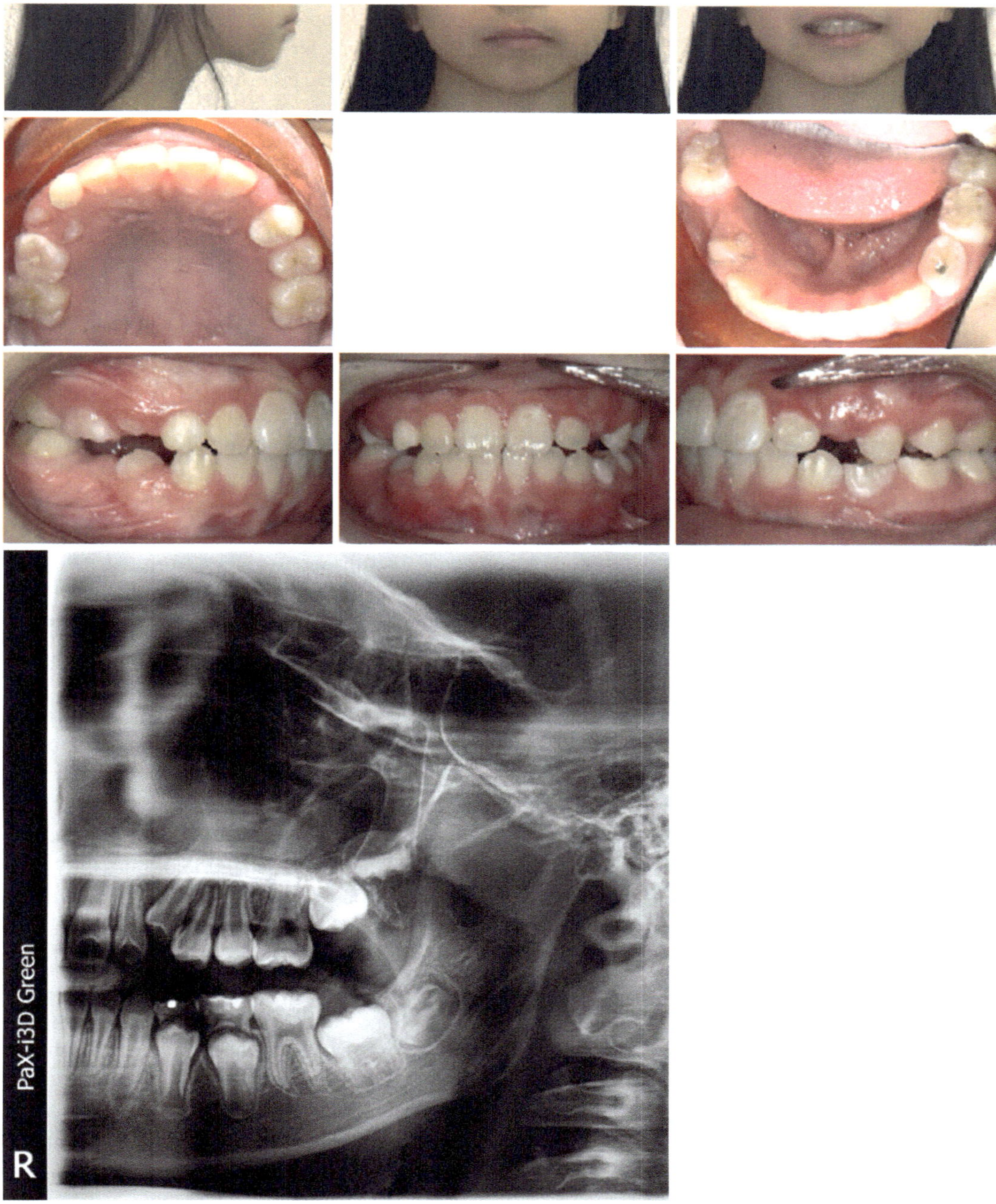

Fig. 2.7 (continued)

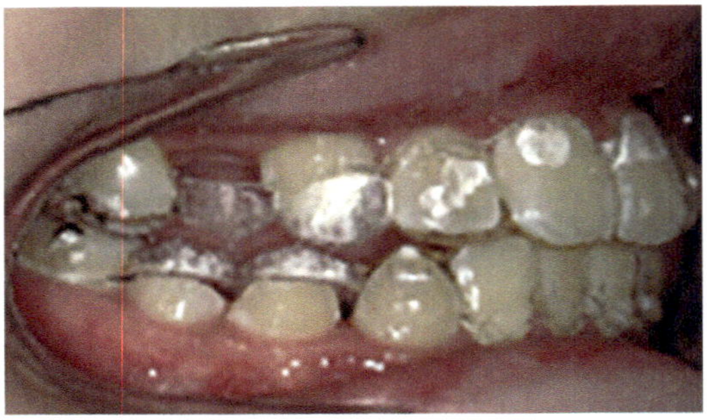

Fig. 2.8 The eruption compensation algorithm occasionally underestimates the space necessary for the eruption of permanent teeth. In this case, the space afforded the erupting maxillary second premolar (both maxillary first premolars have been extracted) is insufficient

Post-Interceptive Treatment Retention

At present, Invisalign First has not developed a form of retention to maintain the results of Phase I treatment. This lack is especially problematic because the outcomes of Phase I treatment are often prone to relapse or becoming undone through natural growth and development. For instance, arch expansion of initially constricted maxillary or mandibular arches tends to relapse toward their original dimensions [19, 20]. Also, without retention, crowding tends to recur and can potentially impact erupting permanent teeth. To prevent such adverse effects, clinicians have to create specialized forms of retention to preserve the outcomes of interceptive treatment with clear aligners.

Solutions to Current Limitations in Clear Aligner Interceptive Treatment

Incorporating Orthopedic Appliances

We have discussed that the Invisalign First appliance allows for RPFM use during a course of aligners. The addition of orthopedic protraction force is essential for the correction of true Class III discrepancies, especially of greater severity. Studies have shown that children with Class III malocclusions who received treatment with protraction facemask demonstrated significant skeletal changes when compared to non-treated controls, including ANB: +3.66°, SNA: +2.10°, SNB: −1.54°, and significant changes in the palatal and mandibular plane angles [21]. The facemask's protraction force can be delivered with elastics directly to the aligner's precision cuts on the maxillary first molars or canines or to buttons bonded onto the maxillary first molars (Fig. 2.9). In this manner, the protraction force can be directed approximately through the center of resistance of the maxilla. These concepts are illustrated in Fig. 2.9, in which patient W. W. was treated during phase I with RPFM and two courses of clear aligners. The protraction force was applied through elastics from the RPFM to precision cuts incorporated into the aligner respective to the first maxillary molars. Therefore, the patient was able to wear the RPFM while the clear aligners corrected other aspects of the malocclusion, including decrowding of the maxillary and mandibular anterior teeth and creation of space for the maxillary lateral incisors. The anterior crossbite was corrected through the combination of RPFM and clear aligner movements through both the normalization of maxillary incisor inclinations and forward movement of the maxilla.

However, the appliance still lacks features for compatibility with other major orthopedic appliances, such as the headgear. At present, the headgear can be incorporated into clear aligner interceptive treatment as a phase prior to a course of Invisalign First aligners. That is, the patient would wear the headgear until Class II molar relationships were improved to Class I and subsequently, the patient would receive a course of aligners to achieve the other objectives of Phase I treatment, such as normalization of overjet or creation of adequate space for erupting permanent teeth. Alternatively, the headgear could be combined with a course of aligners. For instance, the maxillary first molars can be banded, while

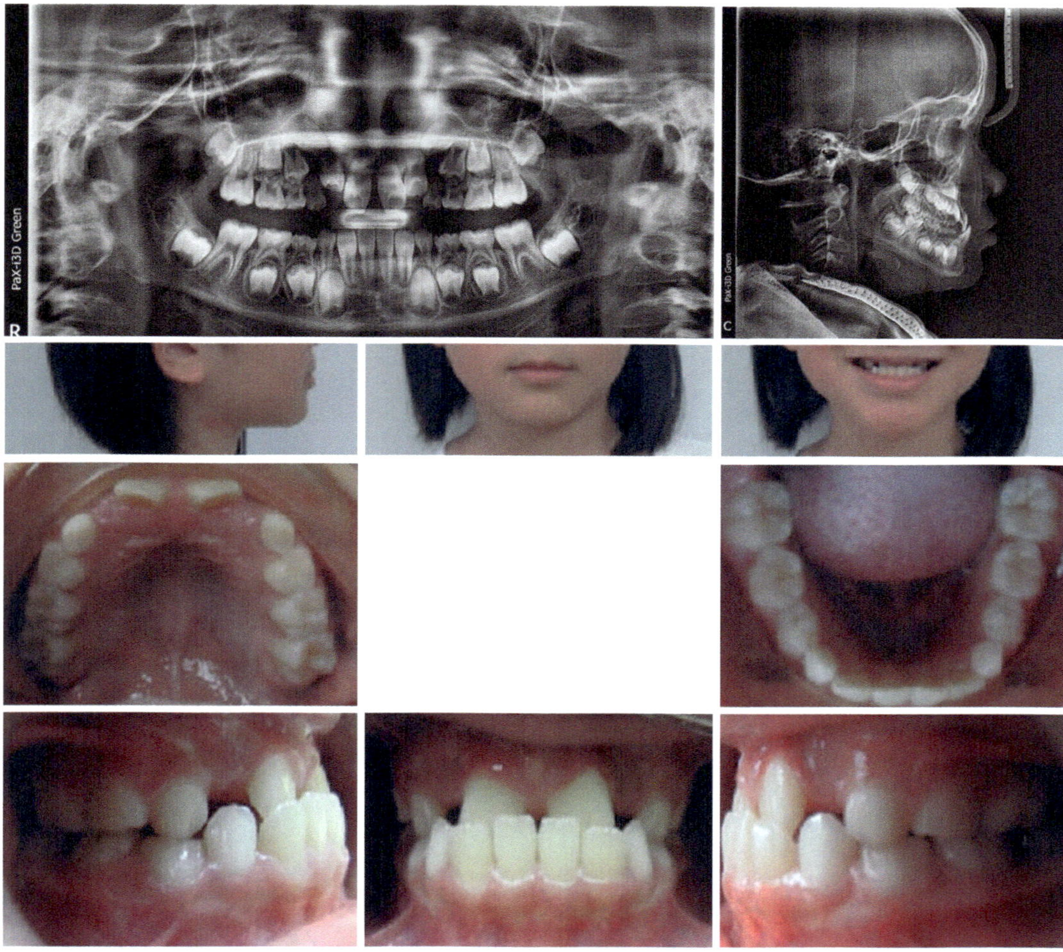

Fig. 2.9 Patient W.W. was treated with a combination of RPFM and clear aligners (Invisalign First). The protraction force aided in jumping the anterior crossbite and promoting the forward movement of the maxilla. The RPFM force was directed via elastics to precision cuts respective to the first maxillary molars. After the initial and single refinement course, we achieved ideal overjet and overbite, Class I molar relationships, and adequate space for erupting permanent teeth

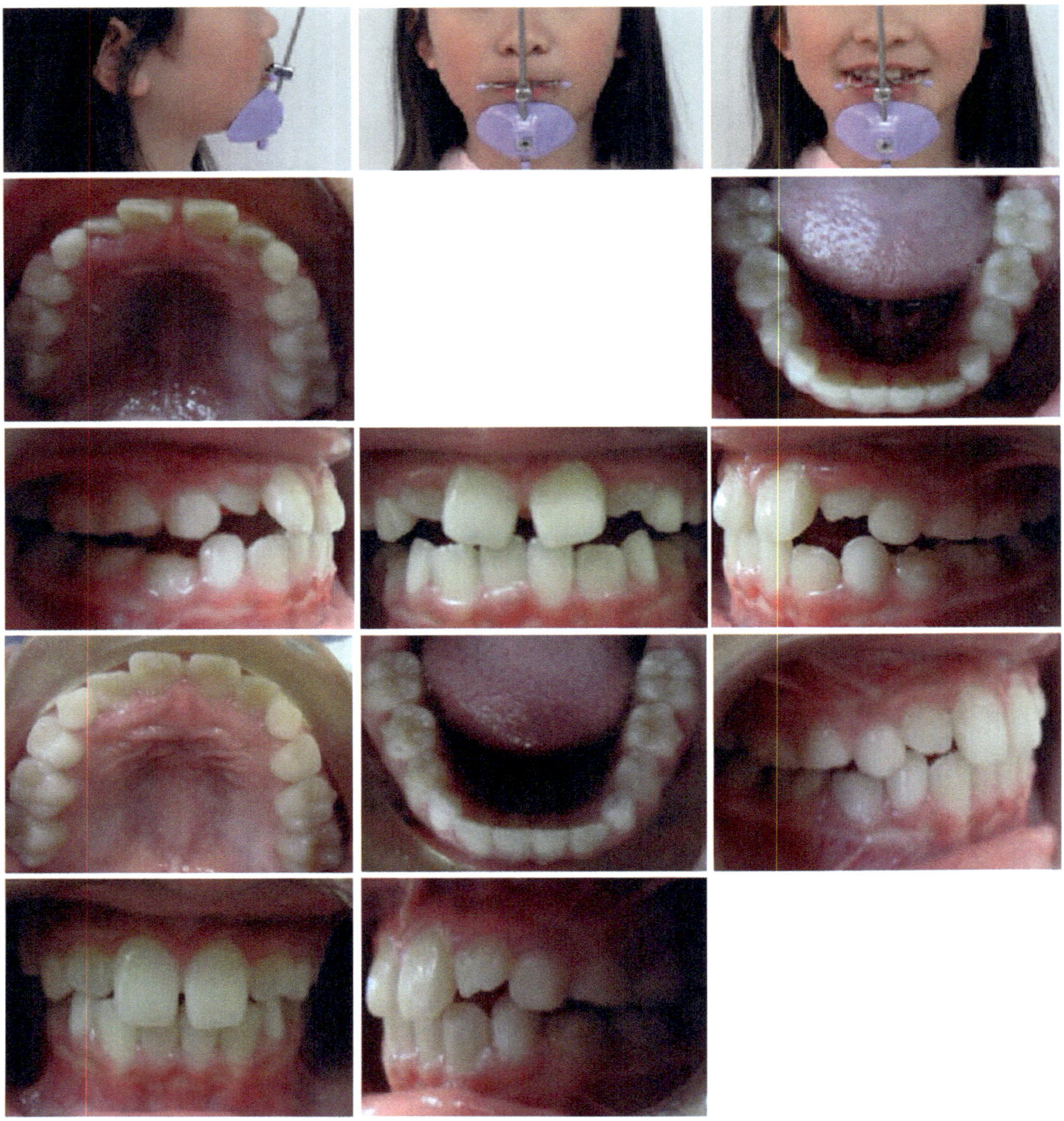

Fig. 2.9 (continued)

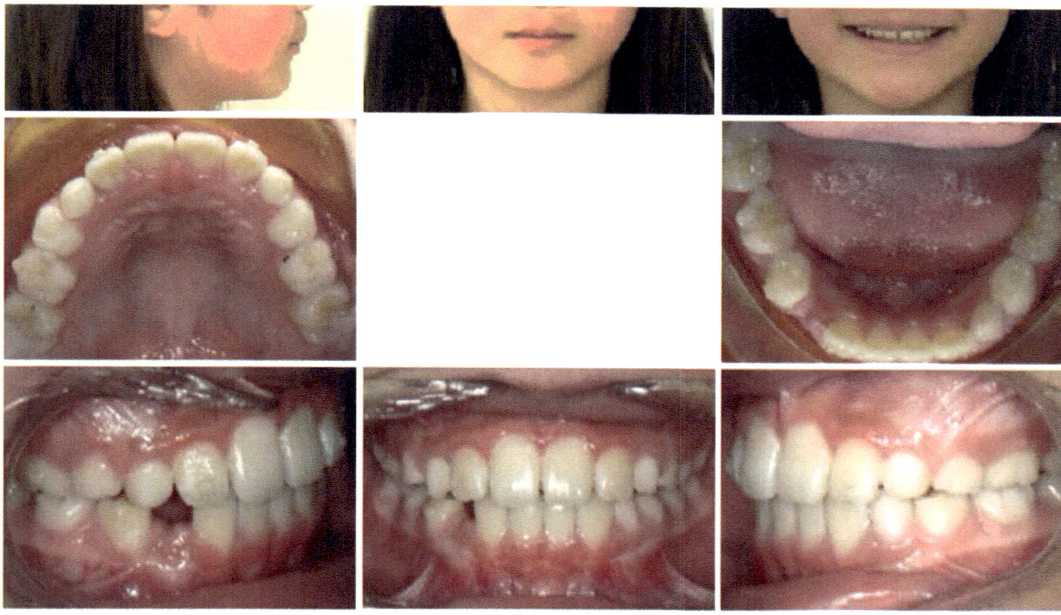

Fig. 2.9 (continued)

the maxillary aligner is cut short immediately distal to the maxillary second premolars so that the patient can wear the headgear during treatment (Fig. 2.10). In Fig. 2.10, patient S.M. received an initial course of cervical headgear treatment prior to a course of clear aligners. The cervical headgear was continued during the course of clear aligners by sectioning the maxillary aligners immediately distal to the maxillary second premolars. In this manner, the distalizing forces of the cervical headgear supplemented those of the clear aligners to maintain the maxillary molars during retraction of the maxillary anterior teeth. The cervical headgear could also continue to provide orthopedic effects during the course of the clear aligners.

Both of the previously mentioned approaches are viable, but theoretically, the most effective solution would be to have the aligner specially fabricated to encapsulate the molar band, while the headgear tube remains uncovered for use (Fig. 2.11a,b). The distalizing effects of the headgear could be incorporated into the Clincheck simulation along with the rest of the tooth movements at an average rate of 0.25 mm of movement per aligner. This design would allow for the combination of the distalizing force supplied by the aligner and the orthopedic effects of the headgear and would be the most effective out of the three approaches in the early correction of Class II discrepancies.

Similarly, other Class II correcting distalizing appliances besides the headgear can be incorporated into the Invisalign First appliance. Traditionally, Class II distalizers may have been employed in a separate initial stage prior to a series of clear aligners. Instead, precision cuts can be incorporated on the distal of the maxillary canine

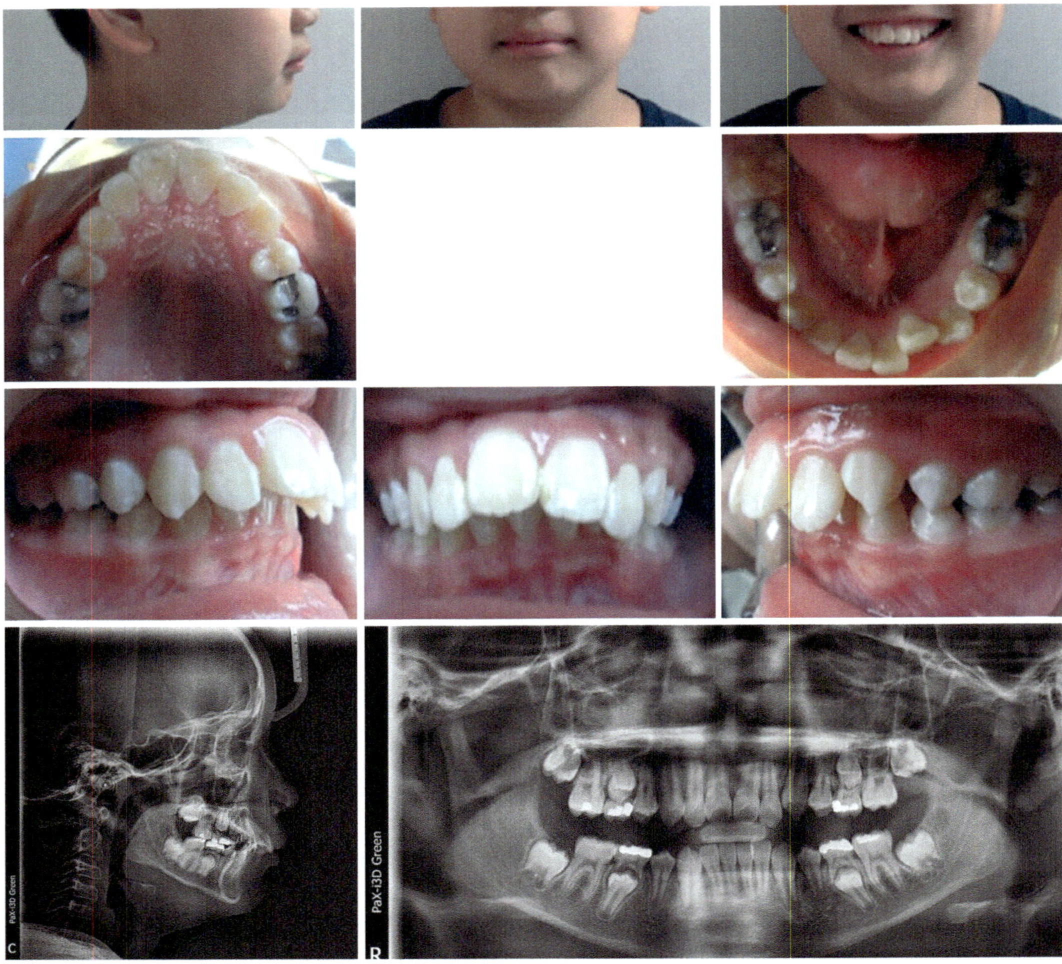

Fig. 2.10 Patient S.M. first received 8 months of Phase I treatment only with cervical headgear. After Class I molars and reduction of overjet were achieved, the patient received two courses of clear aligners. During the first course, bands were kept on the first maxillary molars for continued CHG wear and to maintain Class I molar relationships. The second course of aligners corrected minor discrepancies in alignment (derotation of the left maxillary lateral incisor) and achieved ideal posterior interdigitation

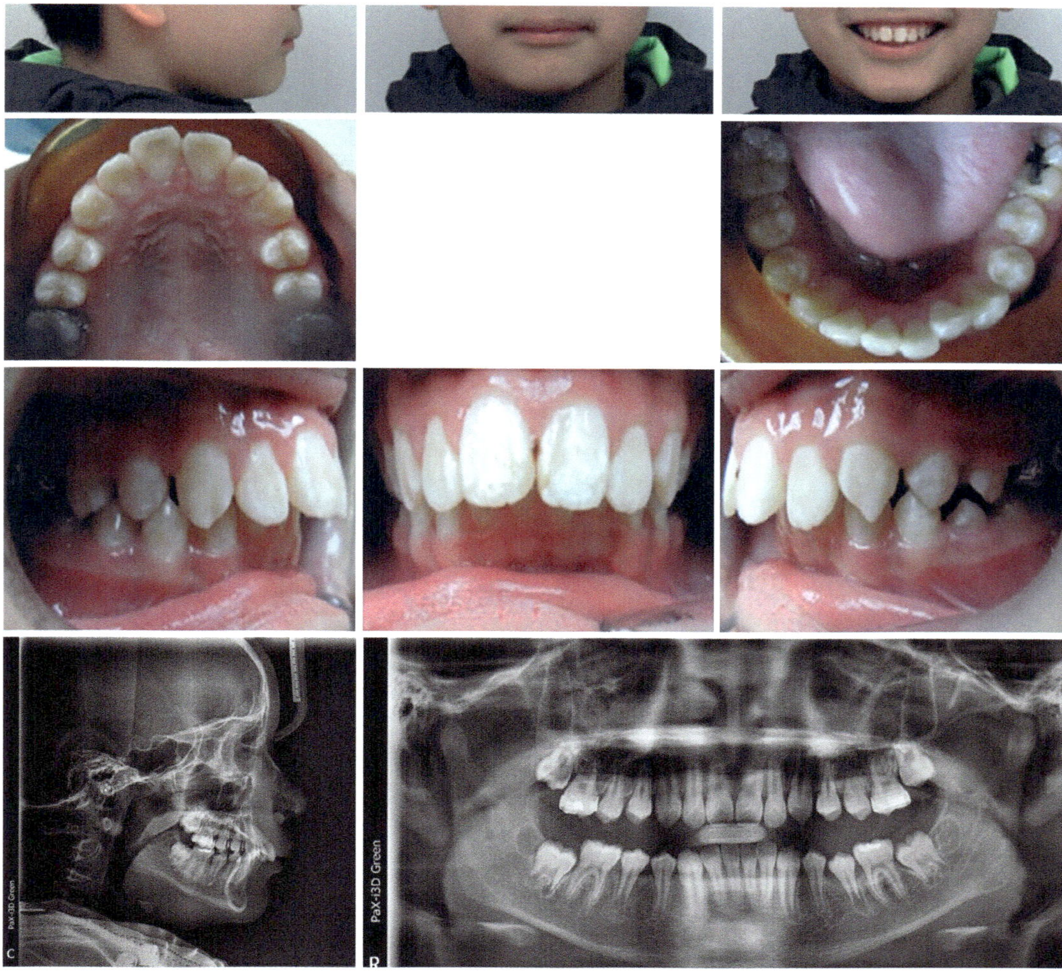

Fig. 2.10 (continued)

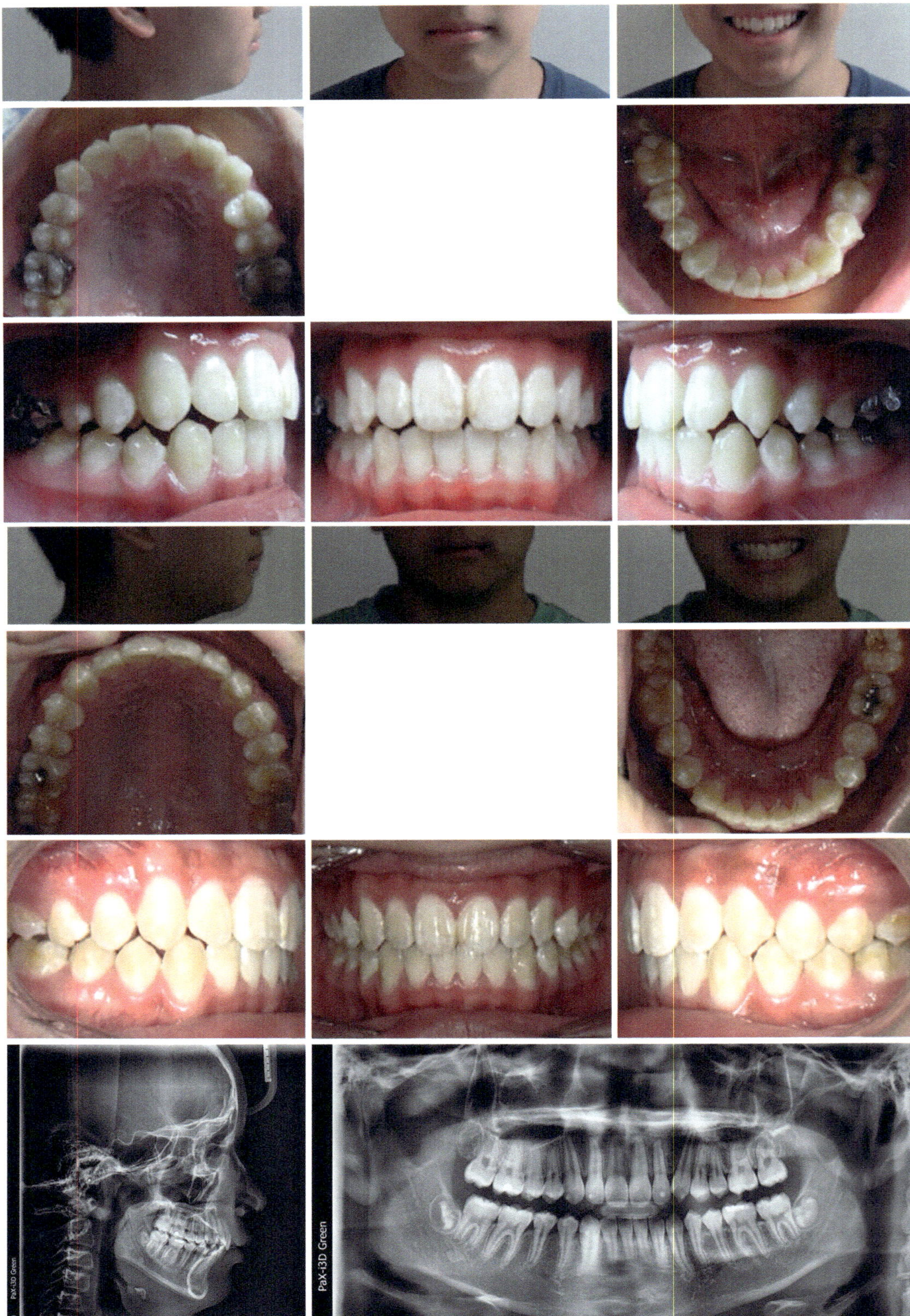

Fig. 2.10 (continued)

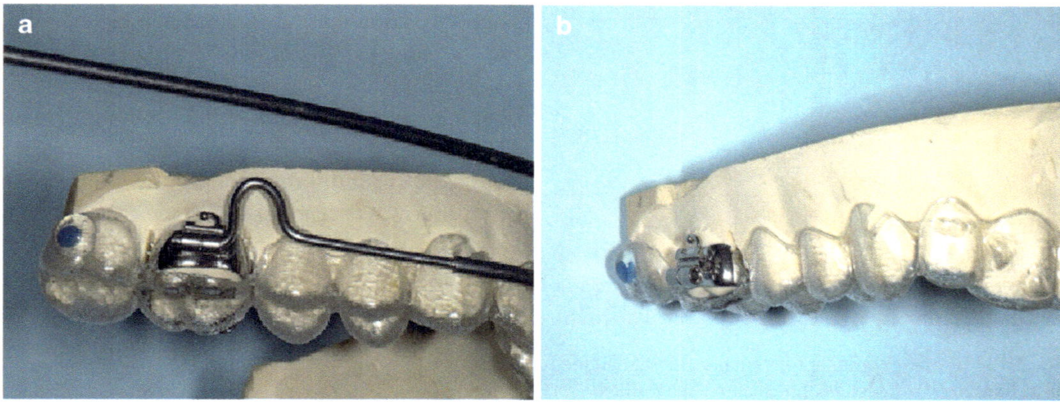

Fig. 2.11 (**a**) The headgear can be functionally combined with the clear aligner to incorporate orthopedic effects into treatment and provide additional distalizing forces to the maxillary arch. (**b**) The clear aligner is cut out for molar band encapsulation around the tooth, while allowing for headgear use

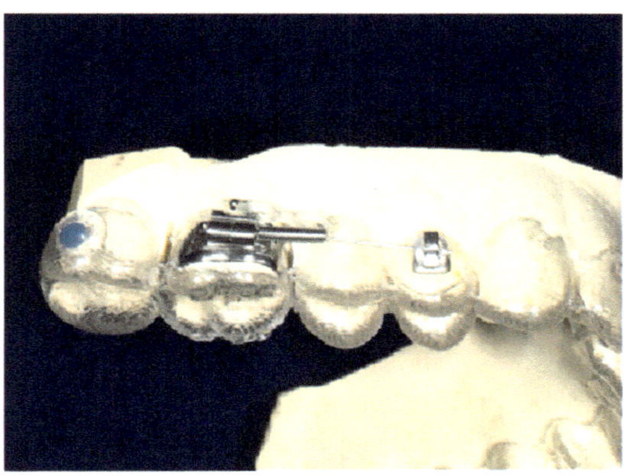

Fig. 2.12 The clear aligner can be cut out to accommodate a bonded distalizer, which can be activated at every appointment

and the first maxillary molar, along with button cutouts for the bonded distalizing appliance (Fig. 2.12). As in the case of the headgear, the distalizing effects of the distalizer can be incorporated into the Clincheck at an average rate of 0.25 mm of movement per aligner. Therefore, the distalizing effect of the bonded distalizer can be supplied to the maxillary arch in addition to other dental movements performed by the clear aligners for greater distalizing forces as well as decreased treatment time.

Retention to Small Clinical Crowns

The small clinical crowns of the deciduous teeth pose difficulties for aligner retention, especially when they receive supplementary forces, whether through intermaxillary elastics or RPFM. Retention can be enhanced on these teeth through a number of methods. Firstly, lingual attachments can be placed on deciduous teeth with small clinical crowns, especially when the aligner encapsulating the tooth will receive additional force from intermaxillary elastics. At present, the clinician can manually add lingual attachments on any of the deciduous teeth. Secondly, clinicians may consider a different type of gingival finish to the aligner when confronted with problems of retention. Though Invisalign only permits a "scalloped" gingival finish, an aligner that finishes slightly on the gingiva would increase retention for teeth with small clinical crowns (Fig. 2.13). As discussed in Chap. 1, 3M's clear aligner currently finishes slightly on the marginal gingiva (Fig. 2.14). The clinician may prefer such an alternative to overcome retention issues with small clinical crowns. Thirdly, the clinician may add retention grooves to the aligner respective to the deciduous tooth

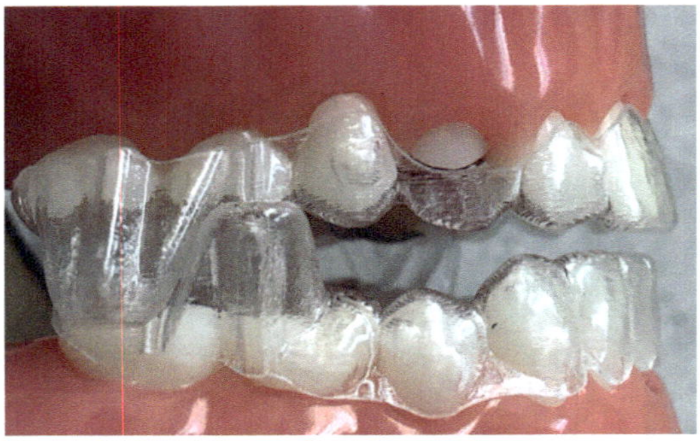

Fig. 2.13 Invisalign aligners invariably use a scalloped gum line finish. This design feature may allow for improved patient comfort compared to aligners that finish on the marginal gingiva. However, the scalloped finish will be a limiting factor for retention to teeth with small crowns, such as the deciduous tooth #A shown above

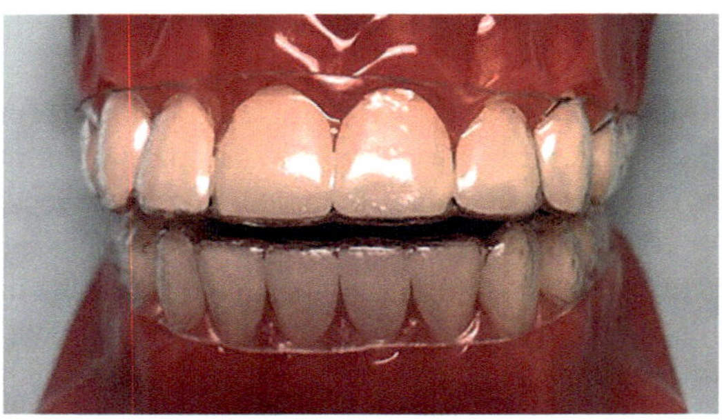

Fig. 2.14 3 M aligners are fabricated with a gum line finish, which would allow for greater retention to teeth with small clinical crowns, such as deciduous teeth

with a small clinical crown (Fig. 2.15a–c). The addition of grooves is not currently available through the Invisalign software. However, the clinician can manually add an indentation onto the aligner with a hand instrument for increased retention. This method can be useful when the clinician decides to initiate intermaxillary elastics or RPFM wear.

Expansion Limits

A number of the options for expansion exceed the recommended limit of 2–4 mm. Expansion beyond these limits could cause future mucogingival problems and recession [22]. Ideally, the software would recognize expansion beyond physiological limits and alert the clinician in a fashion similar to the tooth movement assessment. However, such alerts presently only exist for individual tooth movements with the tooth movement assessment in the current version of Clincheck and not for the extent of maxillary expansion. During clear aligner interceptive treatment, the clinician should be cautious to expand the maxilla within physiological limits.

Software Calibration for Eruption Compensation and Incisor Position

The treatment simulation often fails to accurately predict the space necessary for erupting permanent teeth. The clinician should be mindful of the amount of space planned by the software and modify eruption space as needed. Ideally, the algorithm for eruption compensation will be improved in future generations of Invisalign First.

It is also important that the clinician be mindful of incisor positions that are not accurately modeled on the treatment simulation. The clinician can approximate incisor changes with the tooth movement table, but they have not been calibrated with cephalometric data, which remains a future software solution for accurately planning incisor positions.

Expanding Clinical Preferences

Many of the practitioner's clinical preferences, such as the placement of elastics, the timing for placement of attachments, and limits on expansion of the mandibular intercanine width, remain unavailable during the initial submission of the patient case. These factors are often critical for the success of treatment outcomes and have to be controlled with modifications to the Clincheck simulation.

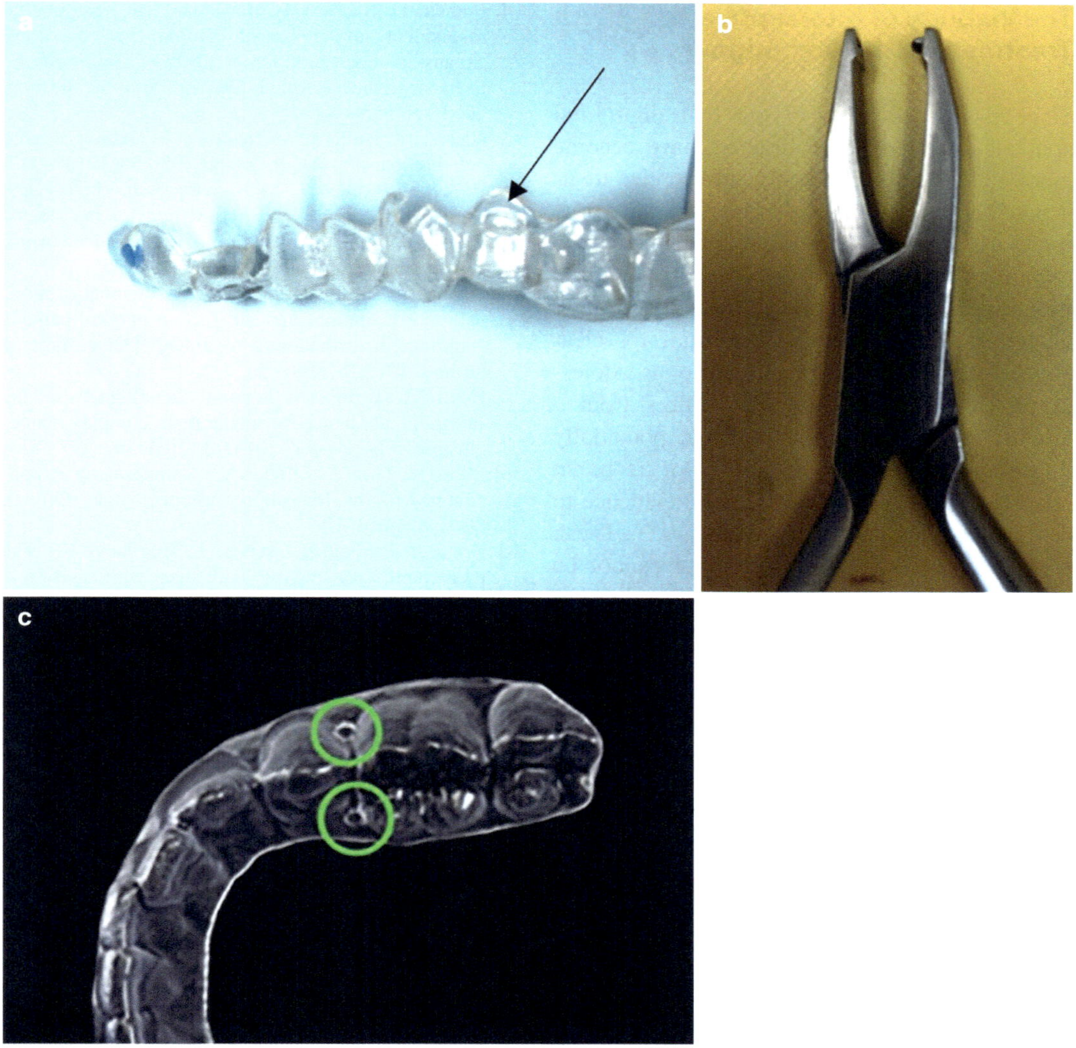

Fig. 2.15 (**a**) The retention groove on the maxillary right lateral incisor can increase retention of the aligner to a tooth with a short clinical crown. (**b**) The retention groove can be created with a 3 mm horizontal dimple plier. (**c**) Retention dimples can also be created on both the facial and lingual surfaces of the aligner in the interproximal areas of posterior segments. These dimples can be created with a 1 mm dimple plier

Post-Interceptive Treatment Retention

As discussed, the lack of explicit clear aligner retention protocols creates issues for patients between Phase I and II treatment. At present, the clinician must either fabricate traditional Hawley retainers or Essix retainers modified with eruption spaces for the permanent teeth. The latter can be a more preferred option for parents who desire for their children a more comfortable form of retention. Ideally, in the future, Invisalign will provide clear aligner retainers with specific eruption spaces or pontics and with more durable material than its SmartTrack for the transition period following interceptive treatment.

The Viability of Interceptive Treatment with Clear Aligners

Since the introduction of the Invisalign First appliance in 2019, clear aligners have become more viable as a modality for interceptive treatment. The appliance's additional features—its force systems and optimized attachments, its eruption compensation algorithm, its retention attachments for short clinical crowns, and other measures—do expand its capabilities for clear aligner treatment in children and young adolescents. However, the appliance suffers from a number of critical deficiencies that potentially limit the success and predictability of treatment outcomes. Most notably, there is no evidence to demonstrate that the current appliance itself can produce orthopedic effects. Also, it cannot be readily combined with many conventional orthopedic appliances with established effectiveness.

In this chapter, we discussed a number of methods by which to modify the current appliance to overcome its inherent limitations. We emphasized the significance of modifying the Invisalign First appliance for the incorporation of traditional orthopedic appliances such as the headgear and the RPFM for maximal use of clear aligners for interceptive treatment. We believe the future development of clear aligner interceptive treatment lies in improved integration of clear aligners with orthopedic appliances for the correction of skeletal discrepancies and more complex malocclusions.

References

1. Align Technology. Invisalign First. 2019. https://info.aligntech.com/lp/Invisalign-First/faq. Accessed 31 Aug 2020.
2. Chiara P, Elisabetta CL, Roberta L, Faltin K, McNamara JA Jr, Cozza P, Franchi L. Treatment timing for functional jaw orthopaedics followed by fixed appliances: a controlled long-term study. Eur J Orthod. 2018;40:430–6.
3. Proffit WR. The timing of early treatment: an overview. Am J Orthod Dentofac Orthop. 2006;129:S47–9.
4. Franchi L, Baccetti T, McNamara JA. Postpubertal assessment of treatment timing for maxillary expansion and protraction therapy followed by fixed appliances. Am J Orthod Dentofac Orthop. 2004;126:555–68.
5. Haas AJ. Long-term posttreatment evaluation of rapid palatal expansion. Angle Orthod. 1980;50(3):189–217.
6. Baccetti T, Franchi L, McNamara JA Jr. The cervical vertebral maturation (CVM) method for the assessment of optimal treatment timing in dentofacial orthopedics. Semin Orthod. 2005;11(3):119–29.
7. Oliveira P, Tavares R, Freitas J. Assessment of motivation, expectations and satisfaction of adult patients submitted to orthodontic treatment. Dental Press J Orthod. 2013;18(2):81–7.
8. Boyd RL. Esthetic orthodontic treatment using the Invisalign appliance for moderate to complex malocclusions. J Dent Educ. 2008;72(8):948–67.
9. Zhou N, Guo J. Efficiency of upper arch expansion with the Invisalign system. Angle Orthod. 2020;90(1):23–30.
10. Houle JP, Piedade L, Todescan R Jr, Pinheiro FH. The predictability of transverse changes with Invisalign. Angle Orthod. 2017;87(1):19–24.
11. Align Technology. Invisalign First. 2019. https://info.aligntech.com/lp/Invisalign-First/faq. Accessed 13 Sep 2020.
12. Brierley CA, DiBiase A, Sandler PJ. Early class II treatment. Aust Dent J. 2017;62(1):4–10.
13. Abbate GM, Caria MP, Montanari P, et al. Periodontal health in teenagers treated with removable aligners and fixed orthodontic appliances. J Orofac Orthop. 2015;76(3):240–50.
14. Align Technology. Mandibular Advancement. 2020. https://info.aligntech.com/MA. Accessed 19 Sep 2020.
15. Spyridon NP, Kutschera E, Memmert S, Gölz L, Jäger A, Bourauel C, Eliades T. Effectiveness of early orthopaedic treatment with headgear: a systematic review and meta-analysis. Eur J Orthod. 2017;39(2):176–87.
16. Podesser B, Williams S, Crismani AG, Bantleon H. Evaluation of the effects of rapid maxillary expansion in growing children using computer tomography scanning: a pilot study. Eur J Orthod. 2007;29(1):37–44.
17. Varlık SK, İşcan HN. The effects of cervical headgear with an expanded inner bow in the permanent dentition. Eur J Orthod. 2008;30(4):425–30.
18. Lee RT, Kyi CS, Mack GJ. A controlled clinical trial of the effects of the twin block and Dynamax appliances on the hard and soft tissues. Eur J Orthod. 2007;29(3):272–82.
19. Myser SA, Campbell PM, Boley J, Buschang PH. Long-term stability: postretention changes of the mandibular anterior teeth. Am J Orthod Dentofac Orthop. 2013;144(3):420–9.

20. Shah A. Postretention changes in mandibular crowding: a review of the literature. Am J Orthod Dentofac Orthop. 2003;124(3):298–308.
21. Cordasco G, Matarese G, Rustico L, Fastuca S, Caprioglio A, Lindauer SJ, Nucera R. Efficacy of orthopedic treatment with protraction facemask on skeletal class III malocclusion: a systematic review and meta-analysis. Orthod Craniofac Res. 2014;17(3):133–43.
22. Handelman CS, Wang L, BeGole EA, Haas AJ. Nonsurgical rapid maxillary expansion in adults: report on 47 cases using the Haas expander. Angle Orthod. 2000;70(2):129–44.

Mandibular Advancement: A Viable Alternative to Functional Appliances?

3

Contents

Class II Functional Correction in Clear Aligner Therapy

Since the introduction of the "bite-jumping" appliance by Norman Kingsley in 1879, functional appliances have developed into a cornerstone of orthodontic treatment for skeletal malocclusions in growing individuals [1]. The first functional appliances and their use were pioneered in Europe during the early twentieth century, in parallel to the growth of fixed appliances in the United States [2]. In 1902, Pierre Robin introduced the simple monobloc appliance for the treatment of mandibular retrognathia and jaw expansion [3]. Robin's monobloc served as a model for Viggo Andresen and Karl Haupl, who modified an upper Hawley retainer with a lingual flange for the treatment of Class II malocclusions by allowing for the forward positioning of the mandible for a more ideal occlusion and an improved maxilliomandibular relationship [4]. Over the next 100 years, the Andresen-Haupl activator was further refined into various bionators and functional regulators, most notably the Twin Block appliance developed by William Clark and an appliance designed by Rolf Fränkel, which employs buccal shields and lip pads to reduce lip and cheek pressure and to normalize abnormal oral muscular activity. Fixed functional appliances were also introduced in the early twentieth century by Emil Herbst in 1905. His appliance was composed of bilateral telescoping pistons extending between the maxilla and the mandible from either orthodontic bands or cobalt chromium caps. The pistons apply a protrusive force to the mandible for its forward repositioning and the correction of Class II malocclusions. The Herbst appliance still remains in use as a Class II corrector and has also been modified into less intrusive forms, such as the FORSUS, which

A. T. Huang, D. Huang, *Controversies in Clear Aligner Therapy*,
https://doi.org/10.1007/978-3-030-92810-0_3

applies a similar protrusive force to the mandible through nickel-titanium springs contained within pistons attached to molar bands [5].

The efficacy of both fixed and removable functional appliances for Class II correction has been extensively researched, with particular attention to their skeletal effects and relationship to mandibular growth. Studies have shown that the use of Class II functional appliances resulted in a statistically significant difference of 1.79 mm in annual mandibular growth compared to a control group, as measured by various cephalometric values [6]. Similarly, a meta-analysis of the mandibular changes during Fränkel-2 (FR-2) treatment of growing patients with Class II malocclusions showed that the appliance had a statistically significant effect on mandibular growth, as measured by mandibular body length, total mandibular length, and mandibular ramus height [7]. However, there is an increasing consensus that though Class II functional correctors do induce an increase in mandibular length compared to untreated subjects, the improvement in mandibular projection is either negligible or insignificant [8]. Nevertheless, though the true skeletal effects of both fixed and removal functional appliances remain undetermined, it has been shown that they are effective in correcting molar relationships and reducing overjets in Class II malocclusions through a combination of dentoalveolar and skeletal effects [9].

In 2017, Align Technology introduced the mandibular advancement modality as a clear aligner alternative to conventional fixed and removable appliances for the correction of Class II malocclusions [10]. The company claimed that their device could function as a "simpler, more efficient, and patient-friendly treatment option than functional appliances to treat teen Class II patients" [10]. The basis of these claims rests on a prospective clinical trial with only preliminary results not published in a refereed orthodontic journal. Align also reports that the preliminary results showed "statistically significant correction of Class II malocclusion," though it remains unclear by what parameter and against what control group this correction was measured [10]. The quality of the trial is also compromised by its high risk of bias, as all the orthodontists involved in the trial are financially tied to Invisalign. Therefore, the trial is questionable evidence for the purpose of evaluating the efficacy of the mandibular advancement appliance. To date, because the mandibular advancement appliance has only recently been made available for clinical use, no controlled clinical trials evaluating its efficacy have been published.

Despite its supposed efficacy, there are significant limitations to the mandibular advancement appliance that require management for successful outcomes. In this chapter, we describe the current state of the modality and its deficiencies. Afterward, we discuss current and future solutions for its effective application in the treatment of Class II malocclusions.

The Mandibular Advancement Appliance: Current Features and Limitations

Mechanism of Bite Repositioning

One of the most significant characteristics of Invisalign's mandibular advancement appliance is the duration of engagement between the precision wings of the maxillary and mandibular aligners. When the precision wings are engaged, the patient's mandible is repositioned forward, typically in cumulative 2 mm increments relative to centric relation, although clinicians are able to program 4 mm or even 6 mm increments. Conventional fixed functional appliances (FFAs), such as the Herbst, also act through a mechanism of mandibular repositioning. The FFAs have been shown to induce both statistically significant dentoalveolar and skeletal changes, though primarily dentoalveolar [11]. Most notably, in Zymperdikas et al.'s systematic review, FFAs induced significant retroclination of the upper incisors and significant proclination of the lower incisors [11]. Also, the same study showed that FFA-treated groups showed slightly greater mandibular skeletal growth, as well as a statistically significant restriction on maxillary growth [11]. However, though Align claims that their mandibular advancement appliance can effectively replace conventional functional appliances, there is no evidence to show that it can achieve similar dentoalveolar and skeletal treatment effects. One of the critical differences between conventional functional appliances and the mandibular advancement appliance lies in their mechanism of mandibular repositioning. The mandibular advancement appliance lacks a mechanism by which to connect the maxillary and mandibular precision wings. Therefore, the patient is not necessarily biting in the forward position, as the wings likely remain disengaged for a significant proportion of time during daily use of the appliance. Similarly, the wings of the appliance are disengaged for a large percentage of the 8–9 hours when the patient is asleep. As a result, the efficacy of the appliance at Class II correction may be compromised because the patient's mandible is only in a protruded position part-time.

This mechanism of bite repositioning differs from conventional functional appliances such as the Fränkel-2 and the Herbst appliance, which functions by keeping the mandible in a continuous protrusive position by connecting the maxillary and mandibular arches through telescopic arms. As a result, this continuous "bite-jumping" is ensured by the appliance, while the patient can still move into lateral excursive movements during functions such as speaking and eating [12]. During mouth closure, the patient must bite into the protruded position. There is evidence that the Herbst appliance's continuous "bite-jumping" induces the stimulation of condylar growth in response to forward positioning of the mandible and may also contribute to the favorable redirection of mandibular growth [13]. Similarly, a conventional removable functional appliance such as the Fränkel-2 also employs a mechanism of continuous bite repositioning through its setup of interconnected lingual flanges, buccal shields, and lip bumper shields (Fig. 3.1). Treatment with the FR-2 has also shown statistically significant enhancement of both mandibular body length, total mandibular length, and mandibular ramus height [7]. The FR-2 can effectively treat severe Class II malocclusions, like the patient in Fig. 3.2, which demonstrates the successful treatment of a severe Class II discrepancy in an adolescent male. Like the Herbst appliance, the FR-2 forces the patient to bite into a protruded position during closure. In contrast to the part-time mechanism of the mandibular advancement appliance, the continuous bite-jumping of the Herbst and FR-2 allows for full-time forward repositioning of the patient's mandible.

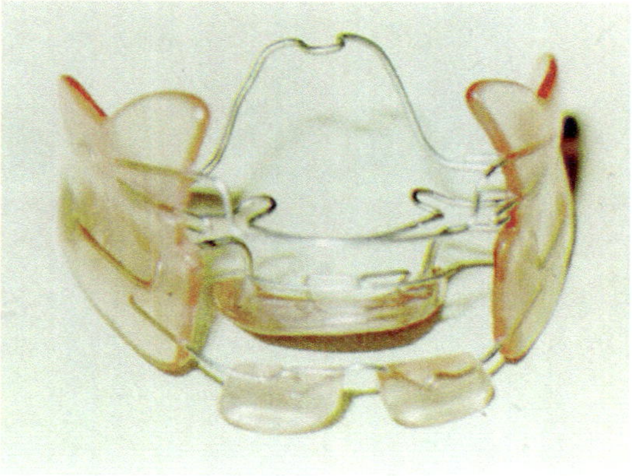

Fig. 3.1 The Fränkel-2 (FR-2) is a removable functional appliance that the patient uses for at least 14 hours/day for mandibular repositioning and retraining of the perioral muscles

Bite Jump Calibration

At present, the mandibular advancement appliance allows for 2 mm incremental bite jumps until an edge-to-edge position (or 1 mm reverse overjet for overcorrection). This mechanism of sequential advancement is similar to that for certain modifications of the Twin Block appliance, as well as for specific FR-2 protocols [14]. In particular, the Twin Block appliance can be adjusted for controlled gradual advancement of the mandible through advancement screws (Fig. 3.3) [15]. This modification allows for increased flexibility of the appliance and accommodation for patients with limitations to significant mandibular protrusion. In contrast, the gradual advancement in the mandibular advancement appliance is not as precisely calibrated as a modified Twin Block, especially because of the former's part-time mechanism of bite repositioning. Therefore, the mandibular

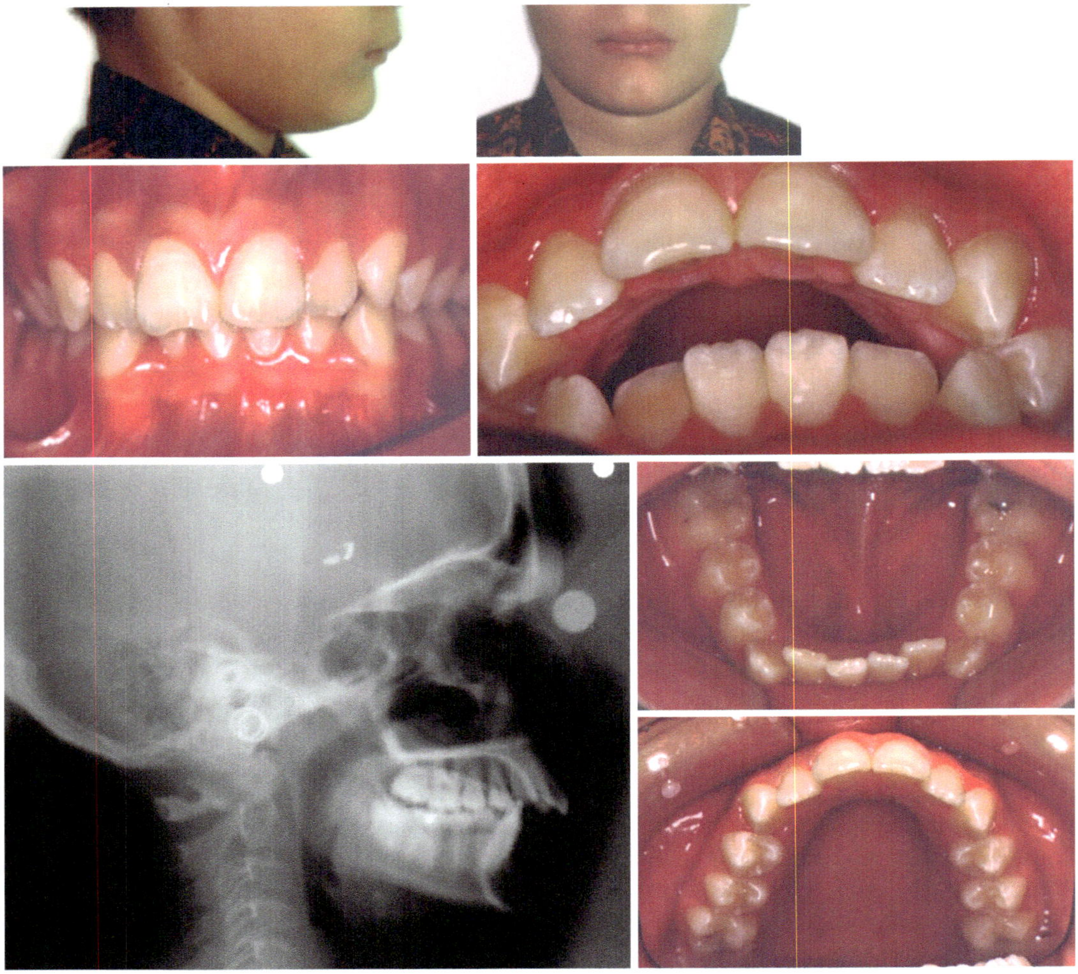

Fig. 3.2 An 11-year-old male with a skeletal Class II malocclusion with a severely prognathic maxilla, retrognathic mandible, 100% overbite, and 14 mm overjet was successfully treated with the FR-2. Cephalometric analysis shows the achievement of ideal overjet and overbite, normalization of the maxillary incisors, control of torque in the mandibular incisors, and Class I relationships bilaterally

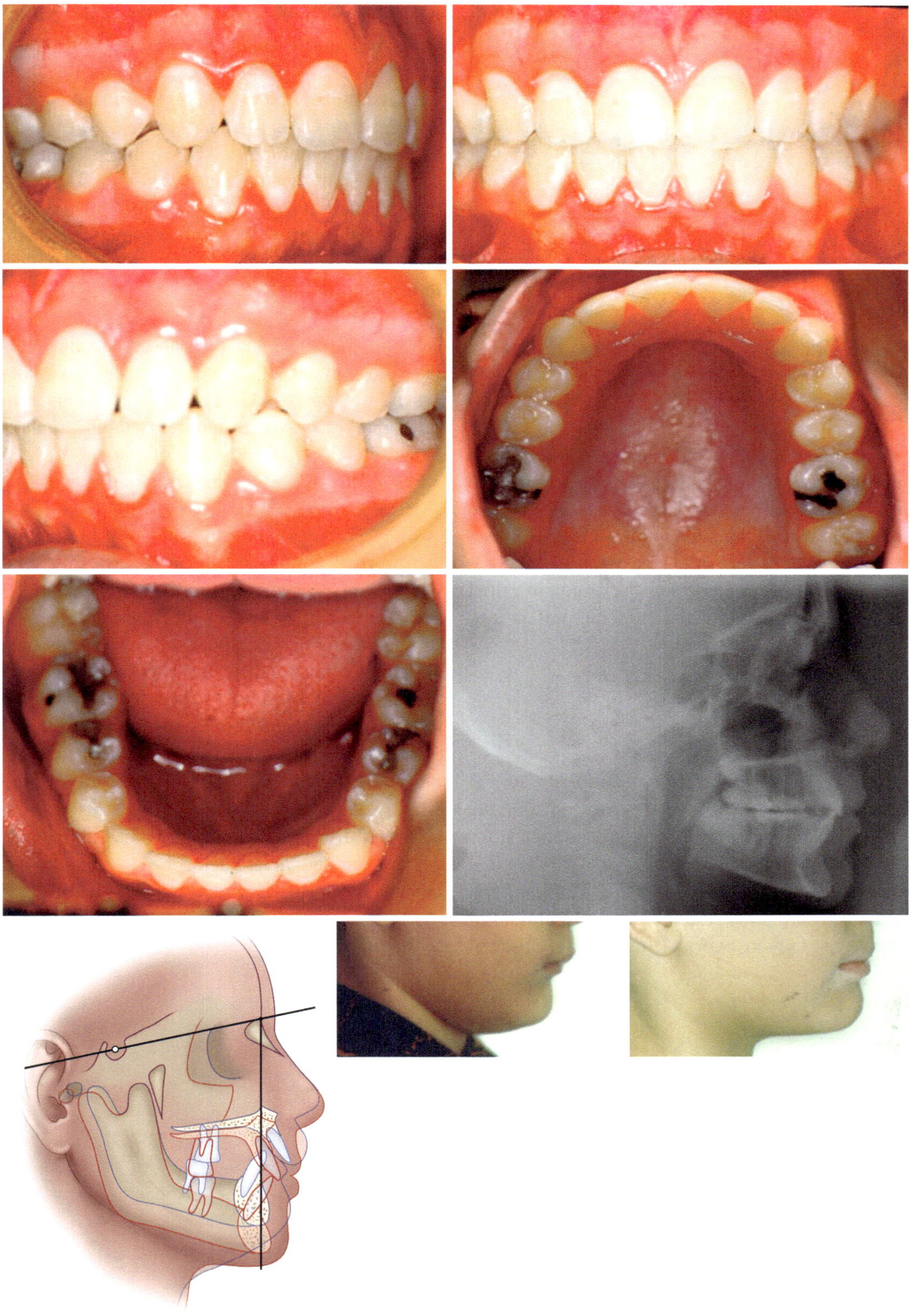

Fig. 3.2 (continued)

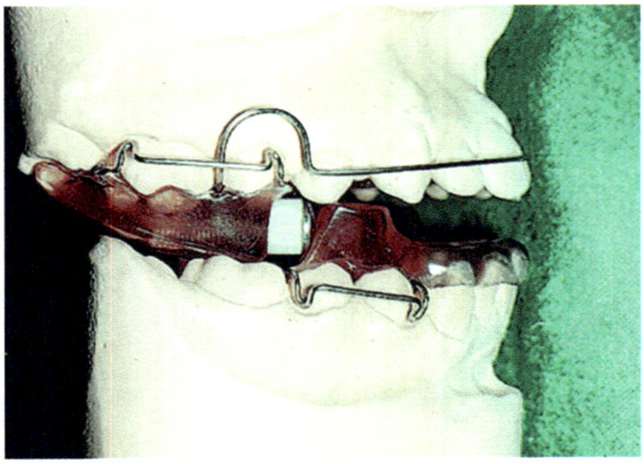

Fig. 3.3 In a version of a modified Twin Block, advancement screws allow for gradual incremental advancement of the mandible during therapy

advancement appliance's bite jumps are often inaccurately calibrated and do not achieve the increments planned by the software. It is also important to note that sequential advancement can be advantageous for patient acceptance and comfort, but Invisalign does offer the option of initial maximum protrusion if the clinician prefers it to incremental bite jumps [16].

Case Selection

Similar to treatment with conventional Class II functional appliances, case selection for the mandibular advancement appliance is critical for successful outcomes. Studies have shown that many of the conventional Class II functional appliances are most suitable for the treatment of moderate to severe overjet (>6 mm), a significant ANB discrepancy, and Class II malocclusions characterized by mandibular retrognathia and orthognathic maxillae. For example, clinicians have recommended the Herbst appliance is most indicated in Class II malocclusions with mandibular retrognathia, an ANB angle ≥4°, and an overjet ≥6 mm [17]. Studies have also shown that optimal timing for Class II correction is during or slightly after the onset of pubertal growth, typically between stages 3 and 4 of cervical vertebral maturation [18].

Clinically, we have observed that similar to conventional functional appliances, the mandibular advancement appliance yields the most successful outcomes in Class II malocclusions with orthognathic maxillae and retrognathic mandibles (Fig. 3.4). In the case of patient K.Z., a 12-year-old female sought orthodontic treatment. She showed a Class II malocclusion, characterized by an orthognathic maxilla and retrognathic mandible, a 6 mm overjet, an 80% overbite, and Class II end-on canines and molars bilaterally. She received clear aligner therapy with a course of mandibular advancement followed by a single course of refinement. At the conclusion of treatment, we achieved ideal overjet and overbite and Class I canines and molars on the left side but were unable to achieve Class I canines and molars on the right, whose canines and molars finished slightly end-on Class II. We attribute this result to a Bolton discrepancy with maxillary deficiency, as well as the deficiencies in the mandibular advancement appliance, which likely did not deliver an adequately aggressive propulsive force to the mandible.

Because the mandibular advancement appliance also relies on mandibular growth to achieve Class II correction, its optimal timing is most likely during or slightly after the onset of pubertal growth, coinciding with that of the Twin Block and other conventional functional appliances. However, we have observed that due to the mechanical limitations of the mandibular advancement appliance, it is most effective for the treatment of Class II malocclusions with an ANB angle <4° and overjet <6 mm and less capable of treating more severe discrepancies (Table 3.1).

Tooth Movement Beneath Precision Wings

During treatment with conventional Class II functional appliances such as the Herbst appli-

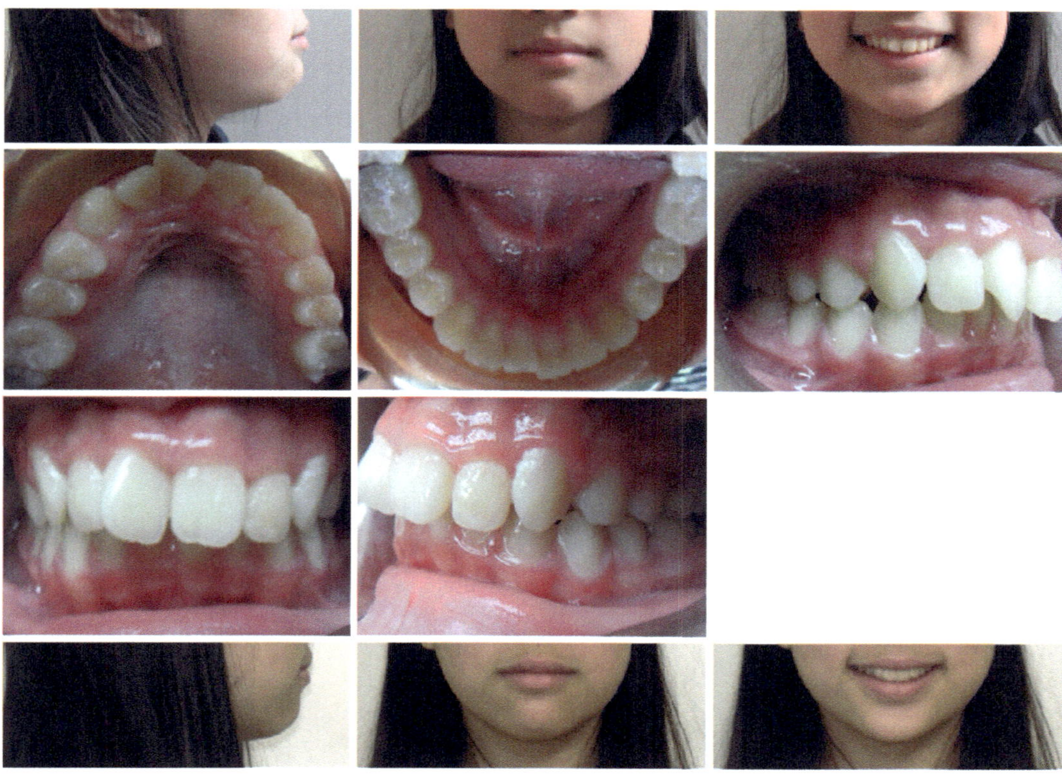

Fig. 3.4 Patient K.Z. was treated with the mandibular advancement appliance. She received an initial course of mandibular advancement followed by a single course of refinement. We achieved ideal overjet and overbite and Class I canines and molars on the left side, but we were unable to achieve Class I relationships on the right side, which we attribute to a maxillary tooth size deficiency (small maxillary lateral incisors) and inadequacy of the appliance in delivering continuous and aggressive protrusion to the mandible. The superimpositions compare the patient's initial and 9 months into treatment following the initial course of mandibular advancement

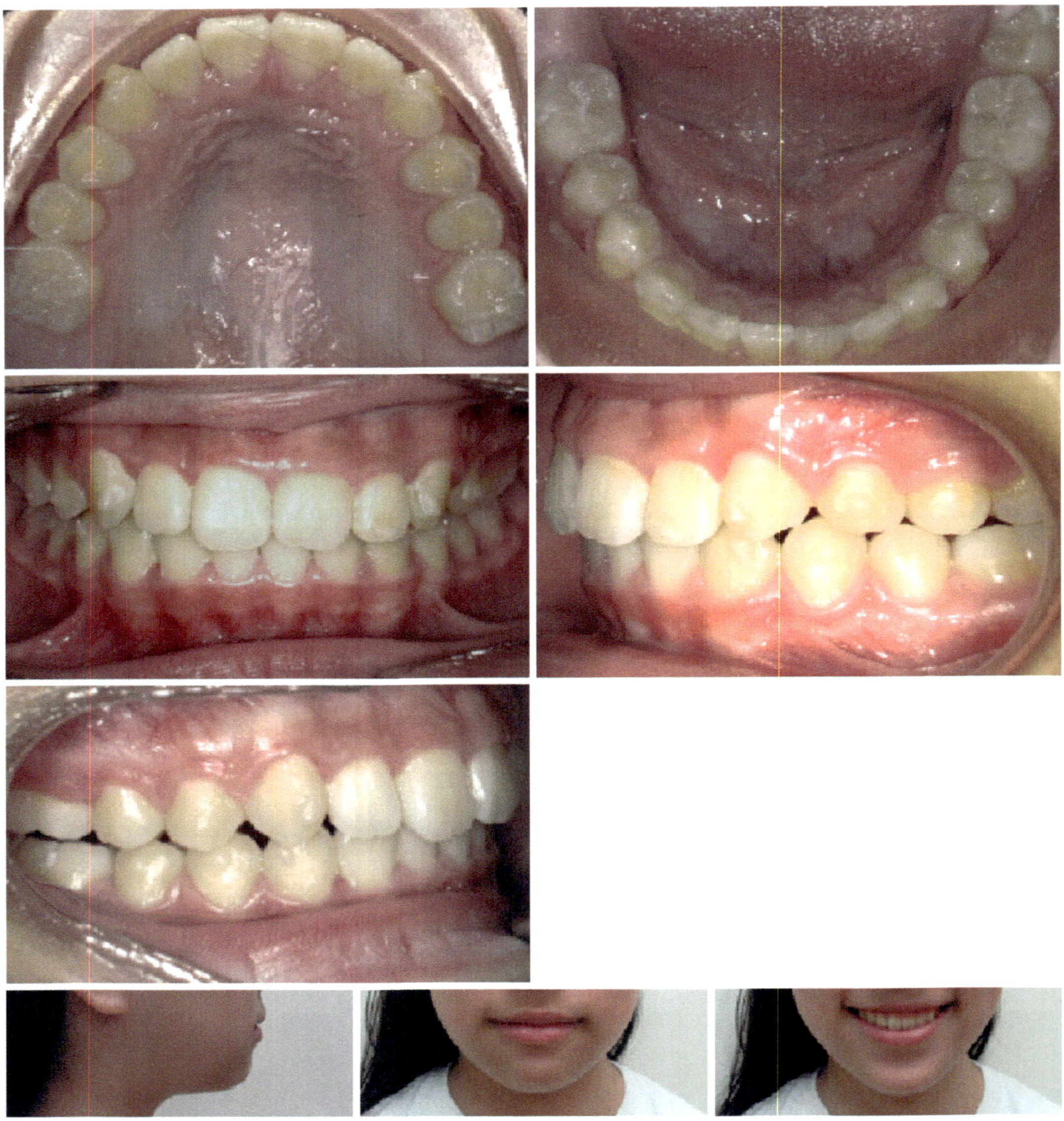

Fig. 3.4 (continued)

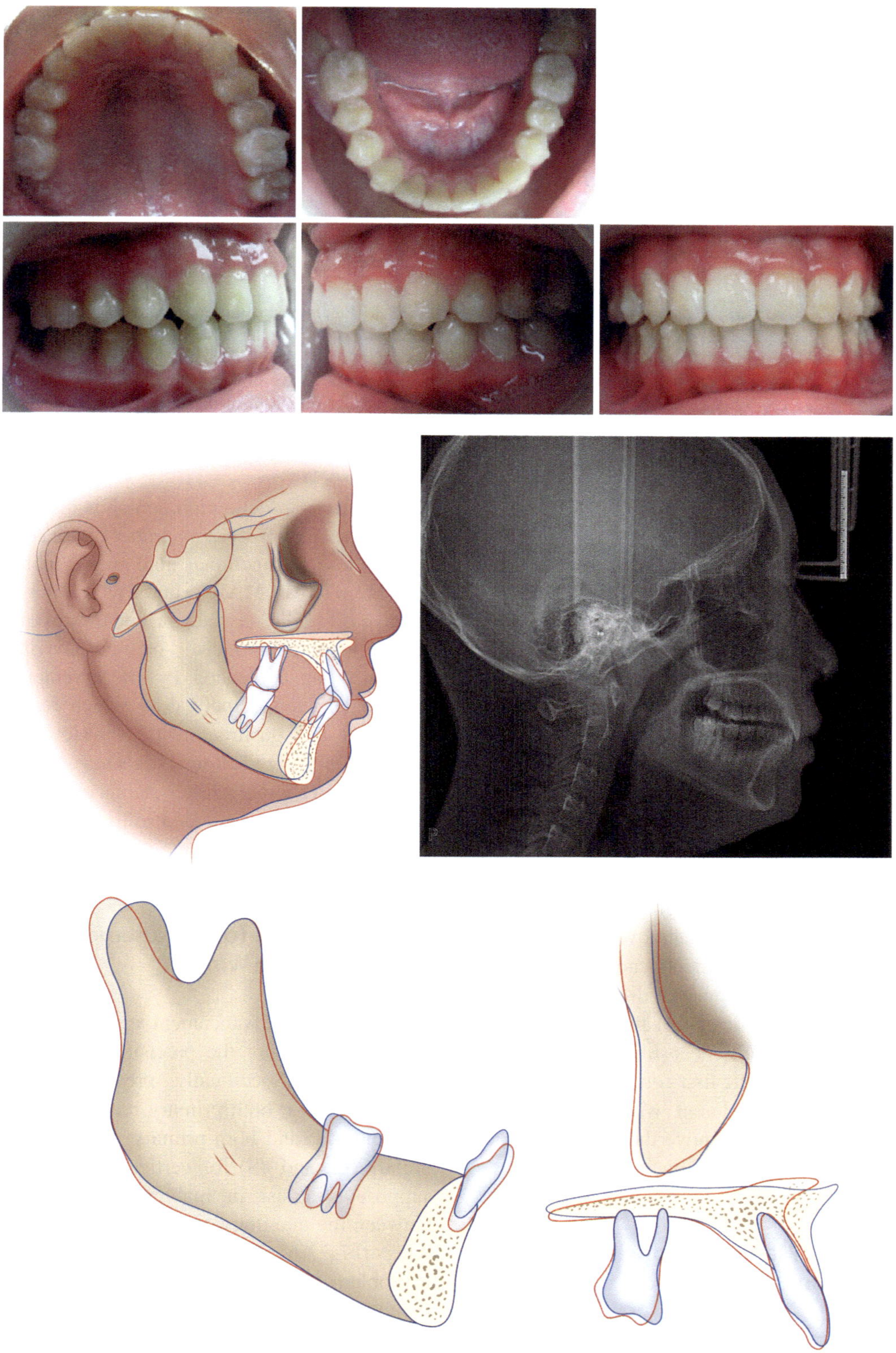

Fig. 3.4 (continued)

Table 3.1 Suggested parameters for use of the MA appliance

Parameter	Diagnosis
Skeletal diagnosis	Mandibular retrognathia
ANB	<4°
Overjet	<6 mm

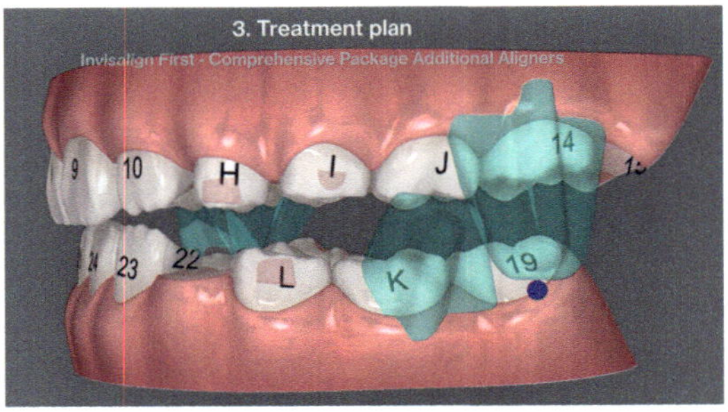

Fig. 3.5 The mandibular advancement appliance's precision wings will encapsulate the maxillary and mandibular first molars and second primary molars on both sides. The precision wings will limit freedom of movement for the encapsulated teeth

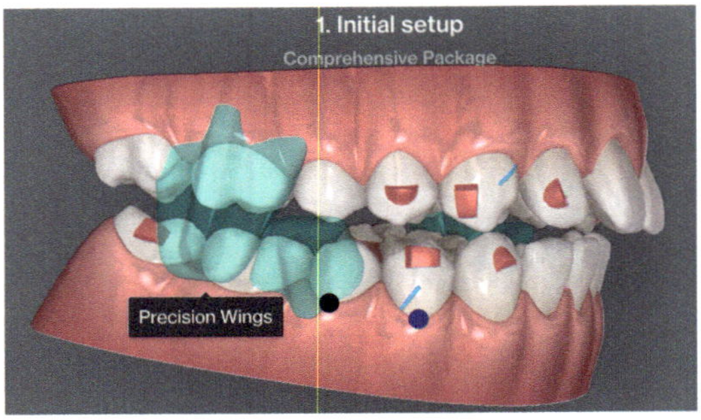

Fig. 3.6 Precision cuts are incorporated on the maxillary canines and mandibular first premolars for vertical elastics wear during mandibular advancement. The use of vertical elastics can be problematic due to frequent dislodging from lack of retention in the maxillary and mandibular posterior segments

ance and the MARA, the teeth encapsulated by the main apparatus are limited in their movements because they function as anchor units for the maxillary and mandibular dental arches. The mandibular advancement appliance likewise limits teeth movement in the segments with the precision wing extensions. Typically, for patients in the mixed dentition, the maxillary and mandibular first molars and the second primary molars are contained within these segments (Fig. 3.5). The efficacy of their individual movements is reduced because firstly, attachments cannot be placed to enhance the performance of difficult movements and secondly, the design of the precision wings does not permit full encapsulation of the anchor teeth. As a result, the first course of aligners with mandibular advancement will often require a refinement course to move the anchor teeth into proper alignment and occlusion.

Control of Mandibular Incisor Inclination

Align Technology has claimed that its mandibular advancement appliance is able to limit mandibular incisor proclination, which is historically an adverse side effect of a number of the conventional Class II functional appliances, including the FR2, Herbst, MARA, and Twin Block [19]. Initial case studies also suggest an improved control of mandibular incisor inclination with the appliance, as evidenced by measurements of mandibular incisor inclination which remained stable pre and posttreatment [20]. However, to date, no randomized clinical trials have been published to corroborate Align's claims regarding the appliance's efficacy in controlling mandibular incisor inclination [20].

Vertical Elastics for Engagement of the Precision Wings

The mandibular advancement appliance includes a feature to secure the precision wings during patient wear. Specifically, precision cuts are incorporated on both primary maxillary canines (#C and #H) and both primary mandibular first molars (#L and #S) for vertical elastics, which supposedly assist in maintaining engagement between the maxillary and mandibular precision wings (Fig. 3.6). This method of vertical elastics is problematic because they frequently cause dislodgment of both maxillary and mandibular aligners, even when the strength of the elastics is low, at ¼″, 2 oz. or ¼″, 3 oz. This frequent dislodging results from the lack of retention of the aligners to the short clinical crowns of the deciduous teeth, which serve as the anchor units for the vertical elastics. Often, these vertical elastics have to be avoided altogether during a course of mandibular advancement because they are counterproductive and dislodge the aligners rather than supplement engagement of the precision wings.

Efficacy in Comparison to Class II Mechanics

Most of the preliminary trials and case studies investigating the efficacy of the mandibular advancement appliance have focused on milder cases of Class II malocclusion, particularly patients whose ANB < 4°. This suggests that the appliance's range of efficacy may be limited to cases of mild severity and not those with ANB > 4°. Though no clinical trials have directly investigated the efficacy of clear aligner therapy for the correction of Class II malocclusions, a number of case studies have shown successful correction of mild cases [21]. Consequently, it is still questionable whether the mandibular advancement appliance is superior in efficacy to the exclusive use of Class II mechanics in the treatment of mild Class II malocclusions.

Maxillary Expansion in Conjunction to Mandibular Advancement

During mandibular advancement, the Invisalign software often plans for significant maxillary posterior expansion. The expansion planned frequently exceeds realistic amounts of physiologically stable molar expansion of 4 mm, which are those achieved by orthopedic appliances, such as the rapid maxillary expander [22]. As a result of this overexpansion, the aligner material in the maxillary posterior segments with the precision wings often tracks poorly and begins to dislodge from its respective teeth (Fig. 3.7). Therefore, the overexpansion compromises not only the movements of the individual maxillary posterior teeth but also the efficacy of the mandibular advancement feature. The clinician should be prudent in monitoring the amount of expansion planned during interceptive treatment, especially when it involves mandibular advancement.

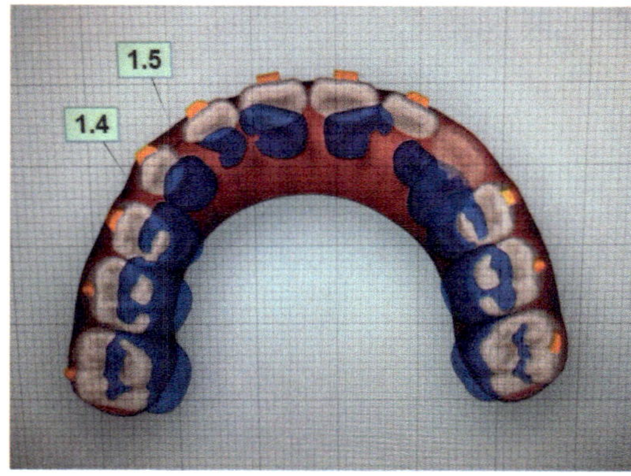

Fig. 3.7 During mandibular advancement, Invisalign frequently programs overexpansion of the maxillary posterior segments, which may lead to poor tracking and dislodging of the maxillary aligners

Solutions to Deficiencies in the Mandibular Advancement Appliance

Improving Engagement of Precision Wings and Mechanism of Bite Repositioning

As previously discussed, one of the major limitations to the current iteration of the mandibular advancement appliance is its method of bite repositioning, which results in disengagement between the precision wings for a significant proportion of time during daily wear. A solution would be to unify the maxillary and mandibular precision wings into a single unit to ensure more regular engagement (Fig. 3.8). This modified mandibular advancement appliance, modeled on conventional Class II correctors such as the FR-2, Herbst, or other activators, would still allow for lateral excursive movements but would force the patient into the desired advanced position during protrusive movements. Therefore, the efficacy of

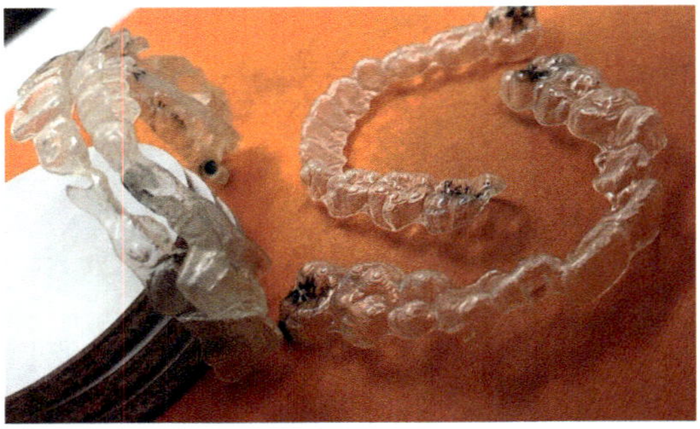

Fig. 3.8 The maxillary and mandibular precision wings can be united into a single unit to ensure more continuous and aggressive mandibular protrusion during patient wear. As shown on the left, the modified aligner with the united maxillary and mandibular precision wings can be worn nightly for bite repositioning. As shown on the right, conventional clear aligners can be worn during the day for optimal tooth movement

the appliance could be potentially improved by more securely tethering the maxillary and mandibular precision wings.

Movement of Teeth Beneath the Precision Wings

The single-unit modified mandibular advancement appliance can be incorporated into an aligner wearing regimen that allows for more accurate movement of the teeth that would be typically encapsulated within the precision wings. The patient can wear the single-unit modified aligner at night for 14–16 hours/day, including during sleep. In the daytime, for 8–10 hours/day, the patient can wear a traditional clear aligner without precision wings to allow for optimal movement of individual teeth. The single-unit aligner and traditional aligner would be coordinated so that the patient would be wearing the same stage of each at any point in time. In this fashion, the patient could receive both optimized movements for individual teeth and the treatment effects of the mandibular advancement appliance.

Is Mandibular Advancement a Viable Alternative to Conventional Class II Correctors?

The mandibular advancement appliance remains largely untested in regards to its efficacy in the correction of Class II malocclusions. Align Technology's early claims of its comparable (or superior) efficacy relative to conventional Class II functional appliances remain unsubstantiated by the scientific literature and rest on a preliminary clinical trial with high risk of bias and questionable conclusions. The current appliance, which is modeled after the Twin Block, is characterized by a number of mechanical limitations, including a bite repositioning method that results in constant disengagement between its parts and a pattern of vertical elastics wear that frequently dislodges the maxillary and mandibular aligners. Early evidence suggests that case selection is pivotal for successful outcomes: the appliance is most ideal for the treatment of mild Class II malocclusions with orthognathic maxillae, retrognathic mandibles, and ANB $< 4^\circ$.

We anticipate that randomized clinical trials in the future will continue to clarify the efficacy of the MA appliance relative to both conventional Class II functional appliances and Class II mechanics with clear aligners. The future optimization of the mandibular advancement appliance likely lies in the improvement of its bite repositioning mechanism for more aggressive and continuous mandibular protrusion.

References

1. Wahl N. Orthodontics in 3 millennia. Chapter 9: functional appliances to midcentury. Am J Orthod Dentofac Orthop. 2006;129(6):829–33.
2. DiBiase A, Cobourne M, Lee R. The use of functional appliances in contemporary orthodontic practice. Br Dent J. 2015;218:123–8.
3. Robin P. Observation sur un nouvel appareil de redressement. Rev Stomatol. 1902;9:42.

4. Levrini A, Favero L. The masters of functional orthodontics. 1st ed. Milan: Quintessence; 2003.
5. Cacciatore G, Ghislanzoni L, Alvetro L, Giuntini V, Franchi L. Treatment and posttreatment effects induced by the Forsus appliance: a controlled clinical study. Angle Orthod. 2014;84(6):1010–7.
6. Marsico E, Gatto E, Burrascano M, Matarese G, Cordasco G. Effectiveness of orthodontic treatment with functional appliances on mandibular growth in the short term. Am J Orthod Dentofac Orthop. 2011;139(1):24–36.
7. Perillo L, Cannavale R, Ferro F, Franchi L, Masucci C, Chiodini P, Baccetti T. Meta-analysis of skeletal mandibular changes during Frankel appliance treatment. Eur J Orthod. 2011;33(1):84–92.
8. Cacciatore G, Ugolini A, Sforza C, Gbinigie O, Plüddemann A. Long-term effects of functional appliances in treated versus untreated patients with class II malocclusion: a systematic review and meta-analysis. PLoS One. 2019;14(9):e0221624. https://doi.org/10.1371/journal.pone.0221624.
9. Jena AK, Duggal R, Parkash H. Skeletal and dentoalveolar effects of twin-block and bionator appliances in the treatment of class II malocclusion: a comparative study. Am J Orthod Dentofac Orthop. 2006;130(5):594–602.
10. Align Technology. Mandibular advancement FAQ. https://info.aligntech.com/MA/faq (2020). Accessed 29 Oct 2020.
11. Zymperdikas VF, Koretsi V, Papageorgiou SN, Papadopoulos MA. Treatment effects of fixed functional appliances in patients with class II malocclusion: a systematic review and meta-analysis. Eur J Orthod. 2016;38(2):113–26.
12. Howe RP. The bonded Herbst appliance. J Clin Ortho. 1982;15:663–7.
13. Valant JR, Sinclair PM. Treatment effects of the Herbst appliance. Am J Ortho Dentofac Orthop. 1989;95:138–47.
14. McNamara JA Jr, Huge SA. The Fränkel appliance (FR-2): model preparation and appliance construction. Am J Orthod. 1981;80(5):478–95.
15. Banks P, Wright J, O'Brien K. Incremental versus maximum bite advancement during twin-block therapy: a randomized controlled clinical trial. Am J Orthod Dentofac Orthop. 2004;126(5):583–8.
16. DeVincenzo JP, Winn MW. Orthopedic and orthodontic effects resulting from the use of a functional appliance with different amounts of protrusive activation. Am J Orthod Dentofac Orthop. 1989;96(3):181–90.
17. Hägglund P, Segerda S, Forsberg C. The integrated Herbst appliance—treatment effects in a group of adolescent males with class II malocclusions compared with growth changes in an untreated control group. Eur J Orthod. 2008;30(2):120–7.
18. Baccetti T, Franchi L, Toth LR, McNamara JA Jr. Treatment timing for twin-block therapy. Am J Orthod Dentofac Orthop. 2000;118(2):159–70.
19. Align Technology. Mandibular advancement FAQ. https://info.aligntech.com/MA/faq (2020). Accessed 17 Nov 2020.
20. Giancotti A, Cozza P, Mampieri G. Aligners and mandibular advancement: a comprehensive option for phase I treatment of class II, division I cases. J Clin Ortho. 2020;54(9):513–24.
21. Bowman SJ, Celenza F, Sparaga J, Papadopoulos MA, Ojima K, Lin JC. Creative adjuncts for clear aligners, part 1: class II treatment. J Clin Orthod. 2015;49(2):83–94.
22. Geran RG, McNamara JA Jr, Baccetti T, Franchi L, Shapiro LM. A prospective long-term study on the effects of rapid maxillary expansion in the early mixed dentition. Am J Orthod Dentofac Orthop. 2006;129(5):631–40.

Problematic Complex Movements: Can Clear Aligners Treat Them Alone?

4

Contents

Have Clear Aligners Improved in Achieving Complex Movements?

Historically, certain complex tooth movements have been problematic for clear aligner therapy. One of the first clinical trials analyzing the efficacy of tooth movement with clear aligners demonstrated that specific movements were lacking in accuracy when predicted tooth positions were compared with actual positions [1]. Notably, the least accurate movement was extrusion, particularly of the maxillary and mandibular incisors [1]. The study also found a low accuracy for the rotation of canines and maxillary lateral incisors [1]. A 2020 follow-up study to the aforementioned clinical trial found that though the overall accuracy of movements improved, rotation was the least accurate movement, especially of maxillary lateral incisors, canines, premolars, and molars [2]. The accuracy of maxillary incisor extrusion was improved to 55%, though the extrusion of maxillary and mandibular molars were less accurate at 40% [2]. Incisor intrusion, at an accuracy of 35% for the mandibular incisors, remained consistently low across both trials [2]. Poor control of overbite due to difficulties with intrusive movements of anterior teeth has been cited as a longstanding limitation of clear aligner therapy [3]. A comparison between these two clinical trials suggests that despite significant advances in clear aligner technology during the last decade, the same teeth movements, including rotation, extrusion (of molars), and incisor intrusion, though improved in accuracy, remain problematic.

Similarly, complex movements such as tooth uprighting remain unpredictable. Studies of extraction treatment with Invisalign indicate that the molars adjacent to extraction spaces do not achieve bodily movement as predicted and are instead characterized by undesired mesial tipping and inadequately controlled root movement despite the incorporation of Invisalign extraction protocols [4]. Tooth uprighting, especially

A. T. Huang, D. Huang, *Controversies in Clear Aligner Therapy*,
https://doi.org/10.1007/978-3-030-92810-0_4

requiring extensive root movement, remains a challenge for clear aligner therapy.

There have been a variety of methods proposed by clinicians to address these deficiencies in clear aligner therapy. Studies have recommended the judicious use of additional attachments for problematic movements, especially for vertical movements in the anterior segments [5]. Clinicians have also observed that the use of overcorrection can be beneficial for achieving difficult movements [3]. Additionally, the use of auxiliaries, such as miniscrew anchorage, elastics, and partial fixed appliances, have been shown to address current limitations in clear aligner therapy and improve the accuracy of problematic movements [6].

In this chapter, we focus on a number of traditionally problematic and complex movements in clear aligner therapy, including control of maxillary lateral incisors, uprighting, intrusion, and extrusion. We discuss the challenges involved in planning and executing these movements, as well as solutions to improving their accuracy and achieving successful and predicted outcomes.

The Challenges of Controlling Maxillary Lateral Incisors

Invisalign G4 and G7 Attachments

Invisalign's G4 and G7 generation features included modifications designed for improving the predictability of maxillary lateral incisor movement. Specifically, the G4 "SmartTrack" features are triggered to automatically incorporate optimized multiplane attachments on maxillary laterals undergoing extrusive movements in addition to rotation and/or crown tipping in the mesiodistal dimension. The G7 generation features, which claimed to enhance detailing and finishing for clinicians, further refined maxillary lateral control through the second generation of optimized multiplane attachments to improve tracking when rotation is combined with either intrusion or extrusion. The G7 generation features also introduced optimized support attachments on maxillary laterals to maintain tracking during intrusion of adjacent teeth, particularly the maxillary central incisors. The G4 and G7 generation optimized attachments have allowed for improved predictability of maxillary lateral movement, as supported by a comparison between the 2009 and 2020 studies on the efficacy of tooth movement with Invisalign [1]. The studies show that the accuracy of maxillary incisor extrusion has improved between 2009 and 2020. This improvement may likely be a result of Invisalign's technological updates, including its G4 and G7 optimized maxillary lateral attachments, which were respectively introduced in late 2011 and late 2016 and specifically target maxillary lateral extrusion [2]. Clinically, we have observed that the incorporation of the optimized lateral attachments have enhanced predictability in correcting displaced lateral incisors, especially when they require the difficult movements of extrusion and derotation. In cases where lateral incisors require significant derotation in addition to intrusion or extrusion, the use of an optimized G4 or G7 attachment is recommended for the accuracy of movement (Fig. 4.1). This is in agreement with the findings of a number of clinicians, who have recommended the use of attachments for improved rotational control [7].

However, we note that despite improvement in maxillary lateral control from earlier generations of clear aligners, the accuracy of their movements remains low, at 53.7% for extrusion and 48.7% for distal rotation, relative to movements such as labial tipping (69.9%) [2]. Consequently, extreme rotations, such as those >15° or significant extrusion, may require further supplementation, in addition to the use of the G4 and G7 optimized attachments, to achieve desired outcomes for maxillary lateral movement.

Another complication in attachment design for maxillary lateral incisors arises when they require significant intrusion, which has been shown to be low in accuracy. Intrusive movements are best performed without attachments. It is recommended that the clinician omit an attachment on the lateral incisor if it requires significant intrusion (without the need for extensive rotational or mesiodistal tipping movements) for improved predictability.

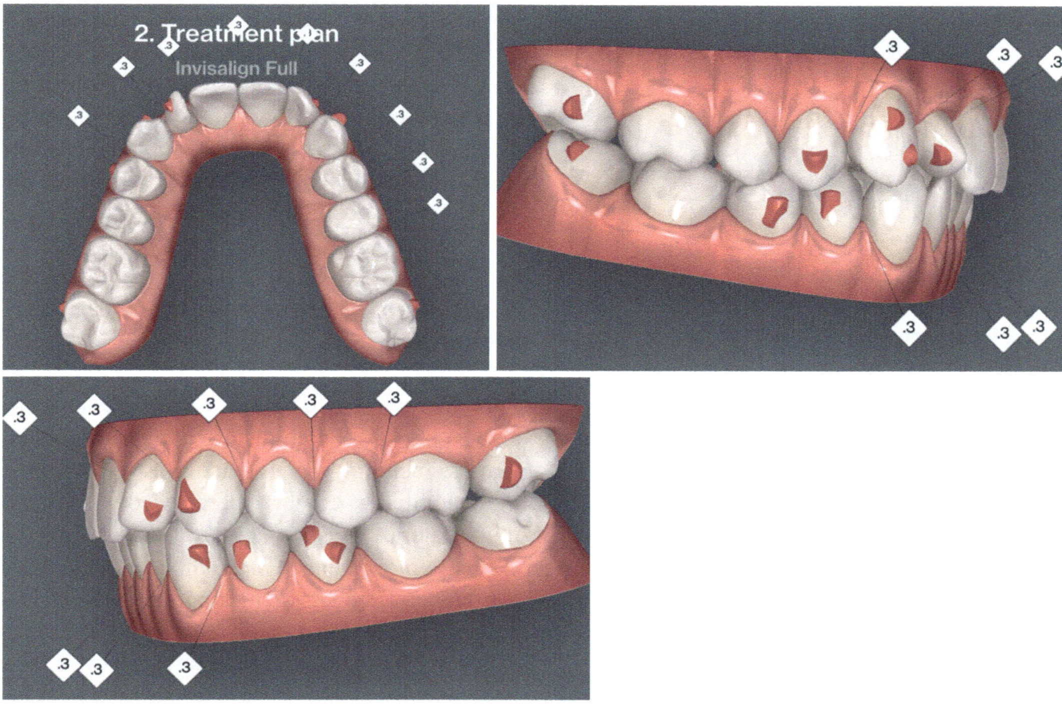

Fig. 4.1 G7 optimized attachments have been placed on the maxillary lateral incisors to enhance the predictability of derotation. When possible, the provider should request optimized G7 attachments for maxillary lateral incisor derotation, especially for significant rotations, such as those >15°

In early 2021, Invisalign introduced its G8 generation features, one of which is designed for the enhancement of incisor intrusion through "aligner activation," which refers to the specific contouring of the aligner to deliver optimal forces and minimize undesirable movements through improved control over location, direction, and amount of force (Fig. 4.2) [8]. The efficacy of the G8 features has not been clinically evaluated. The G8 modifications focus only on optimizing intrusive movements for the anterior teeth and not extrusion or movements in the other orders (though Invisalign claims the modifications will also enhance posterior arch expansion with optimized expansion support attachments).

Alteration in Aligner Geometry for Enhancement of Tooth Movement

Often, cases arise when maxillary lateral incisors fail to track toward the end of a course of aligners, especially when the tooth was initially significantly displaced, whether requiring rotation >15° or in linguoversion. If the necessary derotation of maxillary lateral incisor is minor— <15°—then, the clinician may be able to modify the aligner geometry in order to supplement the forces supplied by the aligner. In such cases, hand instruments can be employed to produce additional forces in either the first or second order. For example, if the maxillary lateral incisor is mesially rotated and requires distal rotation, then the clinician can place dimples with a dimple plier on the mesiolingual and distolabial surfaces of the aligner to create a rotational couple in the distal direction. The patient can wear the modified aligner for an extended period of time, such as 4–6 weeks, to allow for expression of the supplementary forces. It is also prudent for the clinician to verify that there is adequate interproximal space for derotation. Research findings have shown that teeth which received interproximal reduction, when compared to those that did not

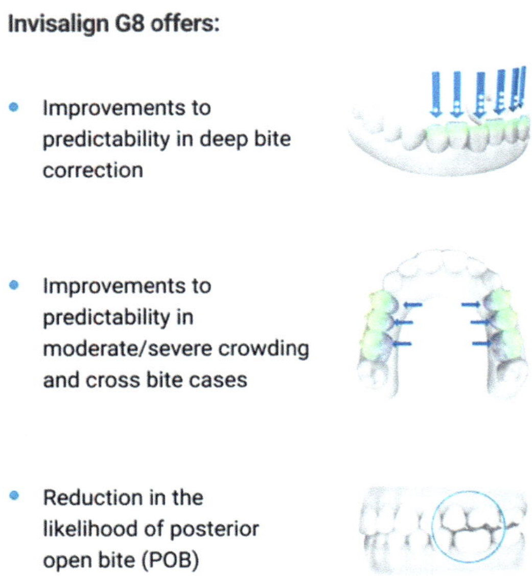

Fig. 4.2 Invisalign G8 generation modifications include “aligner activation” for supposedly improved control over intrusive forces to the maxillary and mandibular anterior teeth. Other features include optimized support attachments designed for more bodily posterior expansion

receive interproximal reduction, show greater accuracy with rotation [9]. (We will further discuss detailing and finishing in Chap. 11). If discrepancies in maxillary lateral incisor position are significant, other measures, such as the use of alternative auxiliaries or a course of refinement, are more adequate.

Combination Treatment with Fixed Appliances

In circumstances when maxillary lateral incisors cannot be fully derotated whether through alterations in aligner geometry or courses of refinement, a short period of partial fixed appliances can be helpful to fully correct discrepancies in tooth position. Partial fixed appliances can be placed on the problematic maxillary lateral incisor and the two teeth immediately adjacent. A light NiTi wire should be able to fully align the lateral incisor in 4–8 weeks (Fig. 4.3). The clinician should be mindful to cut the aligner so that it does not interfere with the fixed appliances, while it still sufficiently encapsulates the adjacent teeth to retain their positions.

Auxiliaries for Enhancement of Tooth Movement

Poor tracking of maxillary lateral incisors can also be improved with the use of alternative auxiliaries, including buttons and elastics. Notably, these auxiliaries can be incorporated when maxillary lateral incisors do not achieve planned extrusive movements. For example, if a maxillary lateral incisor begins to track poorly in the incisogingival dimension and fails to extrude, the clinician can bond a button on the lateral incisor for a vertical elastic to be worn to the opposing canine for a supplementary extrusive force (Fig. 4.4). The elastic can be extended from the button on the problematic lateral incisor to either another button on the opposing canine or a precision cut on the aligner respective to the canine. This supplementary extrusive force can be applied until the lateral adequately tracks or until the completion of the course of aligners (or it can be applied on a final aligner for extended wear to improve tooth position).

Overcorrection for Improved Predictability of Maxillary Lateral Incisor Movement

Overcorrection for improved predictability of tooth movement has been recommended by a number of studies [3]. This method can be applied to the planned movements of maxillary lateral incisors in both first and second orders. For example, for a maxillary lateral incisor that requires significant labialization, the clinician can exaggerate the amount of labialization so that on the Clincheck, the lateral incisor will finish slightly labial to its ideal position relative to the adjacent teeth. Similarly, for a high maxillary lateral incisor requiring significant extrusion, such as >2.5 mm, the clinician can over-engineer the amount of extrusion on the tooth in the Clincheck in order to compensate for the difficulty of the movement. This method can also be useful for addressing severe rotations in maxillary lateral incisors, whose rotational movements can be exaggerated to achieve more ideal outcomes. It is difficult to recommend the precise margin for overcorrection of difficult lateral incisor movements. However, the overcorrections should be applied judiciously so they do not result in adverse effects for the occlusion, such as heavy anterior interferences, anterior open bites, or undesirable changes in overjet and overbite.

Torque Control for Maxillary Lateral Incisors

For severely lingually displaced maxillary lateral incisors, significant labial root torque is often necessary for ideal tooth positioning. As discussed in Chap. 1, most current softwares, from Invisalign to 3M to Suresmile, lack adequate controls for labial root torque. The

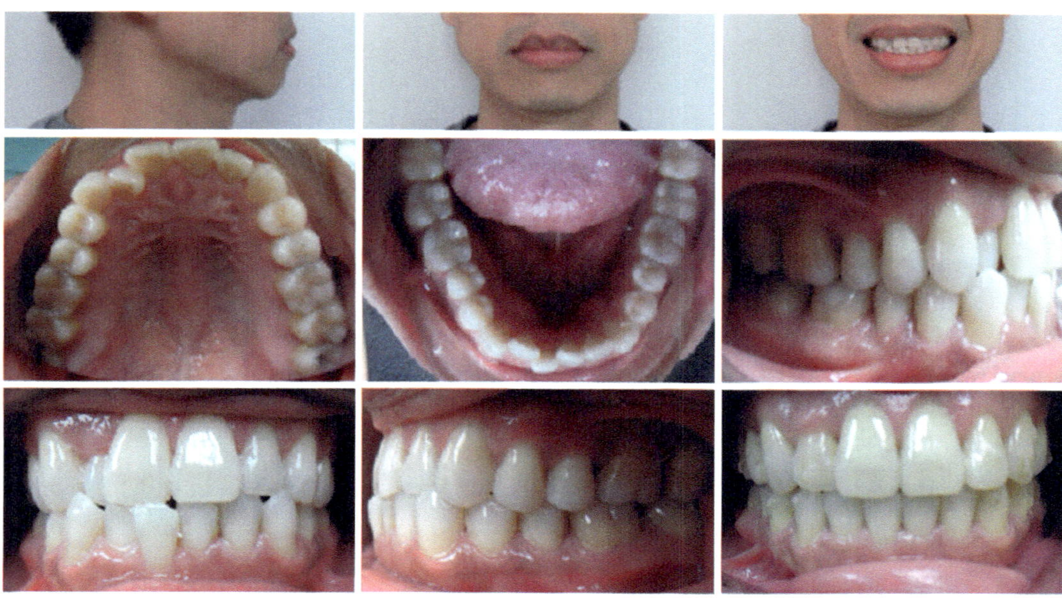

Fig. 4.3 Severe rotations of maxillary lateral incisors may require auxiliary fixed appliances for complete derotation. For patient J.L., an initial and single refinement course of aligners did not completely resolve the rotation of the right maxillary lateral incisor. A short course of partial fixed appliances completely resolved the rotation without the need for another refinement course

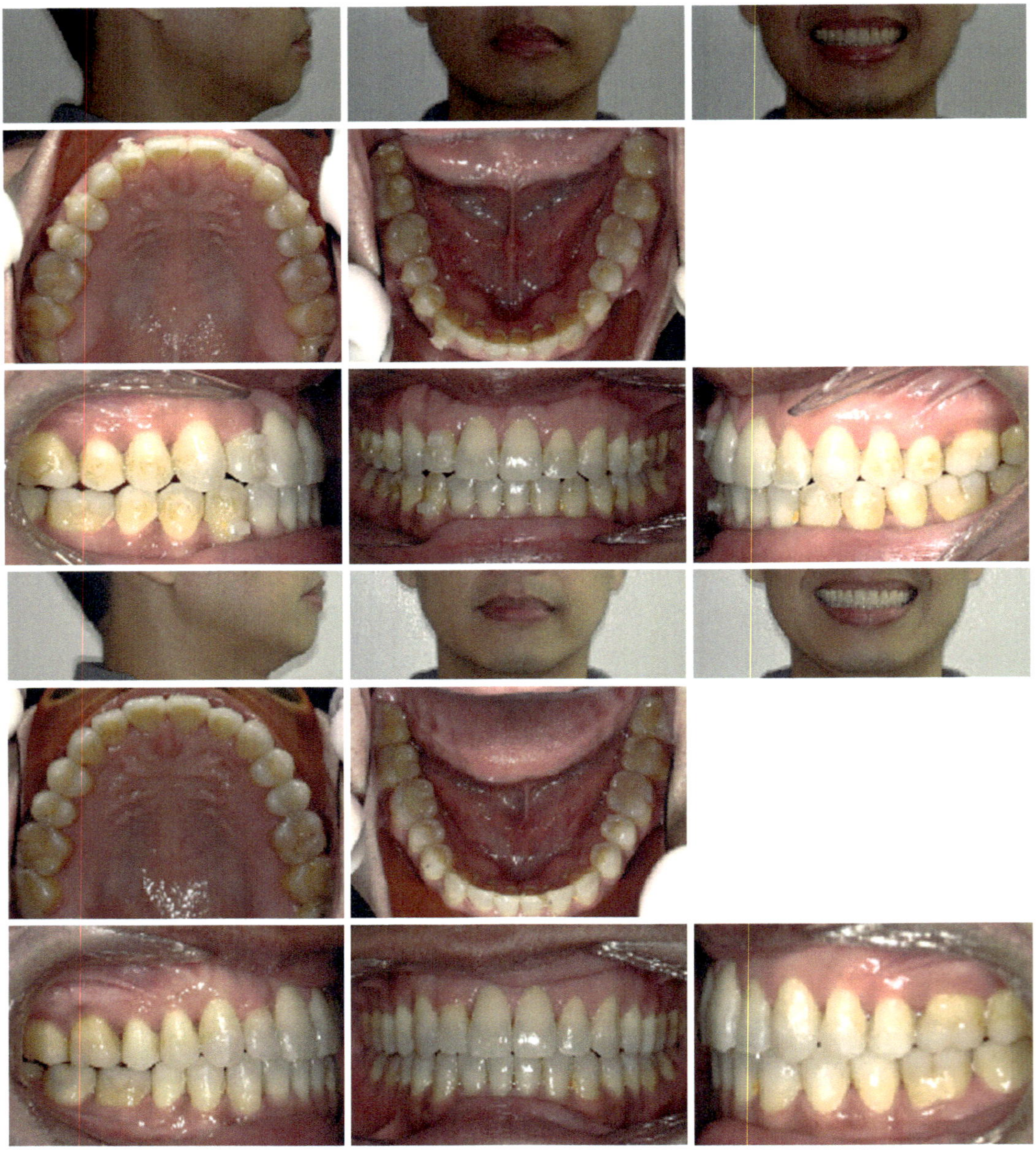

Fig. 4.3 (continued)

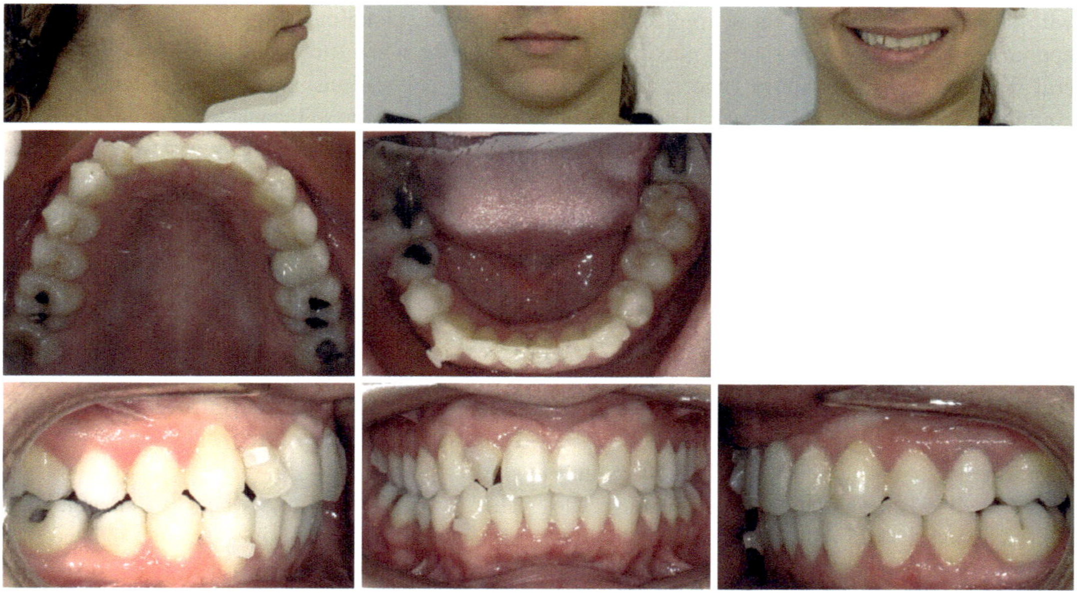

Fig. 4.4 The placement of a button on maxillary lateral incisors allows for the application of a supplementary extrusive force to achieve desired final tooth positions. The button can be bonded toward the end of the initial course of aligners or following the initial course to minimize the duration of refinement

Invisalign software currently does not allow for power ridges on lingual surfaces, nor does it allow for free placement of power ridges by the clinician. As a result, supplementary labial root torque may be programmed through over-engineering in the Clincheck for lateral incisors requiring significant correction. Alternatively, if the lateral incisor fails to track in the third order during a course of aligners, supplementary labial root torque can be incorporated with the use of hand instruments, in the method of a power ridge on the linguogingival surface and pressure point on the labio-incisal surface to produce a torquing couple (see Chap. 1 for more detailed discussion).

Restorative Solutions for Maxillary Lateral Incisors

Maxillary lateral incisors are one of the most commonly congenitally misshapen teeth and the overall prevalence of peg-shaped maxillary permanent lateral incisors has been recently reported to be 1.8% [10]. In addition, 55.5% of individuals with unilateral peg-shaped maxillary lateral incisors exhibit contralateral maxillary lateral incisor hypodontia [10]. Therefore, it is likely the clinician will encounter malformed maxillary lateral incisors that require restorative solutions for optimal occlusion and esthetics. Future restorations can be planned during Clincheck development with the same principles as those applied to fixed appliances [11]. For a peg-shaped maxillary lateral incisor requiring a future veneer, crown, or composite build-up, the clinician can position the final position of the tooth with adequate space for restoration to ideal dimensions (Fig. 4.5). As with fixed appliances, it is recommended that the space allocated for the restoration is determined in an interdisciplinary fashion with the restorative dentist.

Bolton Discrepancies

Abnormally small maxillary lateral incisors may likely result in Bolton maxillary deficiencies. The Bolton analysis tool in the Clincheck can be useful in verifying tooth size discrepancies during treatment planning (Fig. 4.6). Circumstances may arise when the opening of space for lateral incisor restorations are not indicated, such as when the opening of the space for an ideally sized lateral would result in an excessive overjet. In these cases, the clinician may have to close the spaces adjacent to the maxillary lateral incisor, compromise an ideal Class I occlusal relationship, and finish in an end-on Class II relationship on the side with the abnormally small maxillary lateral incisor (Fig. 4.7).

Missing Maxillary Lateral Incisors

There are situations when mesioangulated impacted maxillary canines damage the roots of the adjacent maxillary lateral incisors to such an

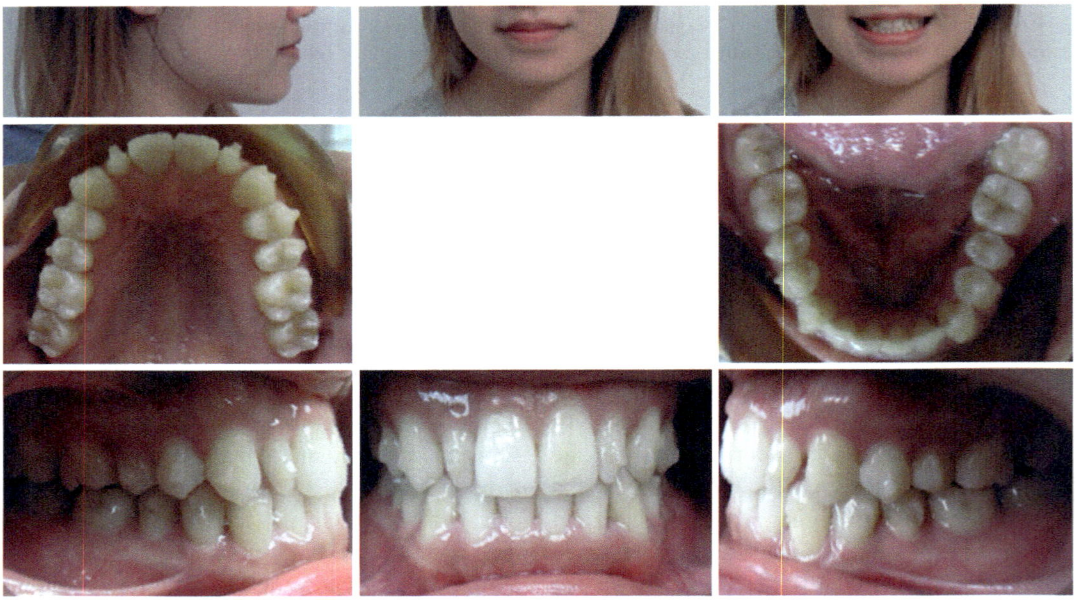

Fig. 4.5 Abnormally small maxillary lateral incisors should be adequately positioned for future restorative treatment, whether in the form of veneers or crowns. The clinician should treatment plan in an interdisciplinary fashion with the restorative dentist for optimal esthetics

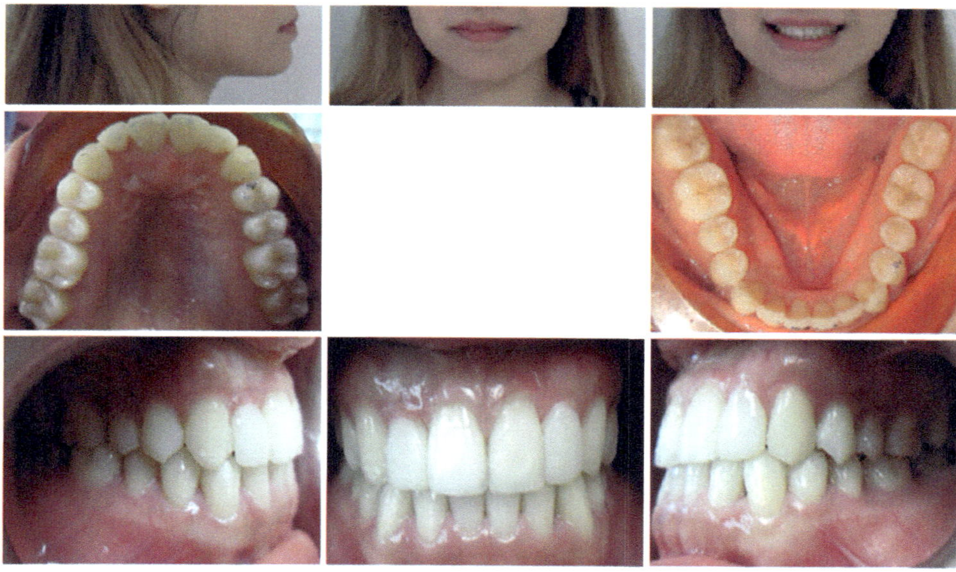

Fig. 4.5 (continued)

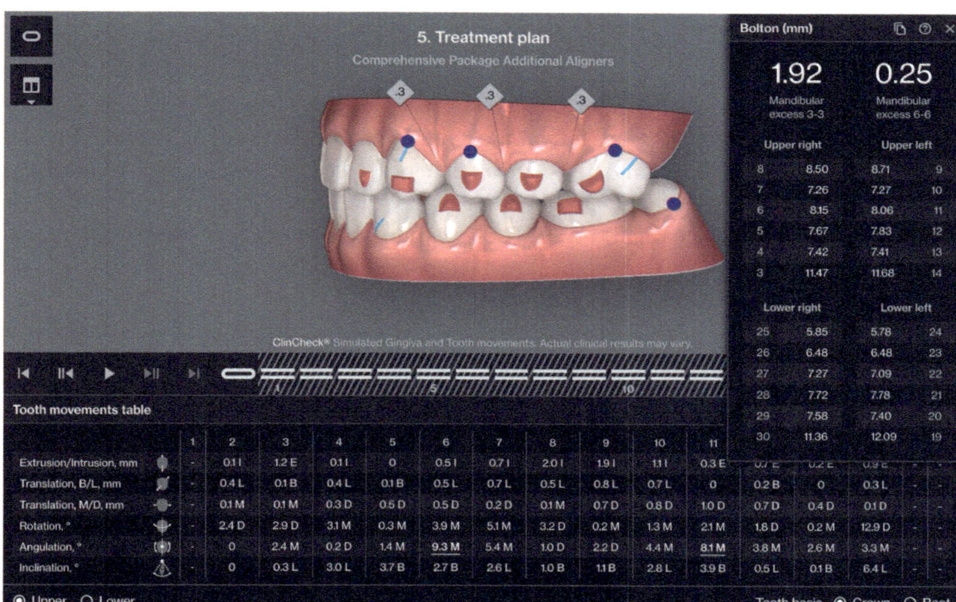

Fig. 4.6 The Bolton analysis feature is a tool during treatment planning that can assist in ideally positioning the maxillary lateral incisors. In certain circumstances, the lateral incisor may need to be positioned for future restorative treatment. It is also useful for planning the correction of sagittal occlusal relationships, which may involve a degree of compromise when Bolton discrepancies exist

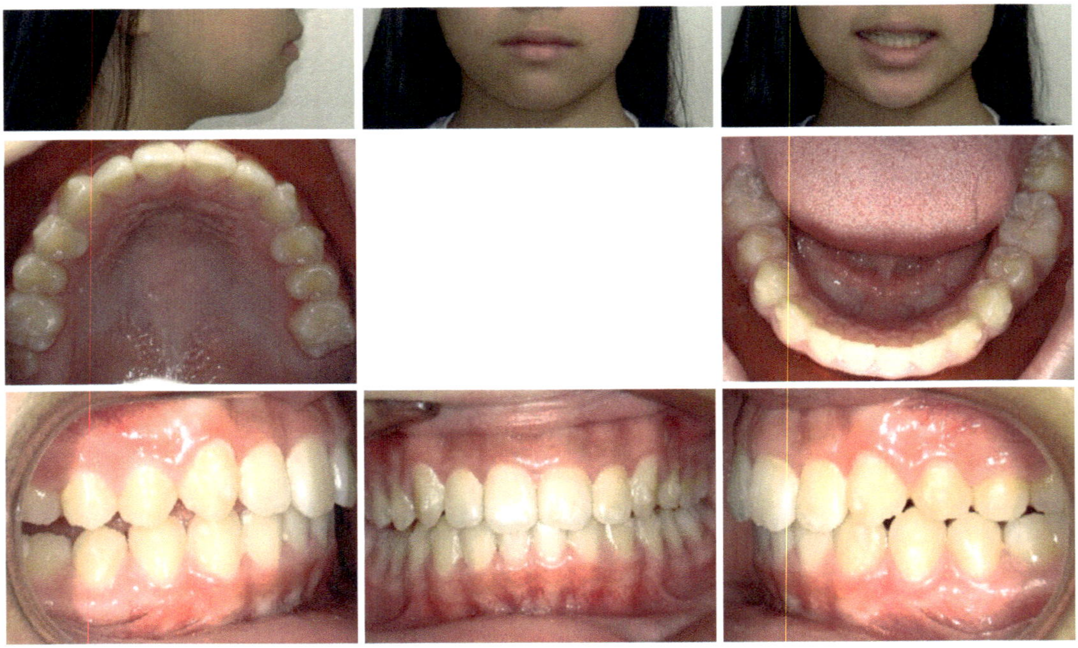

Fig. 4.7 A Bolton maxillary deficiency resulted in Class II end on occlusion on the right side

extent that extraction of the lateral is indicated. In these cases, the clinician can plan in the software for either complete closure of the maxillary lateral space with canine substitution or maintenance of the space for a future implant (Fig. 4.8). Space closure is best when the maxillary incisors are protruded and the posterior teeth are in Class II relationships so that spaces can be reciprocally closed with protraction of the posterior teeth and retraction of the incisors [12]. The substituted canine should be positioned as esthetically as possible with consideration of the canine's shape, color, and gingival level. Ideally, a substituted canine should be of a similar shade to the central incisor, is shaped narrow at the cemento-enamel junction both labiolingually and mesiodistally, and demonstrates a flat emergence profile [13]. To simulate a lateral incisor, the gingival margin of the substituted canine should be slightly incisal to that of the central incisor. For optimal esthetics, after orthodontic treatment, the patient may require crown lengthening for ideal gingival contours and restorative treatment in the form of composite bonding or porcelain veneers.

Root Uprighting

Elements of Successful Uprighting—The Virtual Gable Bend

Studies have shown that clear aligners are not as successful in root control and alignment as compared to fixed labial appliances [14]. Essential elements for the successful uprighting of roots include:

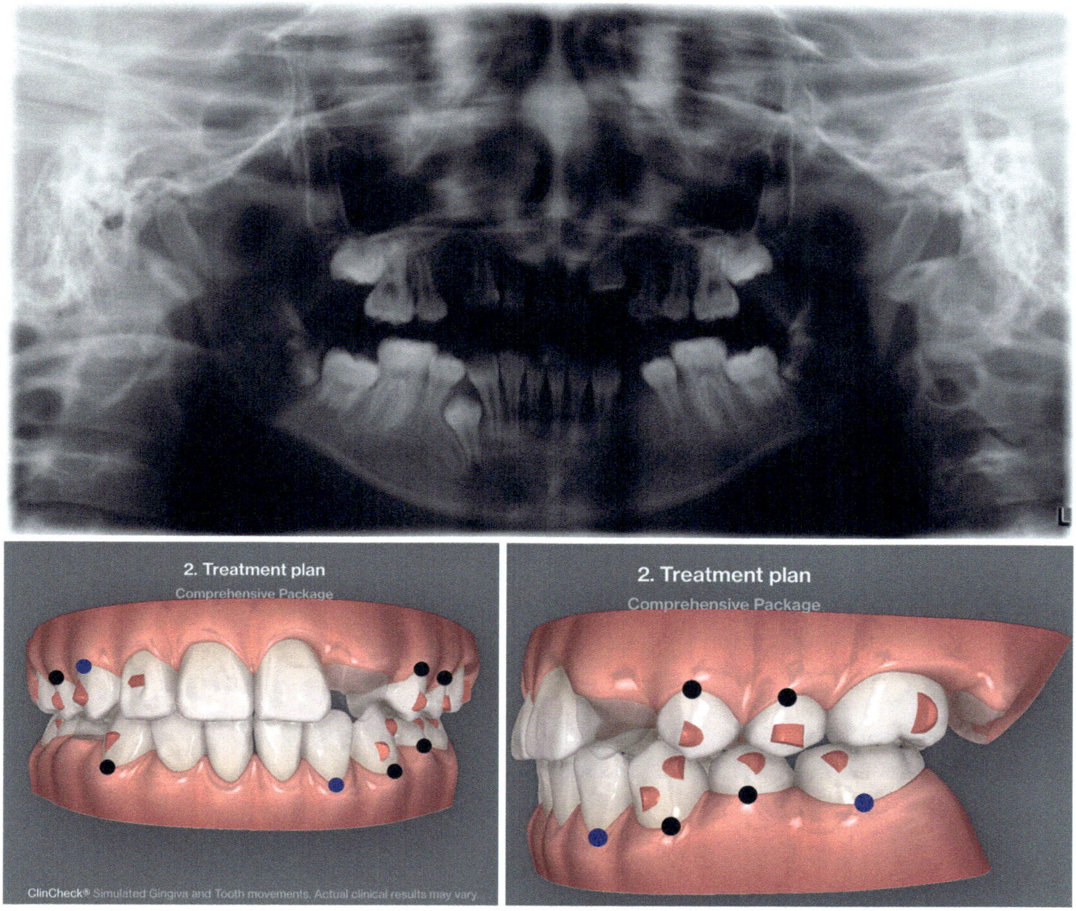

Fig. 4.8 Patient J.L. received two phases of orthodontic treatment. Phase I comprised of rapid maxillary expansion and high-pull headgear. Following phase I, it was observed that the erupting left maxillary canine was resorbing the root of the left maxillary lateral incisor. Because of the damage to the left maxillary lateral incisor, the tooth was extracted and a canine substitution for the maxillary lateral incisor planned

1. The judicious prescription of virtual gable bends.
2. Optimal attachment design.

The virtual gable bend (VGB) allows for simultaneous root movement during crown movement. Though the Clincheck will incorporate root movement for the uprighting of tipped teeth, the clinician frequently has to prescribe a virtual gable bend to supplement uprighting for achieving the desired amount of root movement (Fig. 4.9). The VGB will both increase the amount of root movement and decelerate the velocity of movement by altering the staging and increasing the total number of aligners.

Elements of Successful Uprighting—Attachment Design

The judicious use of attachments on the teeth to be uprighted is also critical for successful outcomes. In the case of uprighting canines or premolars, it is recommended that the clinician either maintain optimized root control attachments or prescribe them if absent. However, the software will often not allow for the placement of optimized root attachments. Consequently, the clinician should design adequately oriented conventional attachments to supplement the uprighting movement. For example, if a mandibular left first second premolar is mesially tipped, then a

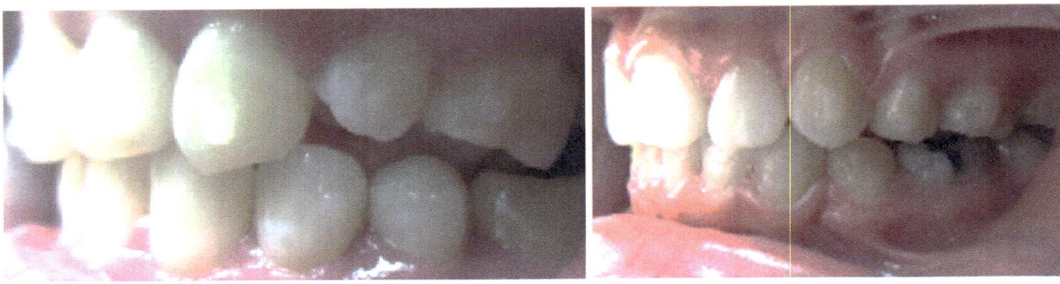

Fig. 4.9 In this case with extractions of maxillary first premolars, the left maxillary second premolar and left maxillary first molar tipped undesirably during space closure. These were uprighted with the addition of a virtual gable bend between the left maxillary canine and the left maxillary second premolar and left first molar. The addition will increase the total number of active aligners but will incorporate greater amount of root movement to the adjacent teeth

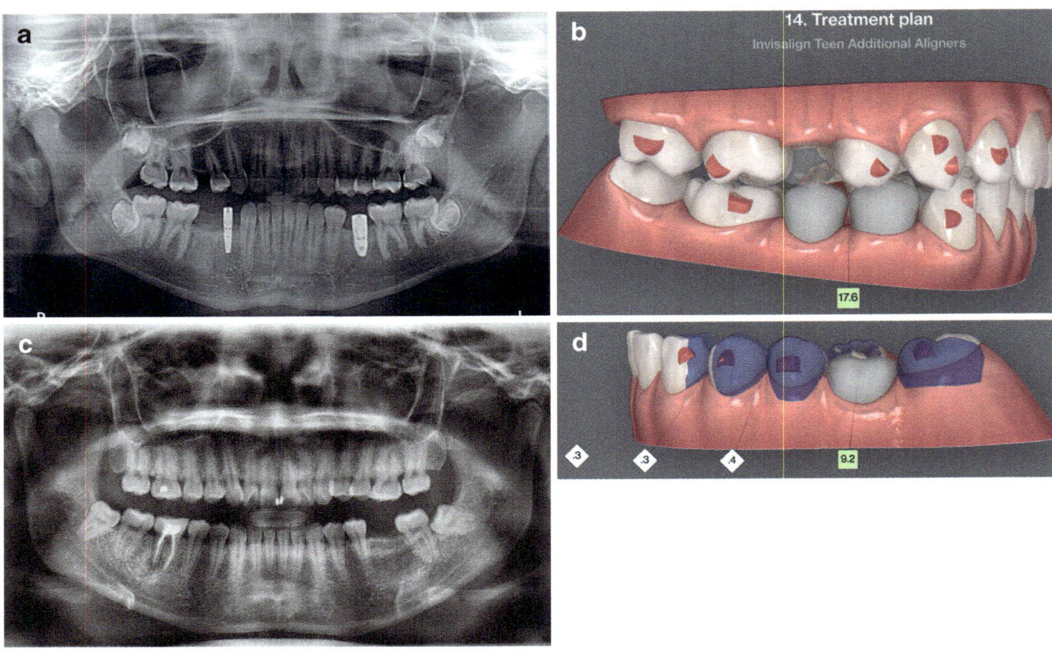

Fig. 4.10 For patient R. W. (**a**, **b**), both the right maxillary first molar and the right maxillary first premolar had to be uprighted to create adequate space for a maxillary second premolar implant. Both attachments were designed with bevels directed mesially to supplement a distal force for mesial movement of the roots. For patient J. X. (**c**, **d**), the left mandibular second molar needed to be uprighted to create adequate space for the left mandibular first molar. An attachment was designed with the bevel (active surface) facing mesially to supplement a distalizing force. The attachment was also directly slightly occlusally to enhance intrusion of the molar

vertical attachment can be placed with its bevel directed mesially. This attachment will supplement a distal force to tip the crown distally and the root mesially. A similar concept can be applied to tipped molars. For a mandibular left first molar tipped mesially because of a missing mandibular left second premolar, a vertical attachment with its bevel oriented mesially can be placed to supplement a distal force to the crown (Fig. 4.10).

Theoretically, the uprighting of a molar would be ideally supplemented with the use of an attach-

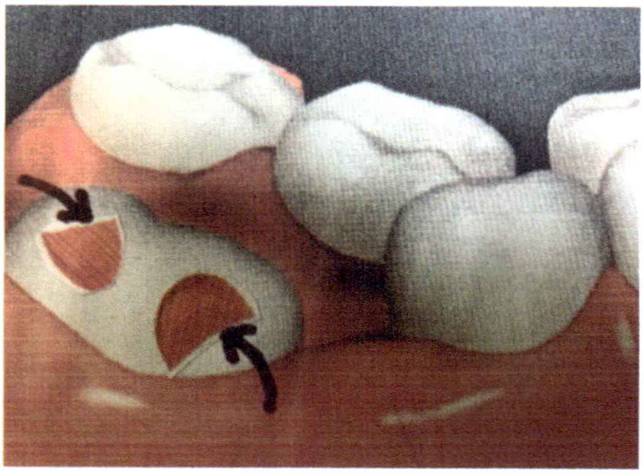

Fig. 4.11 The ideal attachment configuration for the uprighting of a mesially tipped molar would be one that would allow for the delivery of a couple, in the fashion of optimized root control attachments for canines and premolars

ment that allowed for a couple, in the fashion of the premolar optimized root control attachments (Fig. 4.11). At present, these coupled attachments are not available for molars. Instead, the clinician must resort to adjusting the vertical beveled attachments for the proper force systems.

Treatment Duration

For difficult uprighting movements, the incorporation of the virtual gable bend requires an increase in the total number of aligners relative to the same course of aligners without a virtual gable bend (Fig. 4.12). The clinician should appropriately stage the uprighting movement in accordance with current Invisalign software recommendations of 2° tipping/aligner [15]. It has been shown that maintaining forces of less than 2° tipping/aligner is most ideal for delivering optimal forces to the PDL, in accordance with the "optimal force paradigm" of biological tooth movement [16, 17].

Coverage of Aligner Material

It is important for successful uprighting that the aligner material completely embrace the tooth to be moved, especially in that area adjacent to an edentulous site. For example, if a first mandibular left molar, adjacent to a missing mandibular left second premolar, were to be uprighted, then the clinician should ensure the aligner material fully encapsulates the mesial surface of the first molar. This can be achieved by requesting a half-sized pontic for the mandibular left second premolar during the initial setup for the treatment simulation (a full-sized pontic would prevent complete encapsulation of the first molar to be uprighted) (Fig. 4.13).

Auxiliaries for Uprighting

In a similar fashion to achieving difficult maxillary lateral incisor movements, uprighting movements can be supplemented with the use of auxiliaries, whether in the form of partial fixed appliances with sectional mechanics, elastics, or temporary anchorage devices (TADs). For example, for a mesially tipped mandibular right first molar, brackets can be placed on the adjacent mandibular right second molar and mandibular right second premolar and aligned with light wires during clear aligner therapy (Fig. 4.14). Similarly, elastics can be worn from a precision cut of the opposing molar in the maxillary arch for extrusive movement. Alternatively, a TAD can be placed in the buccal shelf mesial to the tooth to be uprighted; a mesializing force can then be applied to the tooth from the TAD to a power arm extending from a band.

Uprighting in Extraction Cases

In extraction cases, the teeth adjacent to extraction spaces often exhibit greater mesiodistal tipping than predicted. For example, in patients receiving maxillary first premolar extractions, maxillary second premolars and maxillary first molars typically demonstrate greater mesial tipping than desired (Fig. 4.15) [4]. As a result, the clinician often has to upright tipped premolars and molars adjacent to extraction spaces (we will further discuss finishing for extraction therapy in Chap. 9). The aforementioned principles for uprighting, including the use of either root con-

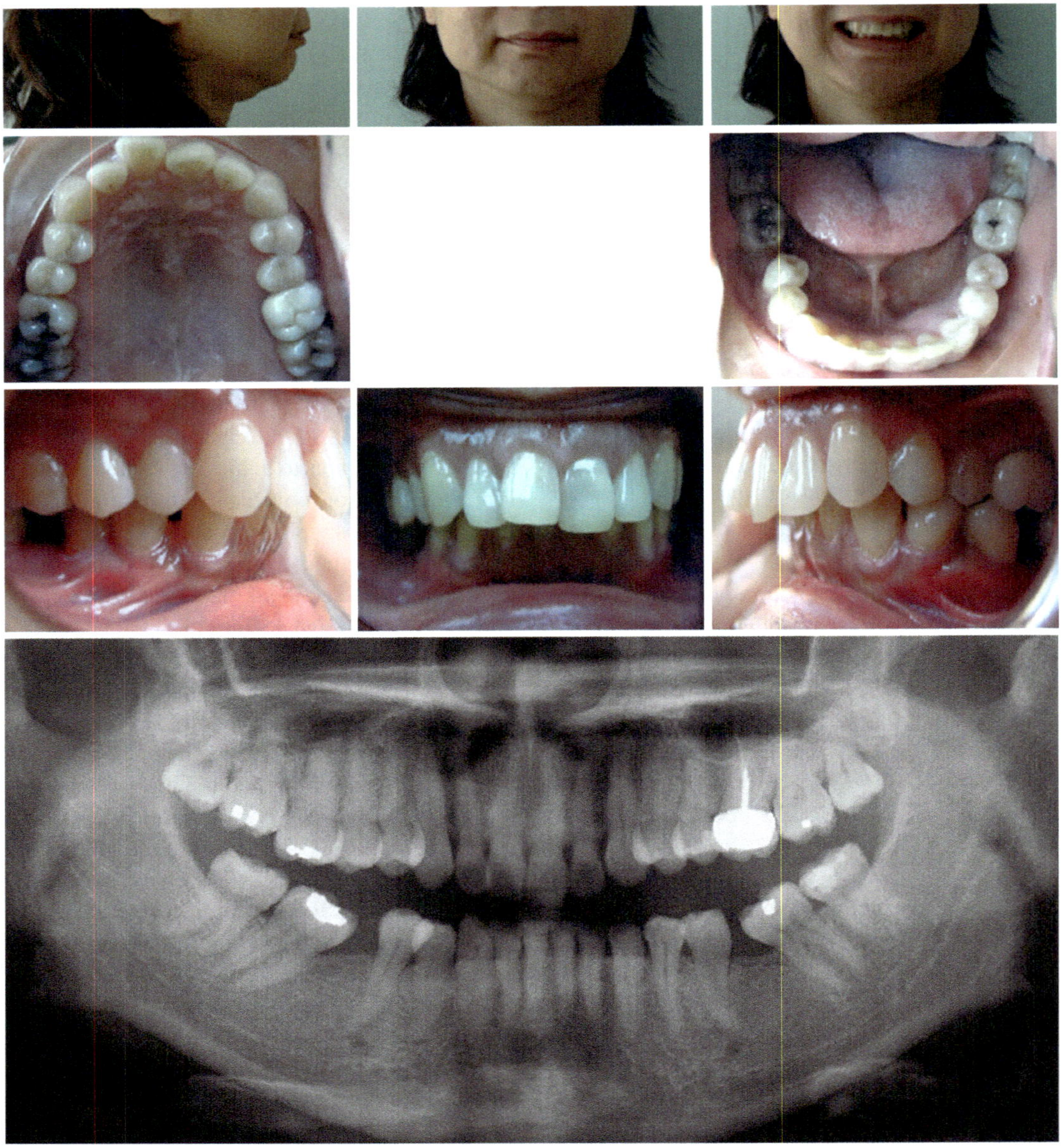

Fig. 4.12 For patient Y. C., the incorporation of a virtual gable bend between the right mandibular second premolar and right mandibular first molar allowed for uprighting of both roots. The increase in amount of root movement with the virtual gable bend also increased the total number of aligners in which the two teeth would be moved to 26. Orthodontic treatment with an initial and single refinement course created an ideal space for a premolar-sized implant restoration. After orthodontic treatment, a premolar-sized implant restoration was placed in the molar's edentulous space

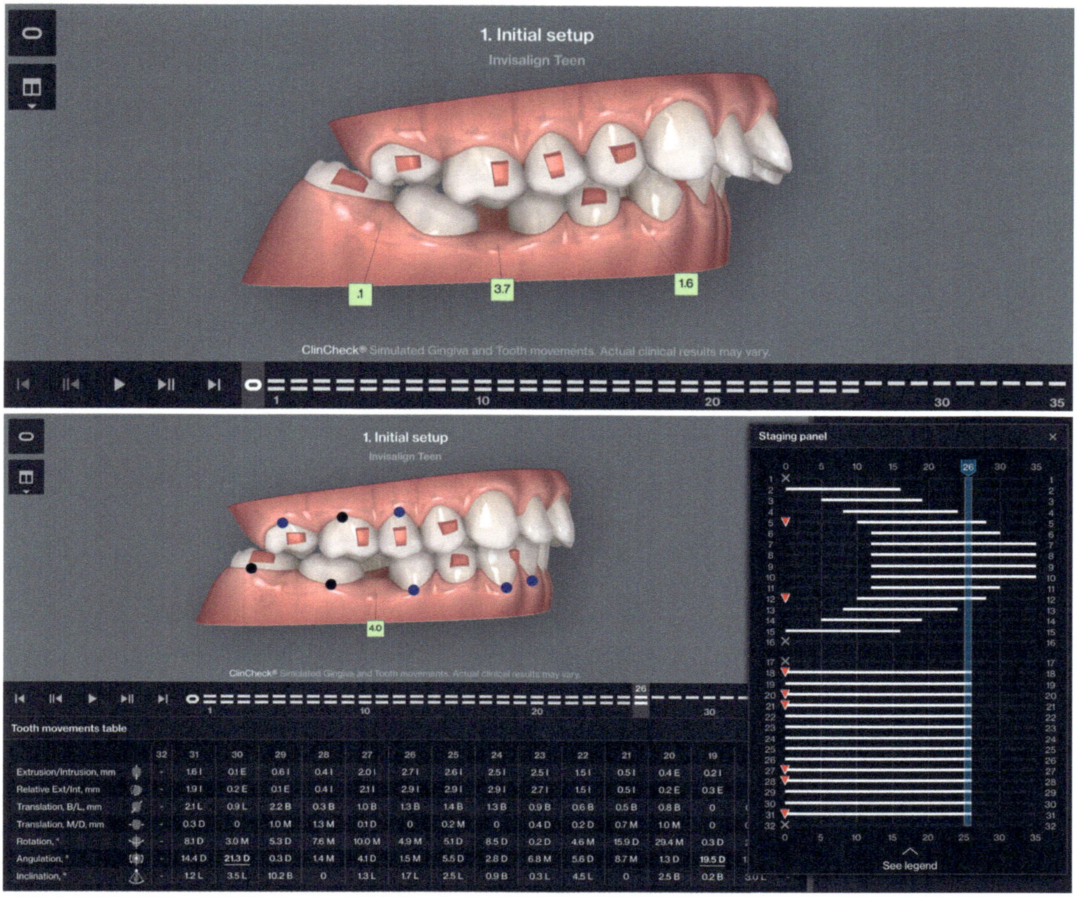

Fig. 4.12 (continued)

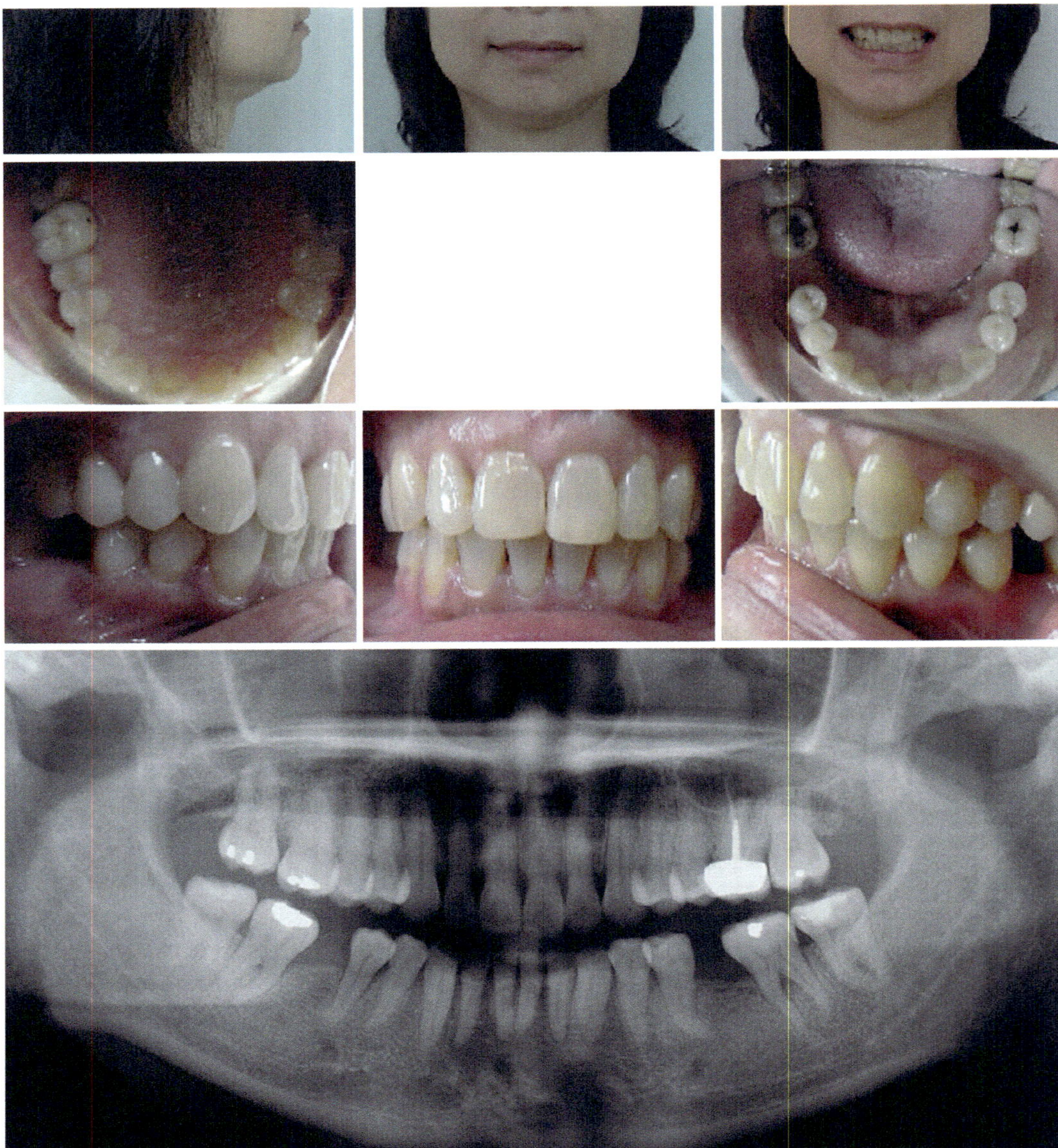

Fig. 4.12 (continued)

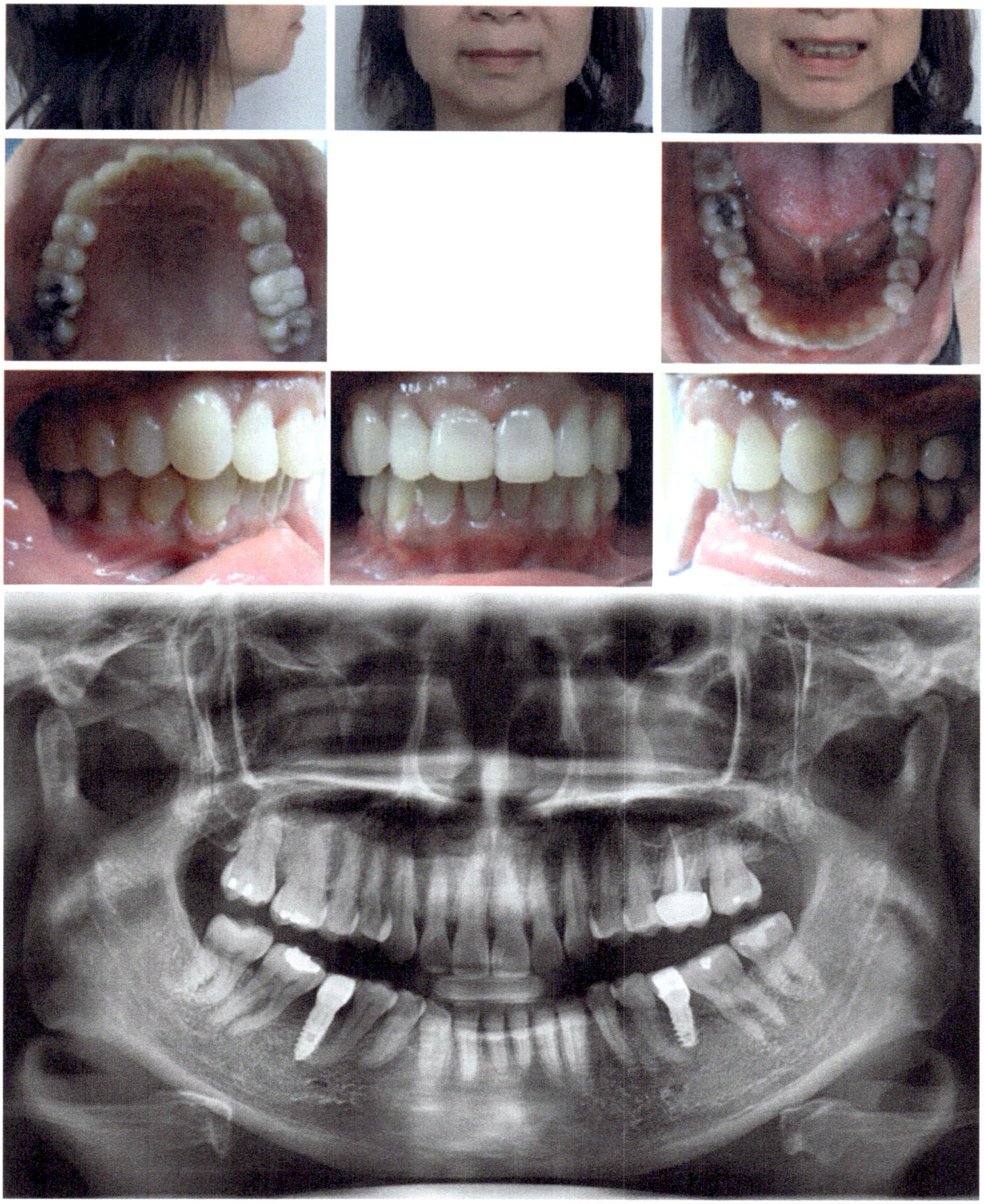

Fig. 4.12 (continued)

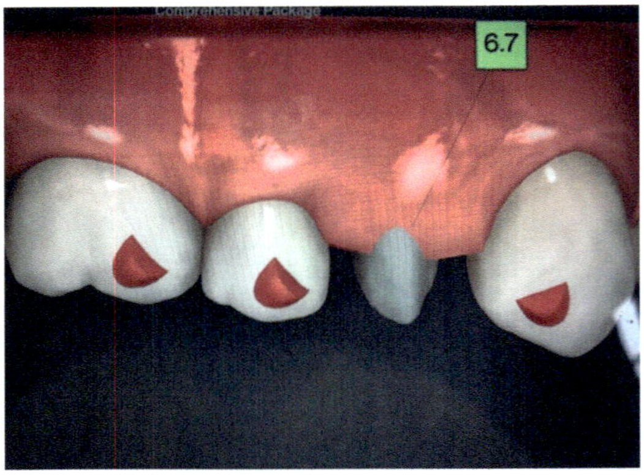

Fig. 4.13 A half-sized pontic adjacent to the premolar that requires uprighting allows for full encapsulation of the tooth with the aligner and more predictable uprighting

trol attachments or properly oriented vertically beveled attachments, should also be applied to teeth that have tipped undesirably during extraction therapy.

Uprighting in Class II Treatment

In the treatment of Class II malocclusions, maxillary canines with crowns that are excessively tipped to the mesial can contribute to posterior end-on Class II relationships. Therefore, it is essential for Class II correction that the maxillary canines be uprighted. This movement can be supplemented with G4 optimized root control attachments and Class II elastics (Fig. 4.16a, b).

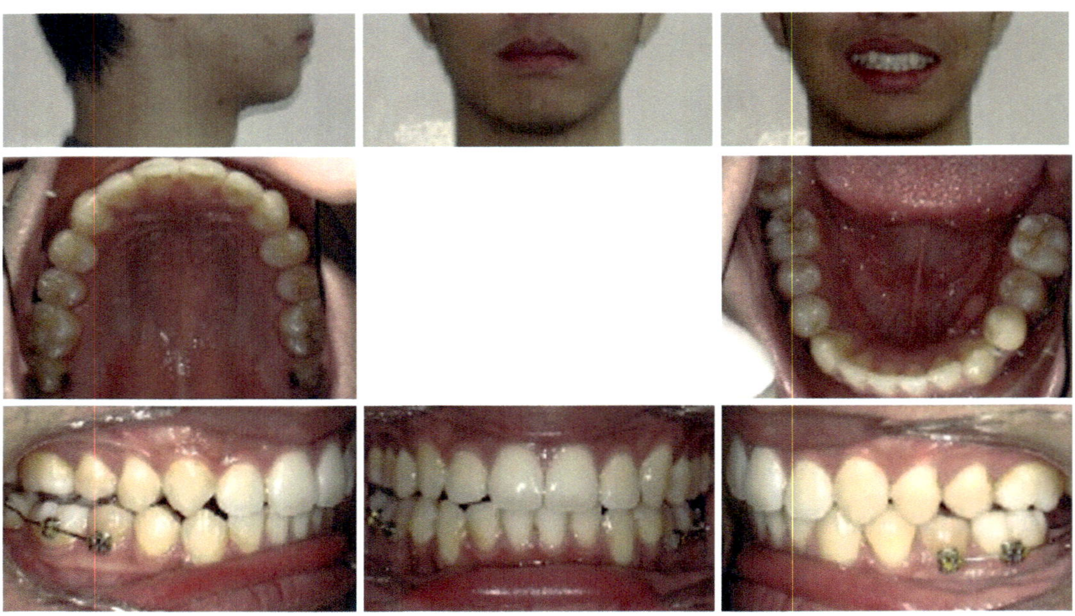

Fig. 4.14 Partial fixed appliances can be combined with clear aligners for complex uprighting movements. In this case, braces were bonded on the second mandibular premolars, mandibular first molars, and mandibular second molars to upright the impacted second molars. Vertical elastics were also worn from lingual buttons on the maxillary second molars to the mandibular second molars to supplement uprighting

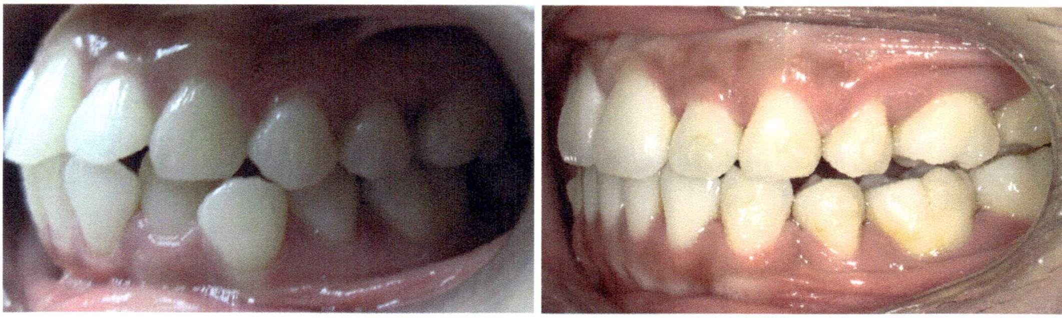

Fig. 4.15 Patient C. Y. was treated with a four first premolars extraction pattern to decrowd maxillary and mandibular arches and reduce their bimaxillary protrusion. After the initial course of aligners, both maxillary and mandibular posterior teeth adjacent to extraction spaces tipped greater than the amount programmed. These premolars and molars will have to be uprighted either with auxiliaries or an additional course of refinement

Similarly, in the treatment of Class II division II malocclusions, inadequately torqued maxillary incisors can result in mesio-occlusion [18]. The incorporation of power ridges has been shown to increase the predictability of incisor torque and therefore would be beneficial in the uprighting of retroclined maxillary incisors [19]. Conversely, the uprighting of proclined maxillary incisors is also critical for successful management of Class II division I malocclusions. The clinician should be cautious not to over-retract the maxillary incisors. Torque can be controlled with the judicious incorporation of power ridges, avoiding overuse of Class II elastics, and sound planning for the degree of incisor retraction.

Simplifying Complex Movements

The control of maxillary lateral incisors and tooth uprighting remain challenges for clear aligner therapy. Recent clinical trials show that they remain problematic despite the technological improvements of the last decade. Both movements consistently show low accuracy compared to simulated outcomes, relative to movements such as lingual tipping.

The clinician can more predictably plan for successful outcomes in these movements through the judicious use of attachments, the incorporation of compensatory mechanics, such as over-engineering and virtual gable bends, and supplementation with auxiliaries in the form of partial fixed appliances, TADs, and elastics. The positioning of maxillary lateral incisors for optimal esthetics and function also depends on a variety of factors, such as tooth size discrepancy, tooth shape, and gingival architecture, which should be considered in the treatment planning phase and Clincheck development.

Tooth uprighting is not only limited to tipped premolars and molars adjacent to edentulous spaces but also to retroclined maxillary incisors, mesially tipped canines, and teeth that have tipped as a result of extraction therapy. The uprighting of tipped canines and lingually inclined maxillary incisors allows for sagittal correction of Class II occlusal relationships and is a cornerstone for the successful treatment of Class II malocclusions.

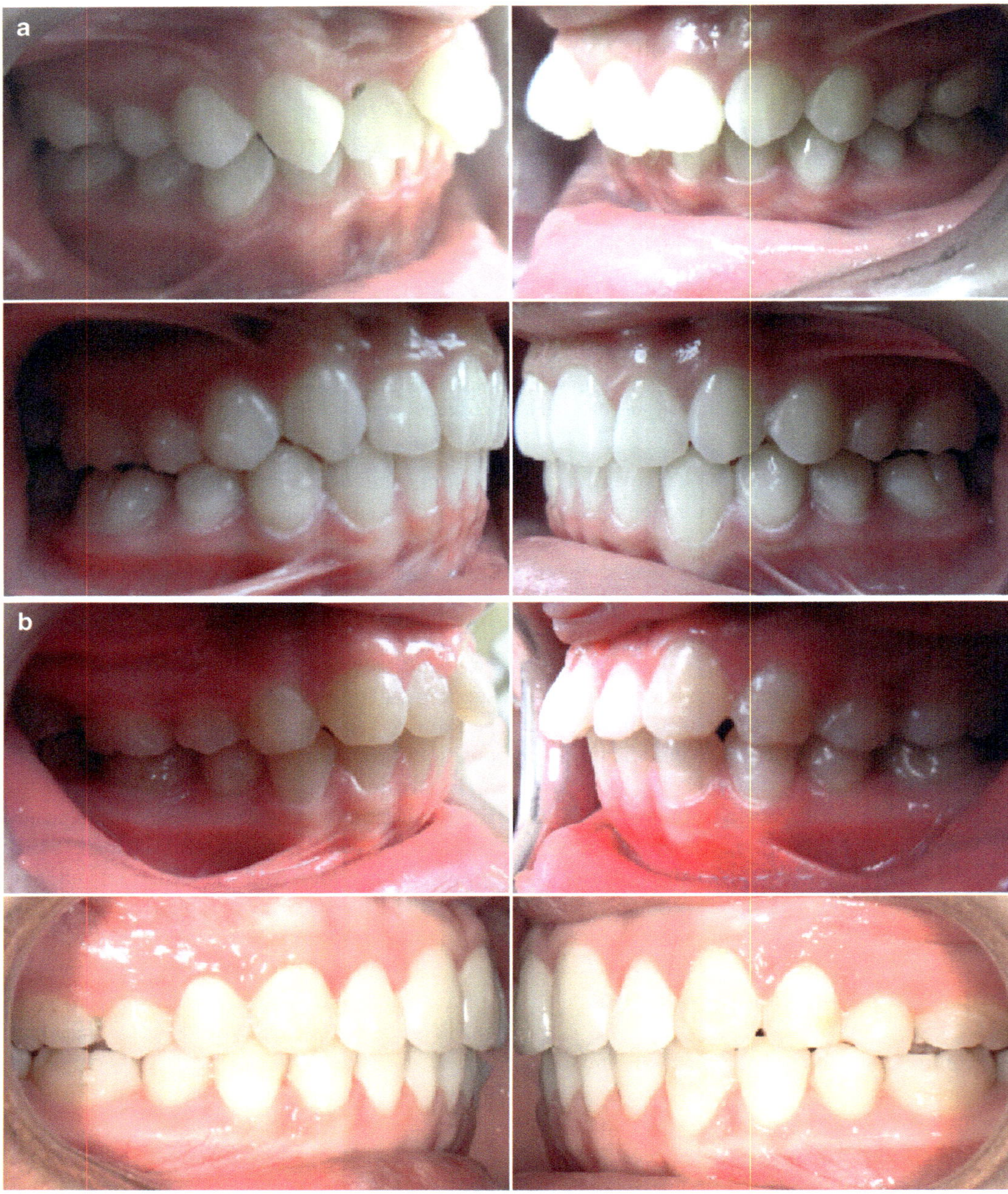

Fig. 4.16 (**a**, **b**) The two cases above demonstrate the uprighting of the maxillary left and right canines allows for uprighting of the posterior teeth. The achievement of proper crown angulations of the maxillary canines is critical for correcting the Class II relationships in the posterior occlusion

References

1. Kravitz ND, Kusnoto B, BeGole E, Obrez A, Agran B. How well does Invisalign work? A prospective clinical study evaluating the efficacy of tooth movement with Invisalign. Am J Orthod Dentofac Orthop. 2009;135(1):27–35.
2. Haouili N, Kravitz ND, Vaid NR, Ferguson DJ, Makki L. Has Invisalign improved? A prospective follow-up study on the efficacy of tooth movement with Invisalign. Am J Orthod Dentofac Orthop. 2020;158(3):420–5.
3. Papadimitriou A, Mousoulea S, Gkantidis N, Kloukos D. Clinical effectiveness of Invisalign® orthodontic treatment: a systematic review. Prog Orthod. 2018;19(1):37.
4. Dai FF, Xu TM, Shu G. Comparison of achieved and predicted tooth movement of maxillary first molars and central incisors: first premolar extraction treatment with Invisalign. Angle Orthod. 2019;89(5):679–87.
5. Krieger E, Seiferth J, Marinello I, Jung BA, Wriedt S, Jacobs C, et al. Invisalign® treatment in the anterior region were the predicted tooth movements achieved? J Orofac Orthop. 2012;73(5):365–76.
6. Bowman SJ, Celenza F, Sparaga J, Papadopoulos MA, Ojima K, Lin JC. Creative adjuncts for clear aligners, part 3: extraction and interdisciplinary treatment. J Clin Orthod. 2015;49(4):249–62.
7. Djeu G, Shelton C, Maganzini A. Outcome assessment of Invisalign and traditional orthodontic treatment compared with the American Board of Orthodontics objective grading system. Am J Orthod Dentofac Orthop. 2005;128:292–8.
8. Align Technology. https://investor.aligntech.com (2020). Accessed 12 Feb 2021.
9. Kravitz ND, Kusnoto B, Agran B, Viana G. Influence of attachments and interproximal reduction on the accuracy of canine rotation with Invisalign. A prospective clinical study. Angle Orthod. 2008;78:682–7.
10. Hua F, He H, Ngan P, Bouzid W. Prevalence of peg-shaped maxillary permanent lateral incisors: a meta-analysis. Am J Orthod Dentofac Orthop. 2013;144(1):97–109.
11. Norris RA, Brandt DJ, Crawford CH, Fallah M. Restorative and Invisalign: a new approach. J Esthet Restor Dent. 2002;14(4):217–24.
12. Profitt WR, Fields HW, Sarver DM. Contemporary orthodontics. 5th ed. St. Louis: Elsevier; 2013. p. 455.
13. Kokich VO Jr, Kinzer GA. Managing congenitally missing lateral incisors. Part I: canine substitution. J Esthet Restor Dent. 2005;17(1):5–10.
14. Pavoni C, Lione R, Laganà PC. Self-ligating versus Invisalign: analysis of dento-alveolar effects. Ann Stomatol (Roma). 2011;2(1–2):23–7.
15. Dickerson TE. Invisalign with Photobiomodulation: optimizing tooth movement and treatment efficacy with a novel self-assessment algorithm. J Clin Orthod. 2017;51(3):157–65.
16. Cortona A, Rossini G, Parrini S, Deregibus A, Castroflorio T. Clear aligner orthodontic therapy of rotated mandibular round-shaped teeth: a finite element study. Angle Orthod. 2020;90(2):247–54.
17. Profitt WR, Fields HW, Sarver DM. Contemporary orthodontics. 5th ed. St. Louis: Elsevier; 2013. p. 295.
18. Andrews LF. The six keys to normal occlusion. Am J Orthod. 1972;62(3):296–309.
19. Simon M, Keilig L, Schwarze J, Jung BA, Bourauel C. Treatment outcome and efficacy of an aligner technique--regarding incisor torque, premolar derotation and molar distalization. BMC Oral Health. 2014;14:68. Published 2014 Jun 11. https://doi.org/10.1186/1472-6831-14-68.

Interproximal Reduction

5

Contents

Interproximal Reduction and Clear Aligner Therapy

Interproximal reduction (IPR) has become an essential method of space creation and arch development in clear aligner therapy. IPR encompasses the reduction and anatomical recontouring of enamel within the interproximal regions of adjacent teeth. It was first employed as a space-gaining procedure by Ballard, who used interproximal reduction for decrowding anterior teeth in 1944 [1]. The method was further developed by practitioners such as Hudson, Paskow, Jack Sheridan with his air-rotor stripping technique, Don Tuverson, and Bjorn Zachrisson, who recommended flexible diamond discs [2]. In contemporary orthodontic practice, the techniques for IPR have evolved to include the use of manual perforated metal strips, IPR burs, rotating discs, and reciprocating strips mounted on a contra-angle handpiece.

IPR was first employed as a means for the resolution of minor anterior dental crowding, but its use has been expanded to a variety of applications. It is now considered a viable alternative to extraction therapy, as the clinician can calculate the removal of tooth structure to generate the specific amount of space necessary for decrowding a dental arch [3]. IPR also functions as an important tool in the correction of interocclusal discrepancies in Class II and Class III malocclusions. It can diminish the effects of Bolton tooth size discrepancies in both the anterior region and full arches [4]. Asymmetric IPR can contribute to the resolution of midline deviations. IPR can also normalize proclined incisors, while in other cases, it can resolve dental crowding while maintaining desirable incisor inclinations and the intercanine distance within dental arches. The method has been shown to reduce the appearance of black triangles by broadening the contact areas

A. T. Huang, D. Huang, *Controversies in Clear Aligner Therapy*,
https://doi.org/10.1007/978-3-030-92810-0_5

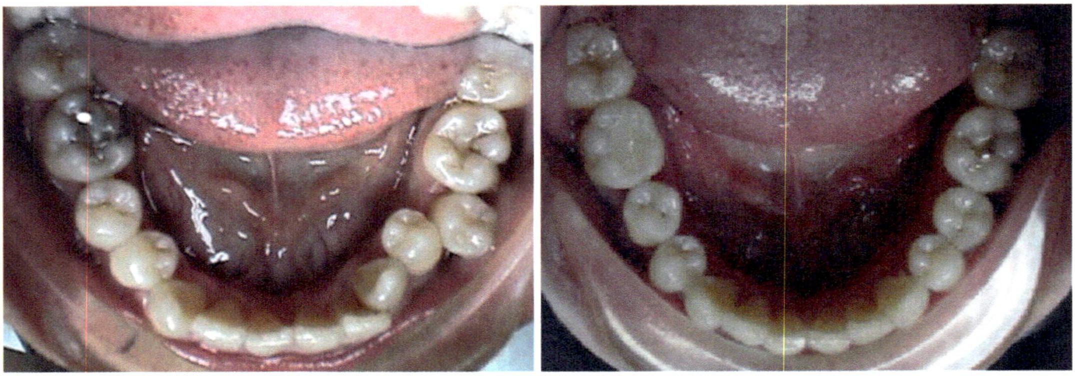

Fig. 5.1 In borderline extraction cases, carefully planned IPR can resolve severe crowding while minimizing undesired expansion of the mandibular intercanine width and maintaining normal mandibular incisor inclinations

and moving them gingivally to minimize gingival embrasures.

The judicious planning of IPR is critical for successful outcomes in clear aligner therapy. The adequate incorporation of IPR is essential for achieving difficult movements, such as canine derotation, predictable treatment of Class II and Class III discrepancies, and decrowding in non-extraction cases, particularly those that lie in the borderline between extraction and non-extraction.

The precise execution of the planned IPR is also essential for sequential fitting of the aligners and the achievement of projected tooth movements [3]. Studies have shown that proper instrumentation and technique are important to performing precise IPR, as well as minimizing unnecessary round tripping of the teeth and adverse sequelae, including root resorption.

In this chapter, we discuss the indications of IPR in the context of clear aligner therapy, ranging from decrowding dental arches to the correction of sagittal discrepancies to midline coordination. Afterwards, we elaborate on techniques for performing precise IPR and conclude this chapter with considerations when planning IPR in the treatment of both simple and complex malocclusions.

The Indications of IPR

Decrowding

One of the primary indications of IPR is the resolution of crowding. In non-extraction cases, the judicious planning of IPR reduces the amount of buccal expansion and proclination of the incisors needed for decrowding a dental arch and therefore diminishes the risk of periodontal problems and stability issues associated with these movements [5]. Current software setups, whether from Invisalign, 3M, Suresmile, or U-Lab, allow the clinician to determine at which site to perform the IPR, the amount of reduction, and the timing of the IPR during the course of treatment [6].

The incorporation of IPR can also reduce the likelihood of extraction therapy, particularly in borderline cases (Fig. 5.1). Arches requiring greater than 8 mm of space would be a contraindication for IPR [2]. In borderline cases, the clinician can digitally simulate extraction and non-extraction treatment plans for comparison prior to committing to a course of therapy.

Treatment of Class II and Class III Malocclusions

One of the modalities for the treatment of Class II malocclusions is the distalization of the upper arch. Rossini et al. have shown that maxillary molar distalization was highly predictable with an 88% accuracy when distalization of 1.5 mm was prescribed (though these results have recently been disputed by a 2021 study on the efficacy of Class II malocclusion correction with clear aligner therapy) [7, 8].The selective incorporation of IPR can improve the predictability of Class II correction by supplementing the distalizing movement, especially when the forecasted translation is not achieved during treatment. Specifically, in a patient where distalization is indicated, the clinician can plan for 0.5 mm of IPR in the posterior segments (distal to the maxillary canines) and 0.3 mm of IPR between the anterior teeth (extending from the mesial contact of the maxillary canine to the contralateral mesial contact of the maxillary canine). This protocol is in accordance with clinical recommendations that have suggested reduction of enamel to a maximum of 0.3 mm per contact point for maxillary incisors, 0.2 mm for mandibular incisors, and 0.6 mm for premolars and molars [2]. This procedure generates a cumulative 4.5 mm from the IPR and 1–2 mm of maxillary distalization on each side for the correction of overjet and Class II sagittal relationships (Fig. 5.2).

In certain cases, significant distalization is necessary, such as translations of greater than

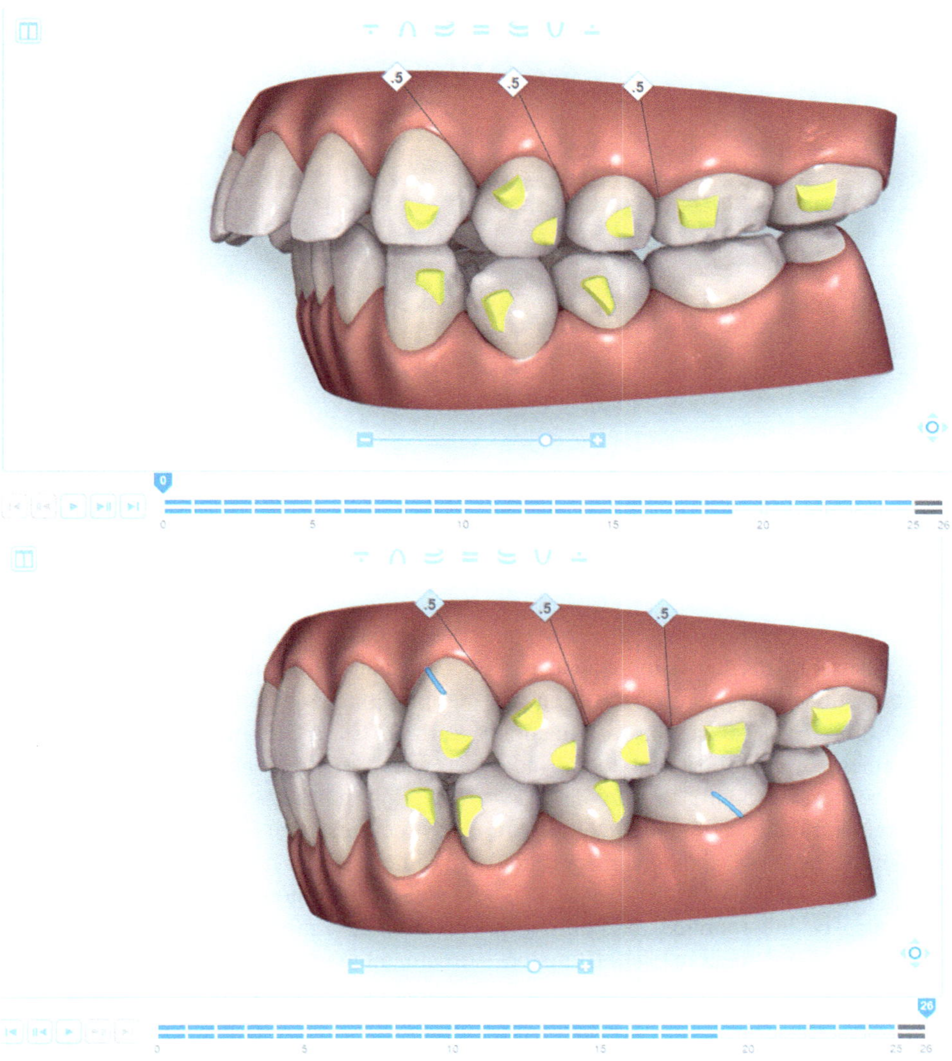

Fig. 5.2 About 1–2 mm of distalization was planned for the left maxillary premolars and left maxillary molars. 0.5 mm of IPR was performed for the interproximal contacts between the left maxillary canine and left maxillary first premolar, left maxillary first and second premolars, and left maxillary second premolar and left first molar. This protocol allowed for the correction of the left canine relationship to Class I, normalization of the maxillary incisors, and the idealization of the overjet

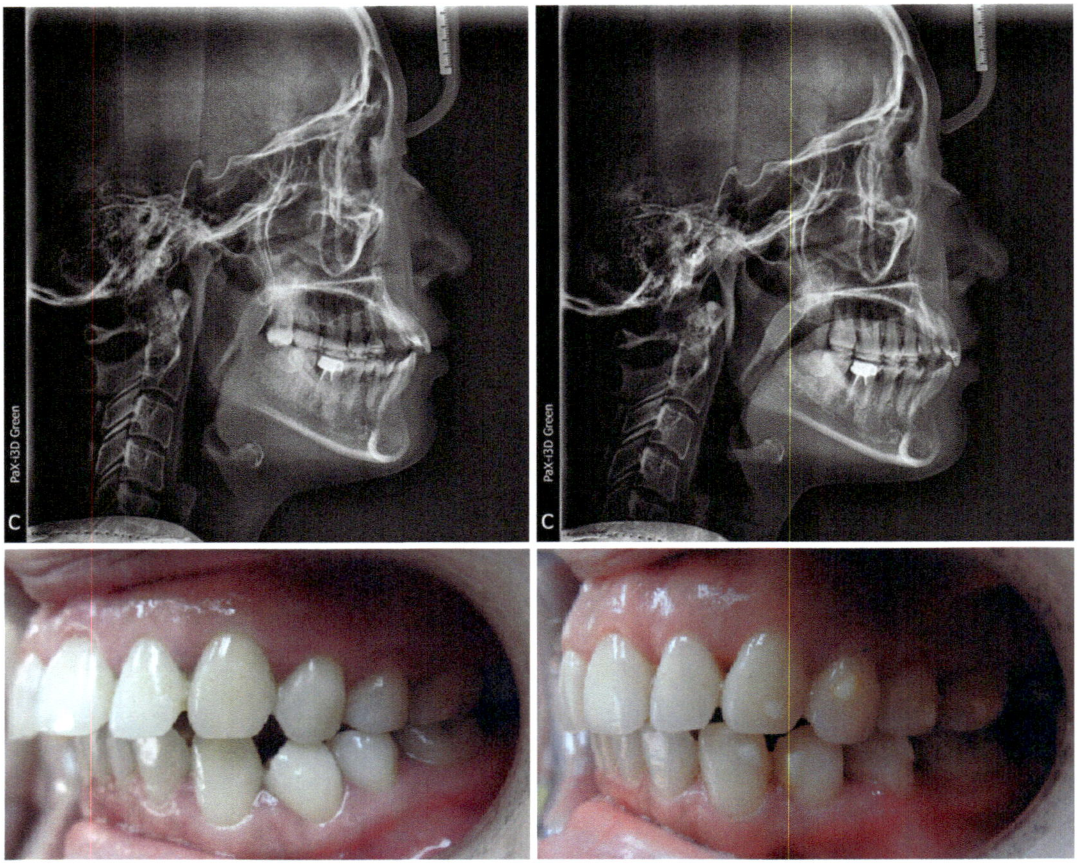

Fig. 5.3 This case was treated with a combination of segmental distalization and posterior IPR to correct the increased overjet and the end-on Class II molar and canine relationships. The treatment duration was 13 months

2 mm. In treatment planning these movements, aggressive posterior IPR can supplement segmental distalization (movement of the segment collectively) in place of sequential distalization (distal movement of each posterior tooth, individually). The former approach can decrease treatment time and increase the predictability of the distal movement of the maxillary arch (Fig. 5.3).

IPR can also be incorporated for improving the predictability of treatment in Class III malocclusions. In cases where non-extraction is indicated, IPR can be employed to supplement retraction of the mandibular premolars and the anterior teeth. For Class III malocclusions of mild to moderate severity, the clinician can adjust according to space required by an IPR protocol of 0.2 mm between the mandibular anterior teeth (extending from the mesial contact of the mandibular canine to the contralateral mesial contact of the mandibular canine) and 0.5 mm in the posterior segments (distal to the mandibular canines). Certain Class III malocclusions with severe crowding or more severe skeletal discrepancies receiving nonsurgical compensatory treatment may require extraction therapy in addition to IPR to achieve successful outcomes. For example, for a patient with moderate mandibular crowding in addition to a moderate reverse overjet, a viable treatment may be the extraction of a crowded out mandibular incisor and maxillary IPR for decrowding and achievement of ideal overjet (Fig. 5.4). Orthodontic camouflage of Class III malocclusions is more likely to be successful in adult patients with an average or short facial pattern, mild sagittal jaw discrepancy, crowding <4–6 mm, normal soft tissue features, and no transverse skeletal discrepancy [9].

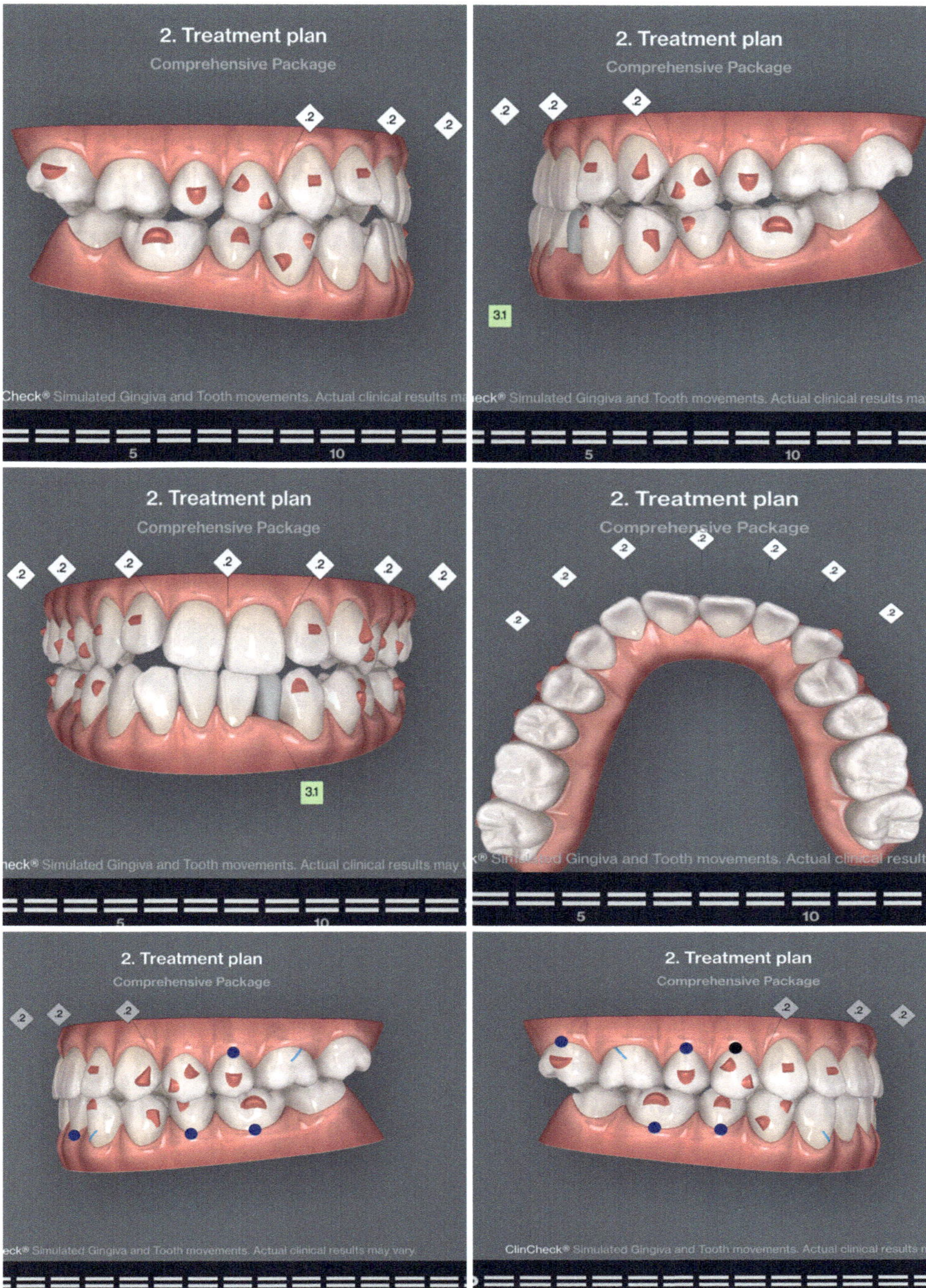

Fig. 5.4 In patients with Class III malocclusions of mild to moderate severity, mandibular crowding, and reverse overjet, the extraction of one mandibular incisor can be combined with maxillary IPR for decrowding of the maxillary and mandibular arches. The maxillary IPR will allow for retraction of the maxillary incisors for the achievement of ideal overjet

Tooth Size Discrepancies

Studies have demonstrated that 20–30% of studied populations present with anterior Bolton discrepancies, while 5–14% of sample populations demonstrate full arch discrepancies [10]. IPR can address Bolton discrepancies, through the removal of enamel in either the maxillary or mandibular arches to compensate for maxillary or mandibular excess, respectively (Fig. 5.5). As previously discussed, the Bolton index can be instantly obtained in the

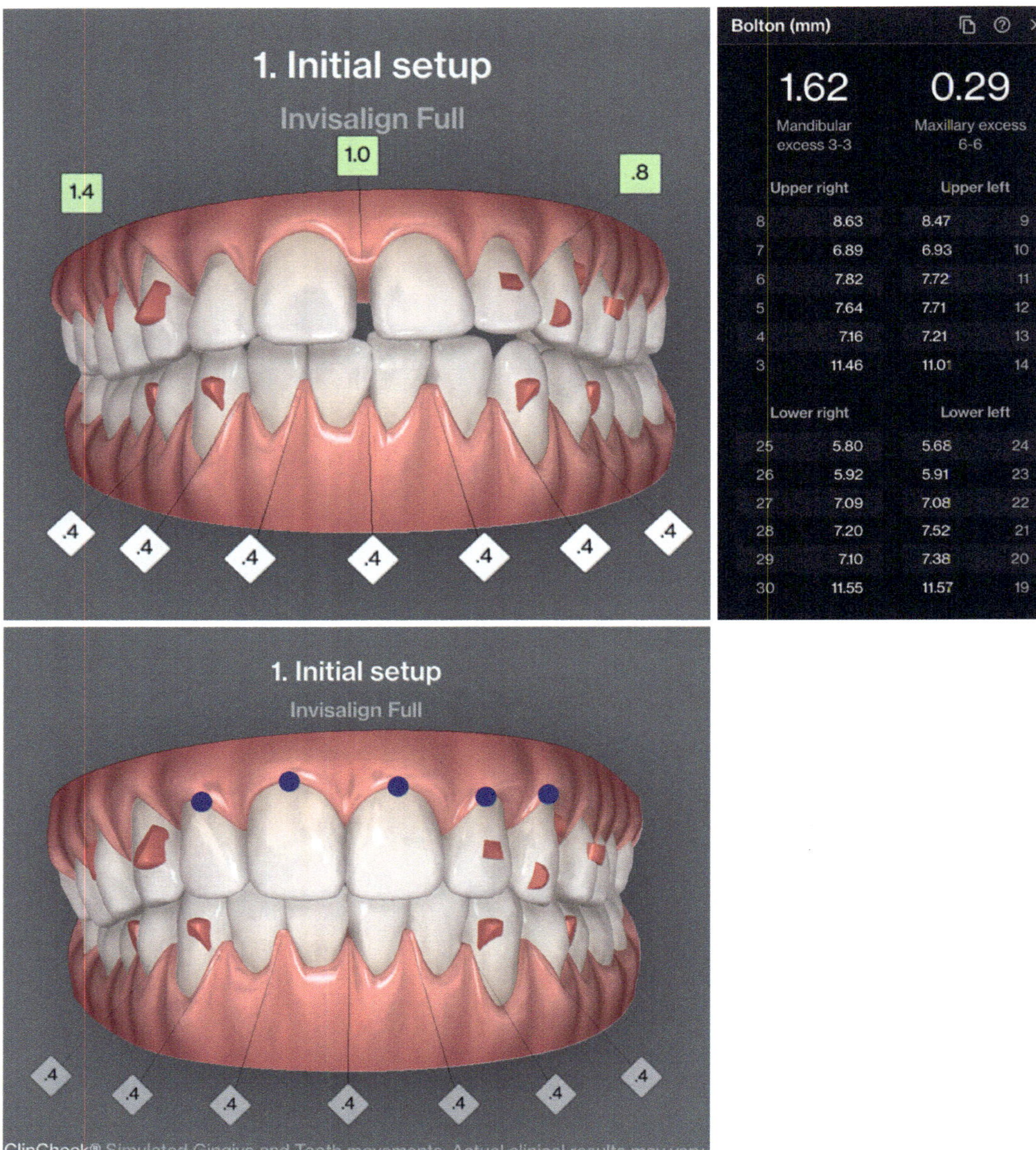

Fig. 5.5 In Patient H. Z., a Bolton maxillary deficiency was addressed with mandibular IPR. Adequate mandibular IPR allowed for decrowding of the mandibular arch, closure of existing maxillary spaces through retraction of the mandibular incisors, and the creation of ideal overjet

Clincheck setup or through most types of cast analysis software. In cases where anterior teeth are abnormally large (macrodontia), the clinician may consider more aggressive IPR to reduce the size discrepancy between the maxillary and mandibular anterior regions and to achieve more ideal overjet and overbite [2].

Incisor Uprighting

IPR is critical for normalizing the inclination of proclined incisors, whether in Class II division 1 malocclusions or cases of bimaxillary protrusion. The normalization can be achieved with an IPR protocol similar to that employed for Class II correction through maxillary arch distalization. For either maxillary or mandibular incisors, the clinician can perform 0.3 mm of IPR per contact in the anterior region and incorporate additional 0.5 mm per contact of posterior IPR, as necessary for incisor retraction. The uprighting of incisors can be supplemented by intermaxillary elastics (Class II elastics for uprighting the maxillary incisors and Class III elastics for uprighting the mandibular incisors). Clear aligners tend to perform buccal-lingual tipping with high accuracy relative to other movements [11]. However, it is important for the clinician to avoid over-retraction of incisors by avoiding excessive IPR and regularly monitoring the use of intermaxillary elastics.

Midline Coordination

Mild midline discrepancies can be resolved with asymmetric IPR on the side toward which the deviated midline must be translated (Fig. 5.6). This translation can be supplemented with asymmetric intermaxillary elastics, a method that has been effectively employed with fixed appliances in nonsurgical treatments of mild asymmetries [12]. Precision cuts can be incorporated on the aligner for either unilateral Class II or Class III elastics or cross-midline elastics.

Gingival Black Triangles

Studies have shown there are multiple factors that comprise the etiology of black triangles, including the interproximal space between teeth, the distance between the bone crest and the contact point between two adjacent teeth, gingival biotype, patient age, periodontal disease, root divergence, and tooth morphology [13]. Orthodontic therapy has been demonstrated to reduce gingival black triangles through a number of applications. Orthodontic movement can close interdental contacts, reduce the distance between the contact point and the crest of bone, and reduce the likelihood of a black triangle. Paralleling converging roots has also been shown to be beneficial in restoring the interdental papillae [14]. IPR can reduce gingival black triangles by reshaping the

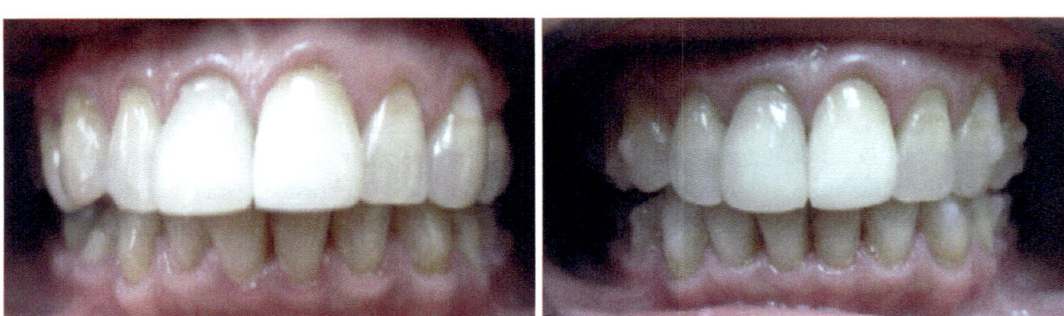

Fig. 5.6 Asymmetric IPR can accurately correct midline discrepancies. In the above case, asymmetric IPR in the mandibular left quadrant allowed for the translation of the mandibular midline to the left. Maxillary IPR also allowed for normalization of the maxillary incisors and overjet

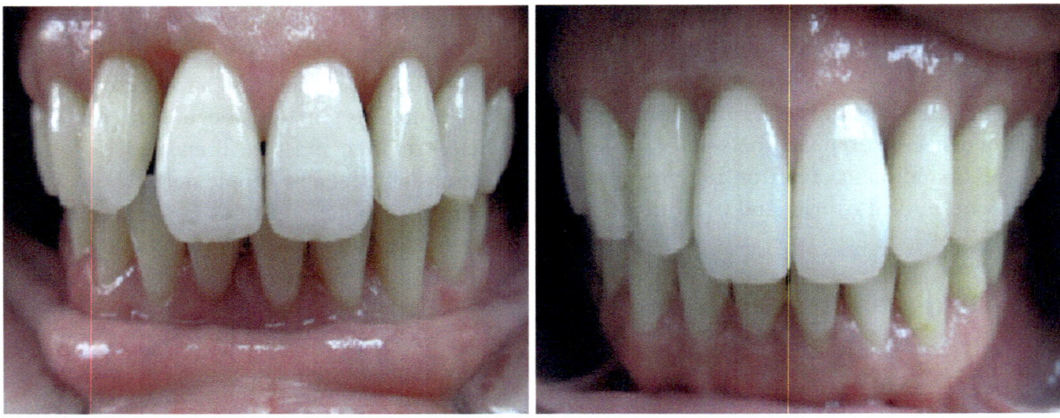

Fig. 5.7 In this case, mandibular anterior IPR was performed to create wider interdental contacts, which allowed for repositioning of contacts more gingivally. This approach can minimize the appearance of gingival black triangles

proximal enamel for broader interdental contacts and repositioning the contact more gingivally (Fig. 5.7).

Retention

There is some evidence that suggests IPR as a means to enhance retention and stability following orthodontic treatment [15]. The improvement in stability may be associated with the broadening of contact point areas and reduction in the amounts of buccal expansion.

IPR Technique

The accurate execution of the planned IPR is critical for achieving desired tooth movements and successful clinical outcomes. Recent studies on the use of IPR in clear aligner therapy suggest that the amount of IPR performed frequently did not correspond to the amount programmed [5]. In most cases, the amount of enamel removed was less than that planned [5]. A recent study on this issue found that there was a greater discrepancy between planned and performed IPR for distal surfaces compared to that of mesial surfaces, while among individual teeth, the mandibular canines showed the greatest discrepancy between planned and performed IPR [16]. The latter discrepancy was attributed by the authors to the tendency of canines to be frequently in difficult to access positions, either in labioversion, distal rotation, or within tight contact areas.

The accuracy of performed IPR is multifactorial, associated with tooth-related factors, such as enamel hardness, tooth morphology, and tooth position, as well as operator-related factors, such as technique employed, the pressure exerted during the procedure, the hardness and particle size of the abrasive, the time taken for the procedure, clinician experience, and accuracy of the space analysis [17]. In particular, studies have suggested the type of technique can influence the accuracy of IPR [16]. At present, there are four common methods of performing IPR [1]:

1. The air-rotor stripping method with tungsten-carbide burs or diamond burs.
2. The air-rotor stripping method with diamond coated strips (Ortho-strips), usually mounted with a handpiece.
3. Diamond-coated disks mounted with a handpiece or contra-angle.
4. Handheld abrasive metal strips used manually.

Research has shown handheld abrasive metal strips (method 4) can be laborious, impractical, and time-consuming, especially for contact points between the posterior teeth. Recent studies have suggested that the discrepancy between performed IPR and predicted IPR was greater for the manual strips technique when compared to that of either burs or handpiece-operated diamond-coated strips [16]. This result may be attributed to the laboriousness of the manual method. Also, the forcing of the abrasive strips into interproximal regions can displace teeth temporarily into periodontal spaces leading to the overestimation of the amount of enamel removed.

The use of burs has gained widespread acceptance because of their advantages of greater precision and painlessness. Burs do have the disadvantage of leaving rough interproximal surfaces after enamel reduction. These surfaces can be subsequently polished with either the handheld abrasive strip or a thin diamond-coated strip. Diamond discs, when operated on a handpiece, can be dangerous intraorally because of their proximity and risk to the patient's lips and cheeks. Discs can also be unpredictable in their removal of enamel. They have the capability of creating ledges, as well as deep cuts into the enamel, resulting in possible complications, such as increased plaque retention, caries risk, and risk of periodontal disease.

Accurate and safe IPR can be achieved through the use of the Ortho-strips in a sequential fashion for anterior segments and the air-rotor stripping method with burs in posterior segments. For an anterior interproximal area, the contact can be broken with a 0.1 mm thick Ortho-strip. Subsequently, the clinician can sequentially remove enamel with a 0.2 mm thick strip, a 0.3 mm strip, until the desired amount has been achieved. In the posterior segment, a 0.5 mm diamond bur can be used for accurate enamel reduction. For both anterior and posterior contacts, a finishing Ortho-strip can be used for smoothing rough interproximal surfaces. Also, an IPR gauge should be used to verify the amount of enamel removed in each site. Naturally, it is less detrimental to perform less IPR than prescribed compared to more than prescribed because if additional IPR is needed, it can be prescribed in a refinement stage. The gauge has been shown to control the amount of IPR performed and improve accuracy (Fig. 5.8). Bitewing radiographs can be taken following IPR to assess for ledges or areas of significant roughness. Lastly, the clinician should provide a type of fluoride treatment after performing IPR, whether in the form of varnish, mouthwash, or solution, such as Gel-Kam, all of which can function as a barrier against the demineralization of reduced enamel [18].

Considerations when Planning IPR

Round Tripping and IPR

A common method of incorporating IPR into a clear aligner treatment plan is programming additional movements and aligners primarily to improve accessibility to obstructed contact areas. In such cases, these additional movements constitute round tripping because they have to be reversed later on in treatment. A recent study showed that though round tripping slightly improved the accuracy of IPR compared to accuracy with lack of round tripping, the difference was not statistically significant [16]. Round tripping can lead to increased treatment times and unnecessary additional movements, increasing the risk for root resorption. It is prudent that the clinician minimize round tripping merely for the sake of performing more accurate IPR. The use of diamond burs and Ortho-strips, which afford a degree of flexibility, more readily allow for enamel reduction in obstructed areas and the minimization of round tripping for the sake of IPR. A viable alternative to round tripping is the use of separators for extremely tight or overlapped contacts prior to IPR, which was advocated by early users of IPR, such as Bjorn Zachrisson [19]. The clinician can place a separator into the tight interproximal space 1–2 weeks prior to the IPR appointment for increased accessibility and greater accuracy.

Timing of IPR

The visit in which the clinician performs the IPR should be considered one of the most critical during the course of treatment because it is a significant factor in the accuracy of the planned tooth movements and the sequential fitting of the aligners. Ideally, all of the IPR should be planned on a

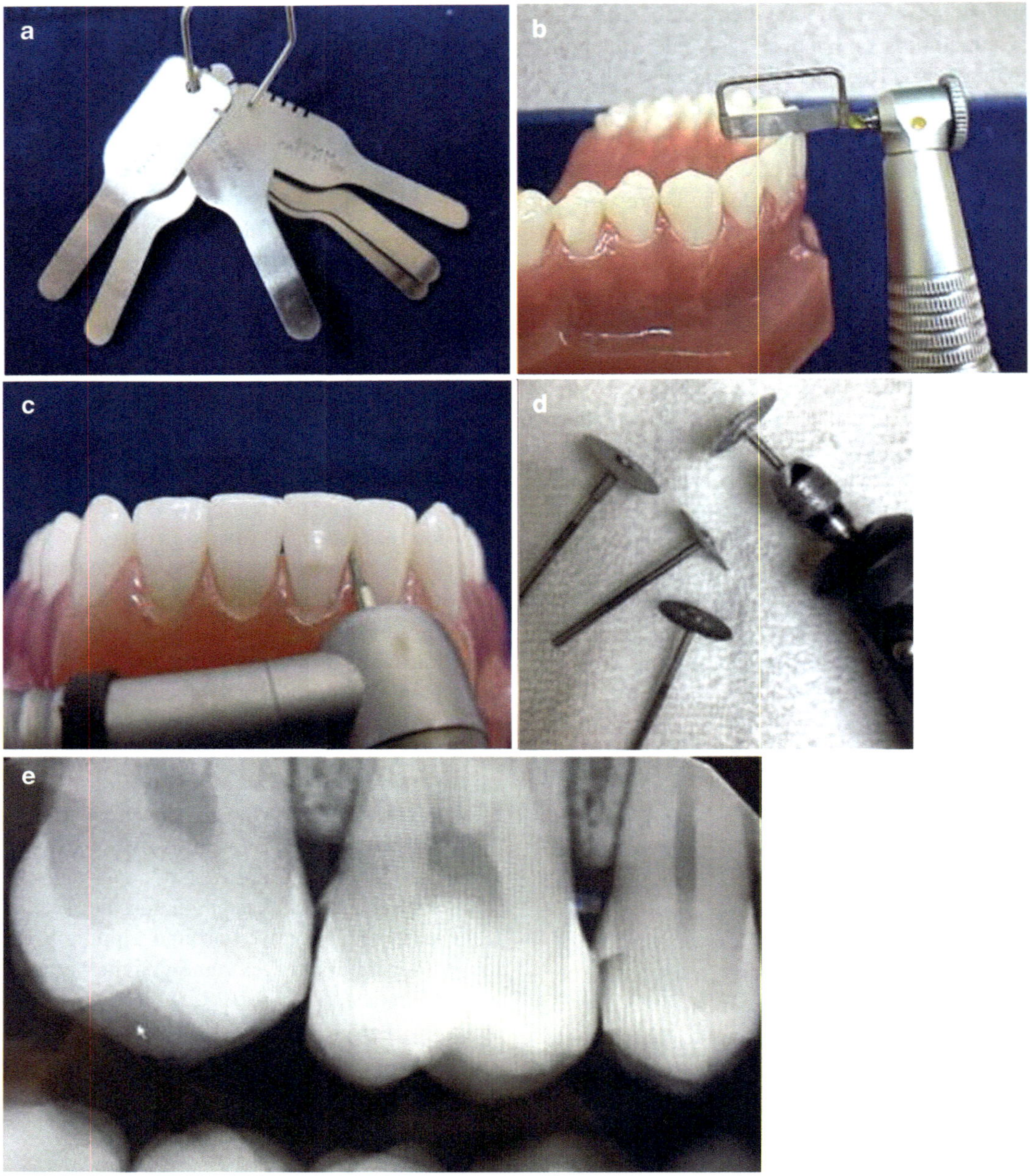

Fig. 5.8 (**a**) IPR gauges can be used to verify that the desired amount of IPR has been achieved. Their use has been shown to improve the accuracy of IPR. (**b**) Ortho-strips mounted on a contra-angle low-speed handpiece allow for precise IPR in both anterior and posterior segments. The strips range from 0.1 mm-0.5 mm in thickness. (**c**) For 0.5 mm IPR in both anterior and posterior segments, a 0.5 mm diamond bur can remove the desired amount of enamel, even in severely crowded segments. The resulting interproximal surfaces can be smoothened either with handheld abrasive metal strips or finishing Ortho-strips. (**d**) Diamond-coated discs can be difficult to operate and risk soft tissue injury to the patient's lips and cheeks. Discs are also prone to creating ledges from improperly angled cuts into the enamel. (**e**) The bitewing radiograph shows ledges were created by inadequately angled cuts with diamond discs during IPR, increasing the patient's risk for periodontal disease and caries

single visit for patient comfort, rather than distributed sporadically over the course of treatment. This can be achieved with a method that allows for access into obstructed areas. The IPR visit should be afforded ample time and be exclusively performed by the clinician, rather than by any dental auxiliaries such as hygienists or orthodontic assistants.

Long Term Consequences of IPR

Some clinicians have expressed concerns over potential damage to the periodontium as a sequelae of IPR. Specifically, Vanarsdall Jr., based on monkey studies, recommended IPR should be avoided in patients with normal attachment, especially in the posterior segments [20]. Vanarsdall Jr. claimed that IPR could lead to loss of attachment, intercrestal bone loss, and poor root proximity. However, a number of studies have contradicted these claims. Notably, researchers observed no deterioration in the periodontium 10 years following IPR [21]. Recent studies have also shown a slight increase in interradicular bone volume following clear aligner therapy and IPR in patients at high risk for periodontal disease (though this increase occurred independently of whether IPR was performed) [22].

There have also been concerns over a possible relationship between increased caries risk and IPR, especially in sites that have been reduced. The current literature suggests that the risk of caries is not affected by IPR [23]. Another review concluded that the incidence of caries on abraded surfaces treated with IPR was statistically the same as that on intact surfaces [24].

Reflections on IPR in Clear Aligner Therapy

We have observed that the amount of IPR performed is significantly greater in clear aligner therapy than fixed appliances (though it is frequently employed in fixed appliances), primarily as a means to compensate for less predictability with distalization and extraction therapy in clear aligners. Nevertheless, clinicians should incorporate IPR with the same pragmatic mindset toward its use in treatment planning, regardless of the appliance. That is, IPR should be planned judiciously and safely, within the limits of healthy amounts of enamel removal and biological tooth movement, and should not be an indication for unnecessary tooth movement and round tripping.

References

1. Rao V, George AM, Sahu SK, Krishnaswamy NR. Surface roughness evaluation of enamel after various stripping methods by using profilometer. Arch Oral Sci Res. 2011;1:190–7.
2. Lapenaite E, Lopatiene K. Interproximal enamel reduction as a part of orthodontic treatment. Stomatologija. 2014;16(1):19–24.
3. Kalemaj Z, Levrini L. Quantitative evaluation of implemented interproximal enamel reduction during aligner therapy: a prospective observational study. Angle Orthod. 2021;91(1):61–6.
4. Pindoria J, Fleming PS, Sharma PK. Inter-proximal enamel. Br Dent J. 2016;221(12):757–63.
5. De Felice ME, Nucci L, Fiori A, Flores-Mir C, Perillo L, Grassia V. Accuracy of interproximal enamel reduction during clear aligner treatment. Prog Orthod. 2020;21(1):28.
6. Kravitz ND, Kusnoto B, BeGole E, Obrez A, Agran B. How well does Invisalign work? A prospective clinical study evaluating the efficacy of tooth movement with Invisalign. Am J Orthod Dentofac Orthop. 2009;135(1):27–35.
7. Rossini G, Parrini S, Castroflorio T, Deregibus A, Debernardi CL. Efficacy of clear aligners in controlling orthodontic tooth movement: a systematic review. Angle Orthod. 2015;15:881–9.
8. Patterson BD, Foley PF, Ueno H, Mason SA, Schneider PP, Kim KB. Class II malocclusion correction with Invisalign: is it possible? Am J Orthod Dentofac Orthop. 2021;159(1):e41–8.
9. Profitt WR, Fields HW, Sarver DM. Contemporary orthodontics. 5th ed. St. Louis: Elsevier; 2013. p. 698.
10. Othman SA, Harradine NW. Tooth-size discrepancy and Bolton's ratios: a literature review. J Orthod. 2006;33(1):45–51.
11. Haouili N, Kravitz ND, Vaid NR, Ferguson DJ, Makki L. Has Invisalign improved? A prospective follow-up study on the efficacy of tooth movement with Invisalign. Am J Orthod Dentofac Orthop. 2020;158(3):420–5.
12. Janson G, de Freitas MR, Araki J, Franco EJ, Barros SE. Class III subdivision malocclusion corrected with

asymmetric intermaxillary elastics. Am J Orthod Dentofac Orthop. 2010;138(2):221–30.
13. Ziahosseini P, Hussain F, Millar BJ. Management of gingival black triangles. Br Dent J. 2014;217(10):559–63.
14. Salama H, Salama M. The role of orthodontic extrusive remodelling in the enhancement of soft and hard tissue profiles before implant placement: a systematic approach to the management of extraction site defects. Int J Periodontics Restorative Dent. 1993;13:312–33.
15. Boese LR. Fiberotomy and reproximation without lower retention, nine years in retrospect: part I. Angle Orthod. 1980;50:88–97.
16. Kalemaj Z, Levrini L. Quantitative evaluation of implemented interproximal enamel reduction during aligner therapy. Angle Orthod. 2021;91(1):61–6.
17. Danesh G, Hellak A, Lippold C, Ziebura T, Schafer E. Enamel surfaces following interproximal reduction with different methods. Angle Orthod. 2007;77(6):1004–10.
18. Vicente A, Ortiz Ruiz AJ, González Paz BM, García López J, Bravo-González LA. Efficacy of fluoride varnishes for preventing enamel demineralization after interproximal enamel reduction. Qualitative and quantitative evaluation. PLoS One. 2017;12(4):e0176389.
19. Tuverson DL. Anterior interocclusal relations. Parts I and II. Am J Orthod. 1980;78:361–93.
20. Bishara SE. An interview with Robert L. Vanarsdall, Jr. World J Orthod. 2004;5:74–6.
21. Zachrisson BU, Nyøygaard L, Mobarak K. Dental health assessed more than 10 years after interproximal enamel reduction of mandibular anterior teeth. Am J Orthod Dentofac Orthop. 2007;131(2):162–9.
22. Hellak A, Schmidt N, Schauseil M, Stein S, Drechsler T, Korbmacher-Steiner HM. Influence on interradicular bone volume of Invisalign treatment for adult crowding with interproximal enamel reduction: a retrospective three-dimensional cone-beam computed tomography study. BMC Oral Health. 2018;18(1):103.
23. Jarjoura K, Gagnon G, Nieberg L. Caries risk after interproximal enamel reduction. Am J Orthod Dentofac Orthop. 2006;130(1):26–30.
24. Koretsi V, Chatzigianni A, Sidiropoulou S. Enamel roughness and incidence of caries after interproximal enamel reduction: a systematic review. Orthod Craniofac Res. 2014;17(1):1–13.

Dilemmas in Bite Opening

6

Contents

The Challenge of Deep Bite Correction

One of the most difficult challenges of clear aligner therapy remains deep bite correction. A 2017 study showed that only 1.5 mm of improvement in overbite could be predictably achieved with clear aligner therapy, which is significantly less than that typically corrected with fixed appliances [1]. Clear aligner therapy's limited capability in bite opening is likely associated with its low accuracy of incisor intrusion and molar extrusion compared to higher accuracy for movements involved in bite closure, such as incisor extrusion and molar intrusion [2]. The control of the vertical dimension can be particularly challenging during extraction therapy, which tends to cause bite deepening. Since its creation, Invisalign has incorporated a number of modifications to address deep bite correction. In 2013, Invisalign introduced its G5 protocol, which included optimized attachments and pressure areas for leveling the Curve of Spee through improved predictability of premolar extrusion and anterior intrusion [3]. Also, the protocol allowed for the addition of bite ramps on the lingual surfaces of maxillary incisors and canines to supplement mandibular incisor intrusion and to disocclude the posterior teeth during bite opening [3]. In late 2020, Invisalign incorporated G8 features, which sought to improve the efficacy of bite opening. Specifically, one of the features targets anterior intrusion with specific contours in the aligners for greater control of force systems and the reduction of unwanted movements [4].

Despite the limitations of the appliance, successful management of the vertical dimension, both during bite closure and bite opening, can be achieved with clear aligner therapy through judicious treatment planning, strategic mechanotherapy during the treatment setup and throughout the course of therapy, and the adequate incorporation of adjuncts such as TADs and intermaxillary elastics. Studies have shown

A. T. Huang, D. Huang, *Controversies in Clear Aligner Therapy*,
https://doi.org/10.1007/978-3-030-92810-0_6

successful outcomes with selective incorporation of the G5 protocol and treatment methods for bite opening such as overengineering the leveling of the Curve of Spee [5]. In this chapter, we discuss the current challenges in controlling the vertical dimension, approaches in treatment planning, and mechanotherapy for the management of mild to severe deep bites.

Factors in Bite Opening

Leveling the Curve of Spee

Like in fixed appliances, the failure of bite opening is often associated with inadequate leveling of the Curve of Spee in either the maxillary, mandibular arch, or both arches. This is attributed to either insufficient intrusion of the anterior teeth, insufficient extrusion in the buccal segments, or a combination. Cephalometric analyses have shown that deep bite correction in clear aligners occurs primarily through the proclination of the mandibular incisors, along with the intrusion of maxillary incisors and the extrusion of mandibular molars [1]. Therefore, it is important that when indicated, these intrusive and extrusive movements are planned for bite opening. In the treatment planning of most deep bite cases, the clinician should confirm that the maxillary and mandibular Curves of Spee have been adequately leveled.

Bite Ramps

Bite ramps were introduced in 2013 as part of Invisalign's G5 protocol and later became available as an option for Invisalign retainers in patients with deep bites (Fig. 6.1). They often have to be prescribed by the clinician during the initial setup for placement on the maxillary central and lateral incisors or all anterior teeth, including the maxillary canines. The G8 modifications incorporated an additional option of the automatic placement of bite ramps when intrusion of the mandibular incisors greater than 1.5 mm has been programmed (Fig. 6.2).

However, one of the weaknesses of bite ramp prescription is the current limitation on the clinician's ability to manipulate both its position and size. At present, in the Invisalign software, once the clinician requests bite ramps, they are automatically placed by the software and cannot be subsequently adjusted. This is problematic because the software frequently places the bite ramps in sites that do not adequately contact the opposing teeth and therefore do not assist in bite

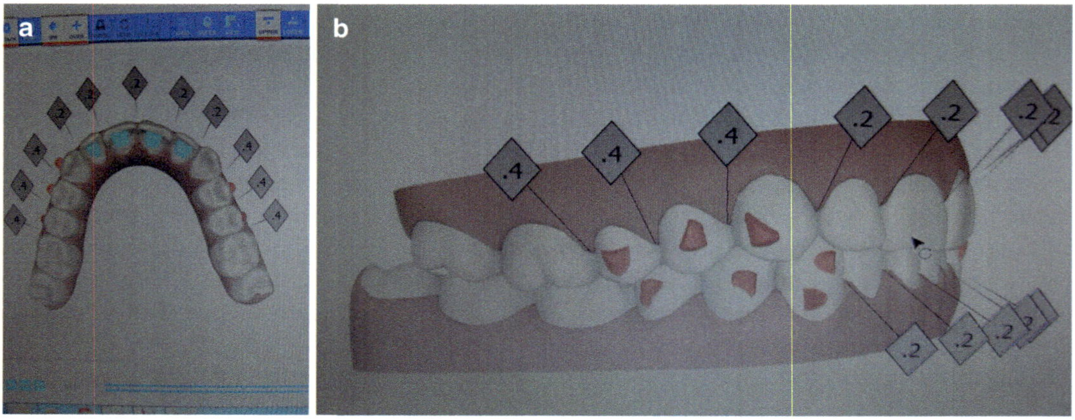

Fig. 6.1 (**a**) The G5 protocol includes the option of bite ramp placement on either the lingual surfaces of the maxillary central and lateral incisors or the lingual surfaces of all maxillary anterior teeth. It also incorporated optimized extrusion attachments for the premolars, as shown on the maxillary right second premolar in (**b**)

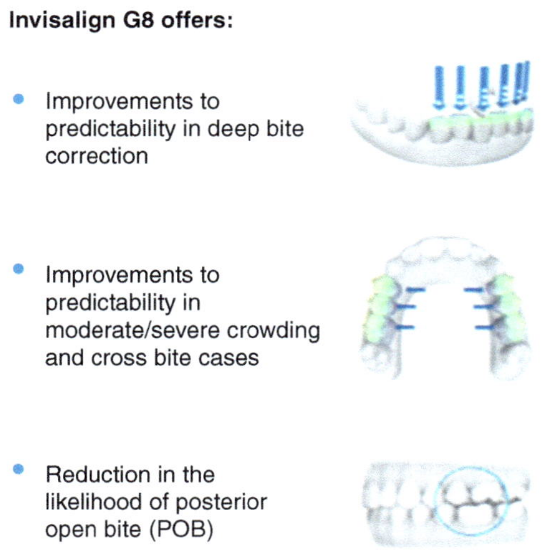

Fig. 6.2 In late 2020, Invisalign introduced the G8 modifications to improve the efficacy of bite opening. When intrusion of the mandibular anterior teeth was programmed to be greater than 1.5 mm, specific aligner contouring would be automatically incorporated to optimize intrusion. The efficacy of these G8 modifications has not been rigorously evaluated in clinical trials

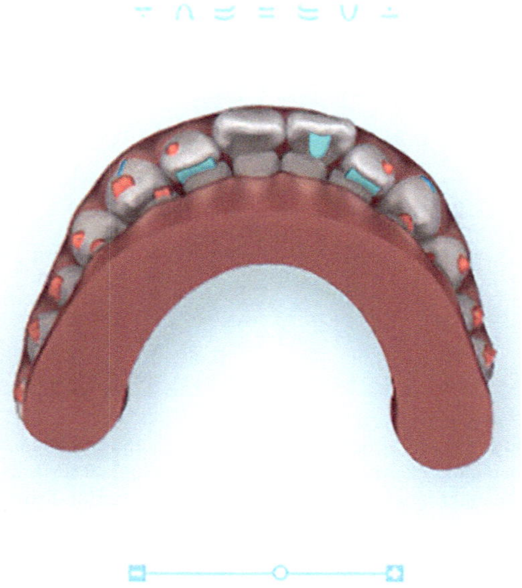

Fig. 6.3 The Invisalign software's default placement of bite ramps may be nonideal, resulting in lack of occlusion with the opposing incisors and poor functionality. Ideally, the clinician should be given free manipulation of bite ramps for proper contact with the opposing incisors and adequate disocclusion of the posterior segments

opening (Fig. 6.3). In other cases, the software delays the placement of the bite ramps due to anatomical limitations. Ideally, the position, size, and timing of the bite ramps should be freely determined by the clinician to optimize the functionality of the bite ramps as early as possible during treatment. Recent studies have shown significant improvement in overbite in deep bite patients with the use of bite ramps and the G5 protocol (though this improvement in overbite was less than that achieved in a group treated with fixed appliances) [5].

Though Invisalign does not permit the free manipulation of bite ramps, the clinician can directly incorporate bite ramps in more ideal positions on the aligner with the use of hand instruments. For example, in severely deep bite cases, the bite ramps on the lingual surfaces of the maxillary incisors and canines may not contact the opposing teeth and be nonfunctional. In these cases, the clinician can manually add bite ramps on the lingual surfaces of the maxillary incisors and canines for contact with the opposing arch to adequately disocclude the posterior segments (Fig. 6.4). Alternatively, certain clear aligner software such as U-Lab allows the clinician the freedom to manipulate bite ramps so that they can be placed on any lingual surface and sized for optimal function during the development of the treatment plan.

G8 Modifications

In late 2020, Invisalign introduced the G8 modifications, which focused on the prevention of posterior open bites and increasing the efficacy of bite opening. In addition to the automatic placement of bite ramps, the aligner in the mandibular anterior teeth would be contoured for the enhancement of intrusion and the control of unwanted movements when mandibular anterior intrusion exceeded 1.5 mm. However, at present, no high-quality studies have been performed on the G8 protocol and its effects on bite opening are still unknown.

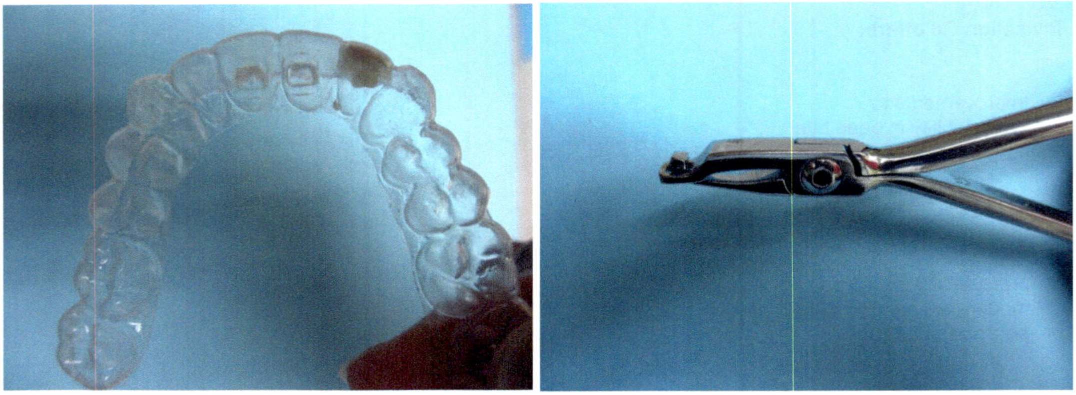

Fig. 6.4 In severely deep bite cases, the clinician can manually incorporate bite ramps on the lingual surfaces of the maxillary teeth for more functional posterior disocclusion. A bite ramp plier can be employed for the placement of a bite ramp in a more ideal location at any time during a course of aligners

Relative Intrusion

Studies have demonstrated that the relative intrusion of the mandibular incisors through proclination constitutes one of the principal mechanics for bite opening [1]. In deep bite cases, it is important to incorporate adequate lingual root torque to upright maxillary or mandibular incisors for relative intrusion and more predictable bite opening. The addition of power ridges or other analogous alterations in aligner geometry in other types of clear aligners have been shown to enhance incisor torque [6]. Therefore, they should be incorporated for lingual root torque and relative intrusion, when indicated (Fig. 6.5). In cases where lingual root torque in the mandibular incisors is required, Class II elastics can be a useful auxiliary.

In the decrowding of an arch, especially anterior segments, the placement of the lingual root torque should be balanced with the appropriate amount of IPR. For example, if the planned IPR is excessive for a segment of crowded anterior teeth, the incisors can be over-retracted, resulting in an undesired deepening of the bite. The recovery of deep bites with over-retracted incisors to normal inclinations can be challenging, requiring significant anterior intrusion and lingual root torque, which have been shown to be problematic movements with clear aligners. The normalization of over-retracted incisors and their associated deep overbites may require auxiliaries, such as TAD-supported intrusion.

Short Clinical Crowns

Short clinical anterior crowns can be a limiting factor in bite opening, even when G5 protocols are applied. In these cases, the limited surface area of the crowns adversely affects the predictability of intrusive movements (Fig. 6.6). The clinician may consider overcorrection of intrusive movements to achieve bite opening in these patients.

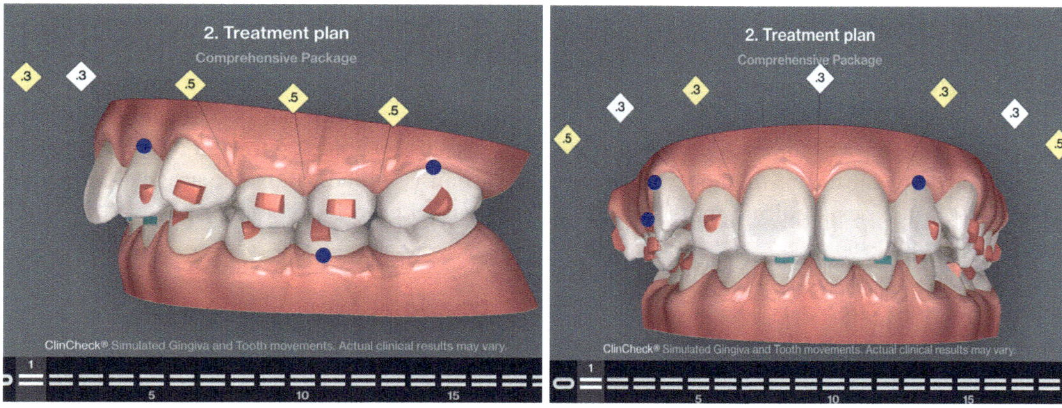

Fig. 6.5 For patient J. L., the placement of power ridges on the mandibular incisors supplements both lingual root torque and bite opening through relative intrusion. This method should especially be considered for the treatment of deep bite cases with upright mandibular incisors

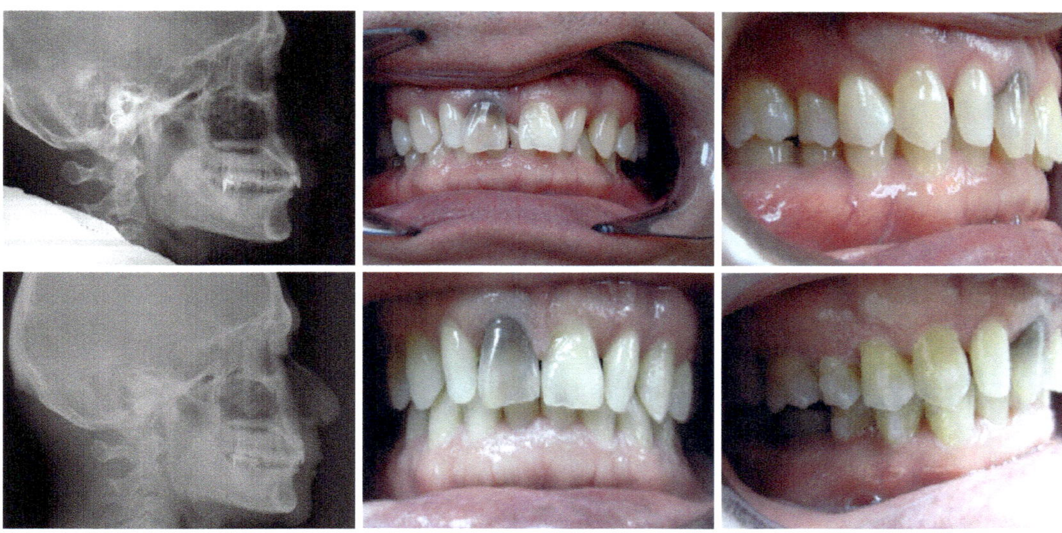

Fig. 6.6 Short clinical crowns with limited surface area for encapsulation by the aligner will adversely affect the predictability of intrusive movements and likely require overengineering to achieve ideal overbite

Treatment Protocols

TAD-Supported Intrusion

Clear aligner therapy has been shown to achieve 1–2 mm of pure intrusion, though with limited accuracy [7]. In cases requiring more significant intrusion of the maxillary incisors, such as 3–4 mm, the clinician can supplement intrusive movements with temporary skeletal devices in the labial bone between the maxillary central and lateral incisors or between the maxillary lateral incisors and canines. Elastics can then be applied bilaterally from the skeletal attachments to precision cuts within the anterior region of the aligner. This form of TAD-supported intrusion can be effective for the reduction of gingival display in patients with vertical maxillary excess (Fig. 6.7). In the design of the Clincheck, the intrusion of the maxillary anterior teeth should be overengineered to a 0 mm overbite or an edge-to-edge position to enhance the bite opening. However, the need for pure intrusion of greater than 3–4 mm is an indication for surgical correction, such as a Lefort I osteotomy.

Extraction Cases

Extraction cases are associated with bite deepening due to the tendency of the maxillary or mandibular incisors to lose torque and extrude during space closure. Studies of clear aligner therapy with first premolar extractions have shown greater lingual crown torque and extrusion in the maxillary central incisors than predicted [8]. The

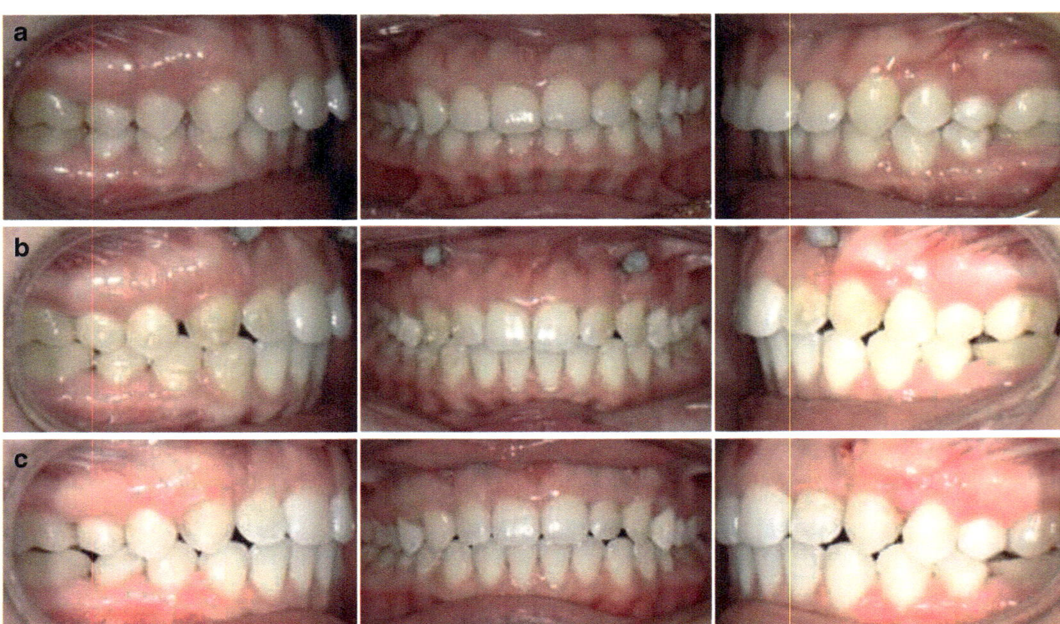

Fig. 6.7 (**a–e**) TAD-supported intrusion can be effective for the reduction of gingival display in patients with vertical maxillary excess when intrusion of 3–4 mm of the maxillary incisors are required. The treatment achieved both ideal overbite and the correction of the Class II relationships on both sides. The maxillary and mandibular incisors were retracted into normal range. Throughout treatment, the patient wore vertical elastics from precision cuts on the upper aligner to the two TADs. (**f–h**) For patient Q. W., progress records show TAD-supported intrusion with clear aligners allowed for significant maxillary incisor intrusion and reduction of gingival display. The patient was instructed to wear full-time vertical elastics (1/4", 4 oz. and 1/4", 6 oz.) from precision cuts on the aligner to the TADs

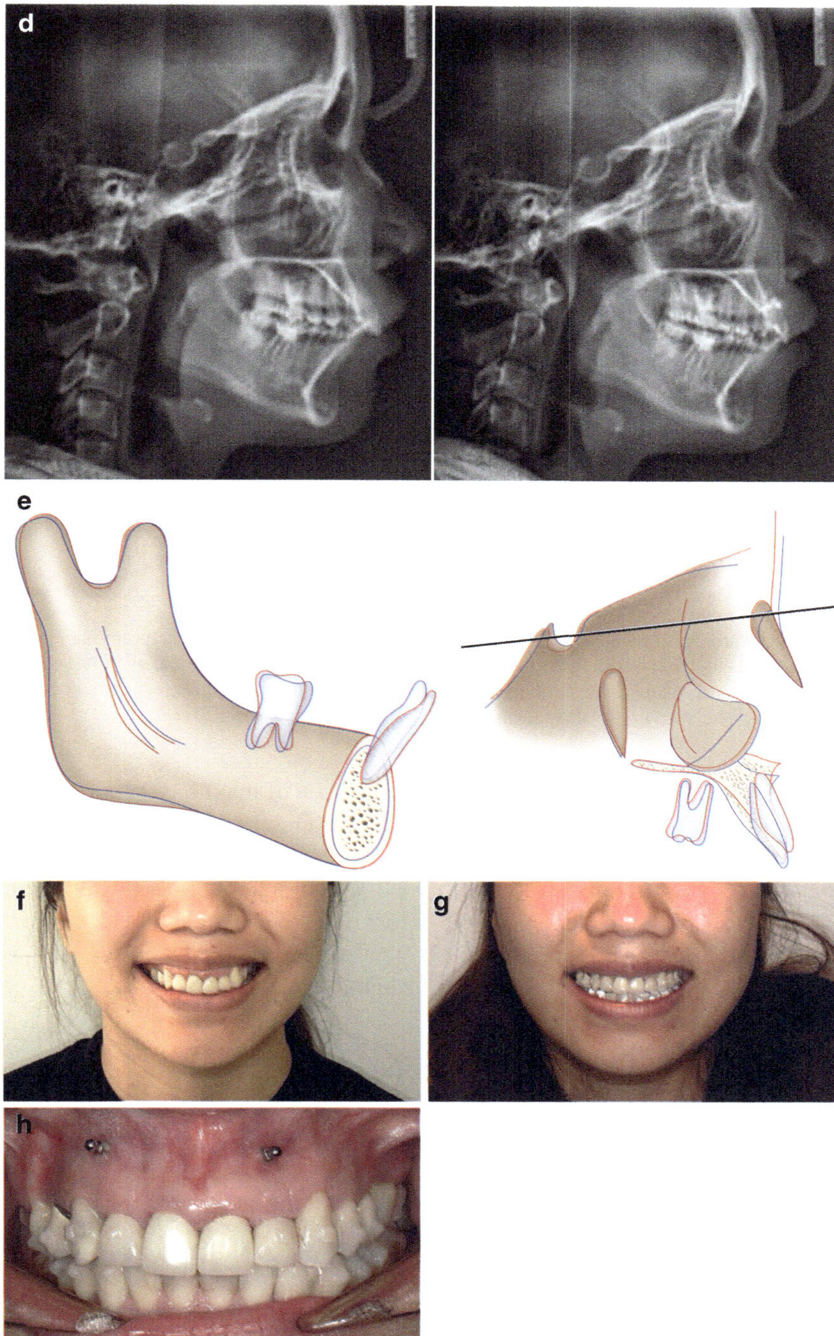

Fig. 6.7 (continued)

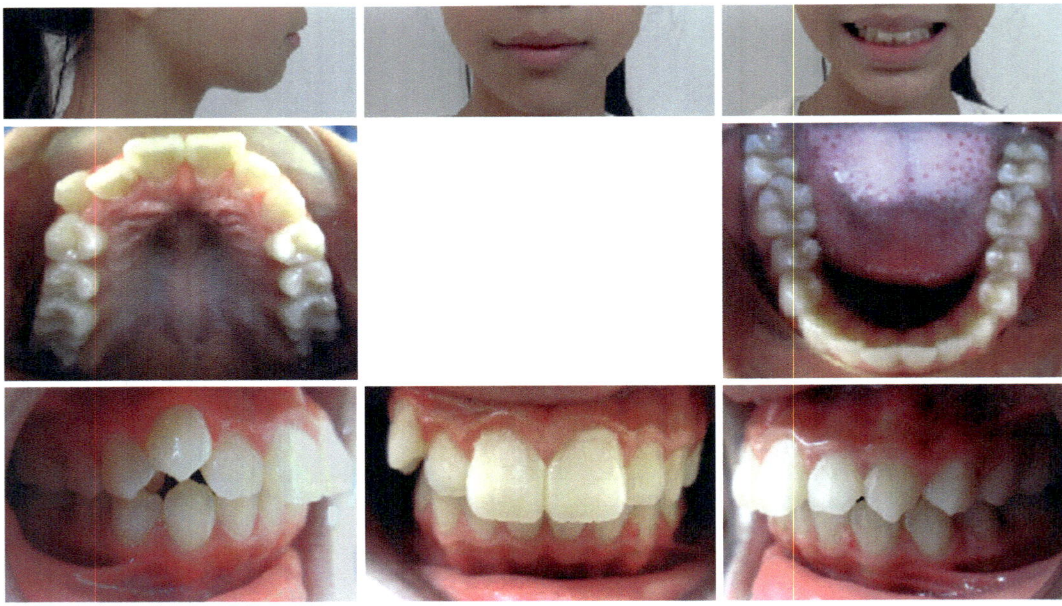

Fig. 6.8 In this case, both maxillary first premolars were extracted, while IPR and slight expansion were performed to decrowd the mandibular arch and control the mandibular incisor inclinations. The extraction of two maxillary premolars rather than four premolars reduced the difficulty of establishing an ideal overbite, which was achieved after an initial and a single refinement course

clinician should especially anticipate bite deepening as a result of loss of torque in the maxillary incisors in cases with maxillary extractions and in the mandibular incisors when mandibular teeth have been extracted. Therefore, the clinician will often have to incorporate the G5 protocol in extraction cases to minimize bite deepening. Also, if intrusive movements are applied to the maxillary or mandibular incisors, the clinician should consider overcorrection to achieve an ideal overbite at the end of treatment.

The limitations of clear aligners in controlling incisor torque may require more conservative approaches toward extraction therapy. In Class II malocclusions with increased overjet and maxillary and mandibular crowding, an extraction pattern of four first premolars may lead to difficulty in bite opening due to loss of torque in the mandibular incisors during space closure. A viable alternative treatment to this type of malocclusion is the extraction of only the maxillary first premolars and judicious IPR and expansion of the mandibular arch (Fig. 6.8). Extraction of maxillary premolars as opposed to the four first premolars may lessen the difficulty of achieving an ideal overbite. A two premolar extraction pattern may be more suitable than a four premolar extraction pattern for hypodivergent patients, in which bite opening is especially challenging.

Molar Extrusion

In patients with extremely deep bites and underlying normodivergent or hypodivergent skeletal patterns, anterior intrusion can be supplemented with molar extrusion for bite opening. This approach is similar to the mechanotherapy produced in fixed appliances by a 2 × 4 setup with tip-back bends mesial to both first molars (Fig. 6.9). Following the use of this protocol, the buccal segments of premolars may require additional extrusion in a course of refinement for ideal interdigitation and complete leveling of the Curve of Spee.

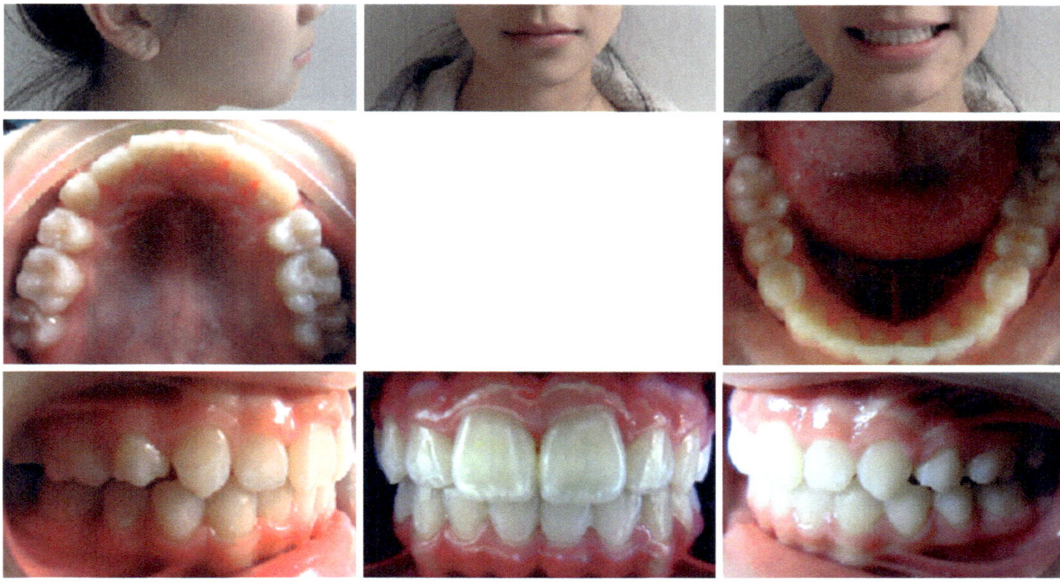

Fig. 6.8 (continued)

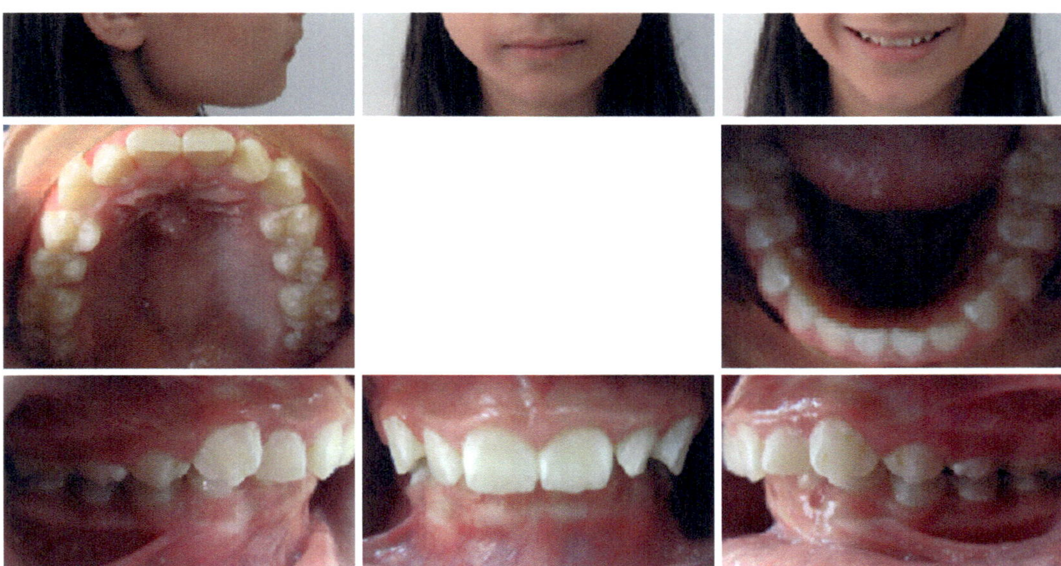

Fig. 6.9 For severe deep bites and normodivergent or hypodivergent skeletal patterns, the clinician should consider molar extrusion for bite opening. Patient C. W. presented with a 100% overbite, hypodivergent vertical pattern, and Class II div II malocclusion. The maxillary right first and second molars were extruded to supplement bite opening. Complete bite opening was also achieved through leveling of the maxillary and mandibular curves of Spee through intrusion of the maxillary and mandibular incisors. Class II canine and molar relationships were corrected with distalization of the maxillary arch and posterior IPR. The final occlusion showed Class I canines and molars, bilaterally, ideal overjet, and ideal overbite

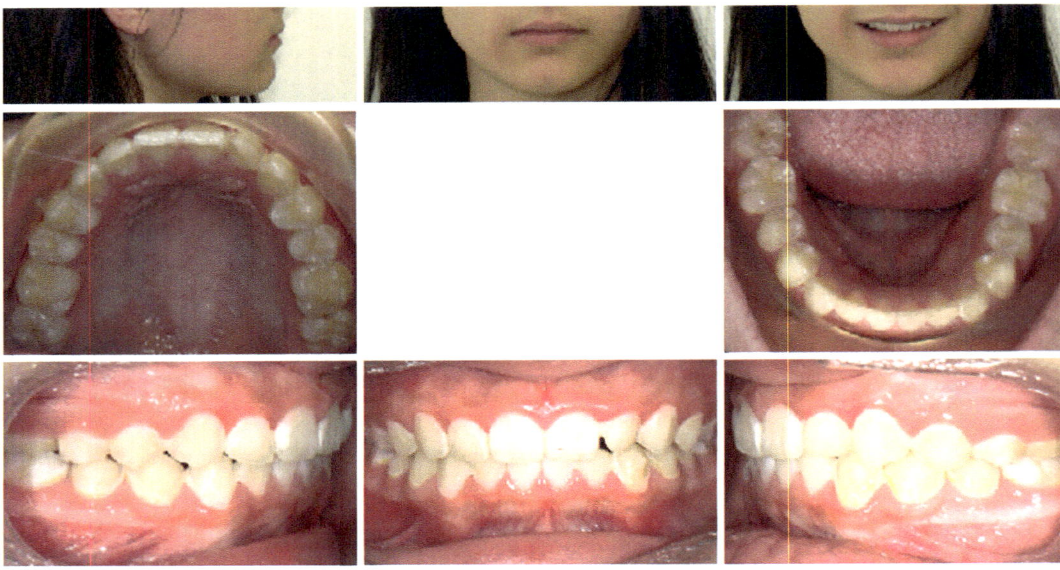

Fig. 6.9 (continued)

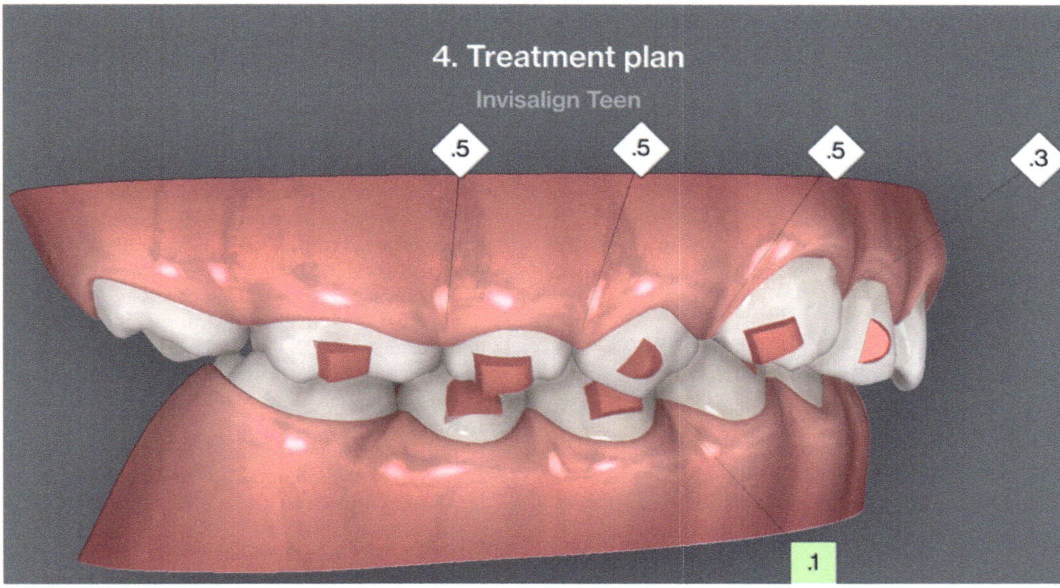

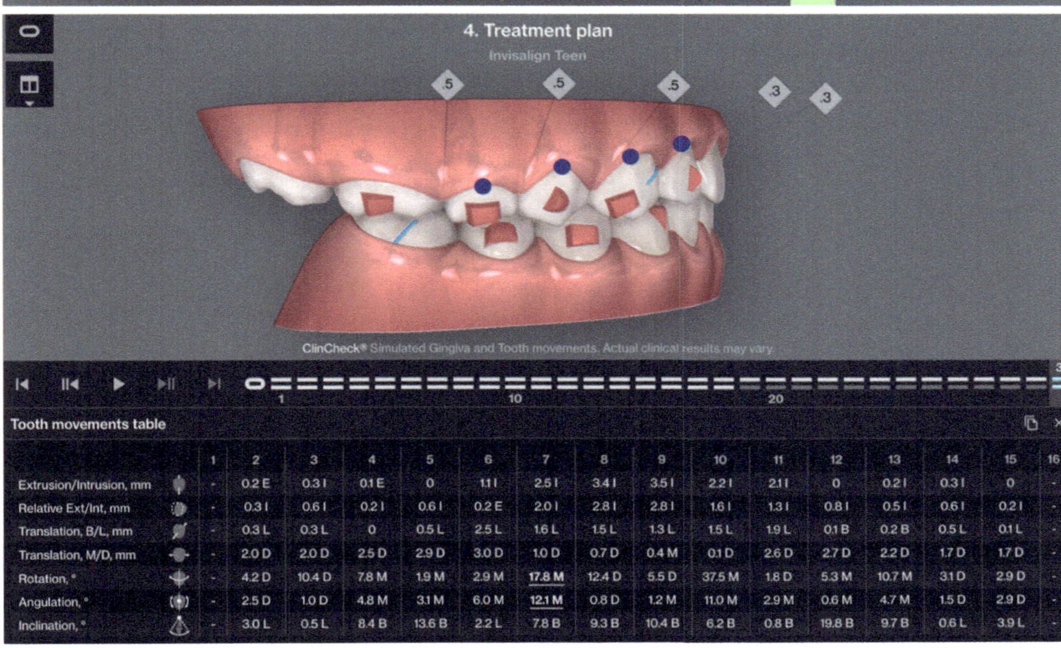

Tooth movements table

	1	2	3	4	5	6	7	8	9	10	11	12	13	14	15	16
Extrusion/Intrusion, mm	-	0.2 E	0.3 I	0.1 E	0	1.1 I	2.5 I	3.4 I	3.5 I	2.2 I	2.1 I	0	0.2 I	0.3 I	0	-
Relative Ext/Int, mm	-	0.3 I	0.6 I	0.2 I	0.6 I	0.2 E	2.0 I	2.8 I	2.8 I	1.6 I	1.3 I	0.8 I	0.5 I	0.6 I	0.2 I	-
Translation, B/L, mm	-	0.3 L	0.3 L	0	0.5 L	2.5 L	1.6 L	1.5 L	1.3 L	1.5 L	1.9 L	0.1 B	0.2 B	0.5 L	0.1 L	-
Translation, M/D, mm	-	2.0 D	2.0 D	2.5 D	2.9 D	3.0 D	1.0 D	0.7 D	0.4 M	0.1 D	2.6 D	2.7 D	2.2 D	1.7 D	1.7 D	-
Rotation, °	-	4.2 D	10.4 D	7.8 M	1.9 M	2.9 M	17.8 M	12.4 D	5.5 D	37.5 M	1.8 D	5.3 M	10.7 M	3.1 D	2.9 D	-
Angulation, °	-	2.5 D	1.0 D	4.8 M	3.1 M	6.0 M	12.1 M	0.8 D	1.2 M	11.0 M	2.9 M	0.6 M	4.7 M	1.5 D	2.9 D	-
Inclination, °	-	3.0 L	0.5 L	8.4 B	13.6 B	2.2 L	7.8 B	9.3 B	10.4 B	6.2 B	0.8 B	19.8 B	9.7 B	0.6 L	3.9 L	-

Fig. 6.9 (continued)

Improving the Accuracy of Bite Opening

It remains unclear how the G8 modifications will affect the predictability of maxillary and mandibular incisor intrusion and the overall efficacy of bite opening. Nevertheless, the accuracy of bite opening in clear aligner therapy can be improved through the incorporation of the appropriate protocols—the G5 protocol or its equivalent in other clear aligner software, the incorporation of relative intrusion when indicated, overengineering intrusive movements, judicious planning of IPR, and conservative approaches to extraction therapy. Adjuncts such as TADs and intermaxillary elastics can supplement movements, such as pure intrusion or relative intrusion through labialization of the mandibular incisors. Ultimately, these treatment methods work toward adequate leveling of the maxillary and mandibular Curves of Spee, which is the central tenet to successful bite opening.

References

1. Khosravi R, Cohanim B, Hujoel P, Daher S, Neal M, Liu W, Huang G. Management of overbite with the Invisalign appliance. Am J Orthod Dentofac Orthop. 2017;151(4):691–699.e2.
2. Haouili N, Kravitz ND, Vaid NR, Ferguson DJ, Makki L. Has Invisalign improved? A prospective follow-up study on the efficacy of tooth movement with Invisalign. Am J Orthod Dentofac Orthop. 2020;158(3):420–5.
3. Align Technology. Align Technology announces Invisalign G5 innovations for treatment of deep bite. 2013. https://investor.aligntech.com/index.php/news-releases/news-release-details/align-technology-announces-invisalign-g5-innovations-treatment. Accessed 16 Mar 2021.
4. Align Technology. Align Technology announces Invisalign G8 with new Smartforce aligner activation features. 2020. https://investor.aligntech.com/news-releases/news-release-details/align-technology-announces-invisalign-g8-new-smartforce. Accessed 18 Mar 2021.
5. Henick D, Dayan W, Dunford R, Warunek S, Al-Jewair T. Effects of Invisalign (G5) with virtual bite ramps for skeletal deep overbite malocclusion correction in adults. Angle Orthod. 2021;91(2):164–70.
6. Simon M, Keilig L, Schwarze J, Jung BA, Bourauel C. Treatment outcome and efficacy of an aligner technique--regarding incisor torque, premolar derotation and molar distalization. BMC Oral Health. 2014;14:68.
7. Al-Balaa M, Li H, Ma Mohamed A, Xia L, Liu W, Chen Y, Omran T, Li S, Hua X. Predicted and actual outcome of anterior intrusion with Invisalign assessed with cone-beam computed tomography. Am J Orthod Dentofac Orthop. 2021;159(3):e275–80.
8. Dai FF, Xu TM, Shu G. Comparison of achieved and predicted tooth movement of maxillary first molars and central incisors: first premolar extraction treatment with Invisalign. Angle Orthod. 2019;89(5):679–87.

Dilemmas in Open Bite Correction

7

Contents

Current Strategies for Open Bite Closure

Anterior open bites constitute one of the most challenging malocclusions for orthodontic management. The difficulty lies in the multifactorial etiology, the complexity of the treatment mechanics, and the high rate of relapse. Open bites can be composed of dental, skeletal, respiratory, neurological, or functional components [1]. They are often categorized as dental, skeletal, or a combination of both. Skeletal dysplasias characterized by excessively vertical patterns of growth can result in anterior open bites. They are also associated with oral habits, such as digit sucking, and the soft tissues, such as lip incompetence, abnormal swallowing patterns, and abnormal tongue positioning. Hypertrophic lymphatic tissues, either the tonsils or adenoids, can lead to airway obstruction, followed by long-term mouth breathing, and resulting in maxillary constriction and a vertical growth pattern [2]. Untreated open bites are associated with functional and psychological issues in patients, including difficulties incising food, speech issues, and facial appearance [3].

A variety of modalities has been employed for bite closure, including habit appliances such as the tongue crib, functional appliances with orthopedic forces such as the high-pull headgear, occlusal equilibration, orthodontic camouflage with or without extraction, the use of skeletal anchorage devices in the forms of mini-implants and miniplates, and surgical forms of correction [4]. A meta-analysis on the long-term stability of open bite correction found 75% stability in open

A. T. Huang, D. Huang, *Controversies in Clear Aligner Therapy*,
https://doi.org/10.1007/978-3-030-92810-0_7

bites treated nonsurgically, while a stability of 82% for surgical treatments [5]. In nonsurgical treatment, the mechanics usually involves extrusion of the anterior segments, intrusion of posterior segments to facilitate autorotation of the mandible, or a combination of both. In certain cases, clinicians have shown successful closure of severe skeletal open bites with the intrusion of maxillary and mandibular molars with mini-implants as a viable alternative to major orthognathic surgery [6].

Clinicians have successfully achieved open bite correction with clear aligners, especially for the treatment of mild anterior open bites [7]. Clear aligners have been claimed to allow for both vertical control and a bite block effect, factors helpful for bite closure [8]. Invisalign's G4 modifications targeted extrusion of the anterior segments through optimized attachments on the maxillary incisors [9]. Clear aligners have also demonstrated efficacy with movements associated with bite closure, including posterior intrusion and the extrusion of anterior segments. Recent clinical trials have shown that open bite closure with clear aligners occurs through a combination of posterior intrusion, extrusion of the anterior segments, and slight mandibular autorotation [10]. A number of clinicians have also supplemented clear aligner treatment with mini-implants for greater control over posterior intrusion movements [11].

As with fixed appliances, the success of open bite treatment with clear aligners depends foremost on the accurate diagnosis and management of the etiologic factors causing the open bite. With respect to clear aligner mechanotherapy, the predictability of bite closure can be improved with strategic planning of posterior intrusive and anterior extrusive movements and the selective incorporation of mini-implants for enhanced control over posterior intrusion. In this chapter, we describe the principles for treatment planning and optimizing the mechanotherapy involved in bite closure.

Efficacy of Movements Associated with Bite Closure

Absolute Extrusion vs. Relative Extrusion

Studies have observed the accuracy of pure extrusion of the maxillary central and lateral incisors to be 55% [12]. This represents a marked improvement over that of previous generations of aligners, which demonstrated an accuracy for extrusion of 18.3% for maxillary incisors and 24.5% for mandibular incisors. However, it remains difficult to achieve pure anterior extrusion of greater than 1 mm in either the maxillary or mandibular arch and greater than 2 mm collectively in both arches (Fig. 7.1). Studies show that during open bite closure, the average absolute extrusion of the maxillary and mandibular incisors remains less than 1 mm per arch [8].

One of the essential strategies for open bite closure is the prescription of *relative extrusion* of the maxillary and mandibular incisors, or extrusion of the incisors achieved through the combination of extrusion with lingual crown tipping during incisor retraction. Relative extrusion, when compared to absolute or true extrusion, allows for greater and more predictable extrusion of the maxillary and mandibular incisors (Fig. 7.2) [13]. However, relative extrusion can only be achieved when spacing is present in the respective arch, either through IPR, extractions, or existing spaces. When relative extrusion is prescribed through retraction, whether through IPR or extractions, the amount of extrusion achieved can be up to 2 mm per arch and up to 4 mm in combination from both arches.

Invisalign's G4 modifications targeted open bite closure by incorporating optimized extrusion attachments for the maxillary and mandibular incisors (Fig. 7.3). Clinical trials have suggested that the addition of optimized extrusion attachments enhanced the accuracy of incisor extrusion compared with the accuracy in aligners prior to

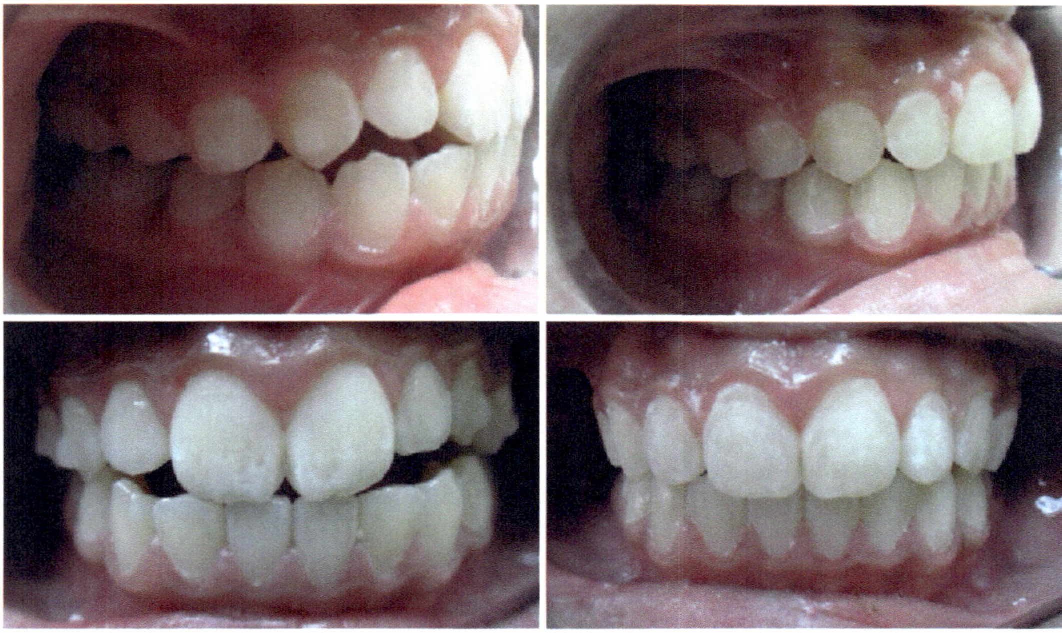

Fig. 7.1 In the treatment of mild anterior open bites, absolute extrusion can be programmed for the maxillary and mandibular incisors. Typically, in the Invisalign system, these extrusive movements can be supplemented with G4 optimized attachments

the G4 modifications [12]. Therefore, it is recommended that G4 attachments be placed on incisors when absolute extrusion is planned, while their placement is optional for relative extrusion. This is because, during relative extrusion, the predictability of the extrusive movement has already been enhanced by lingual crown tipping.

Molar Intrusion

Studies have demonstrated that clear aligner therapy is able to induce significant intrusion of both the maxillary and mandibular molars, even without the supplementation of TADs. One of the most effective methods of open bite closure is the combination of molar intrusion and both absolute and relative extrusion of the maxillary and mandibular incisors. 1 mm of molar intrusion has been shown to result in approximately 2–3 mm of anterior open bite closure [14]. Molar intrusion has been shown to result in mandibular autorotation, which allows for the reduction in the vertical dimension, the closure of the mandibular plane, decreases in the lower anterior facial height, and increased stability [10]. Therefore, it is recommended that when indicated, such as in high-angle patients or over-erupted posterior teeth, the clinician couple anterior extrusive movements with programmed intrusion of the maxillary and mandibular molars for more predictable bite closure (Fig. 7.4).

There have been claims of a "bite block effect" associated with clear aligners due to the thickness of the aligner along with the forces exerted by the patient during mastication [15]. Studies have shown that intrusion of the molars of up to 0.5 mm can occur even when intrusive movements have not been programmed by the clinician [16]. However, it is questionable that clear aligners can simulate the bite block effects produced by conventional functional appliances with posterior bite blocks of greater than 3 mm thickness, which allow for much greater and long-term

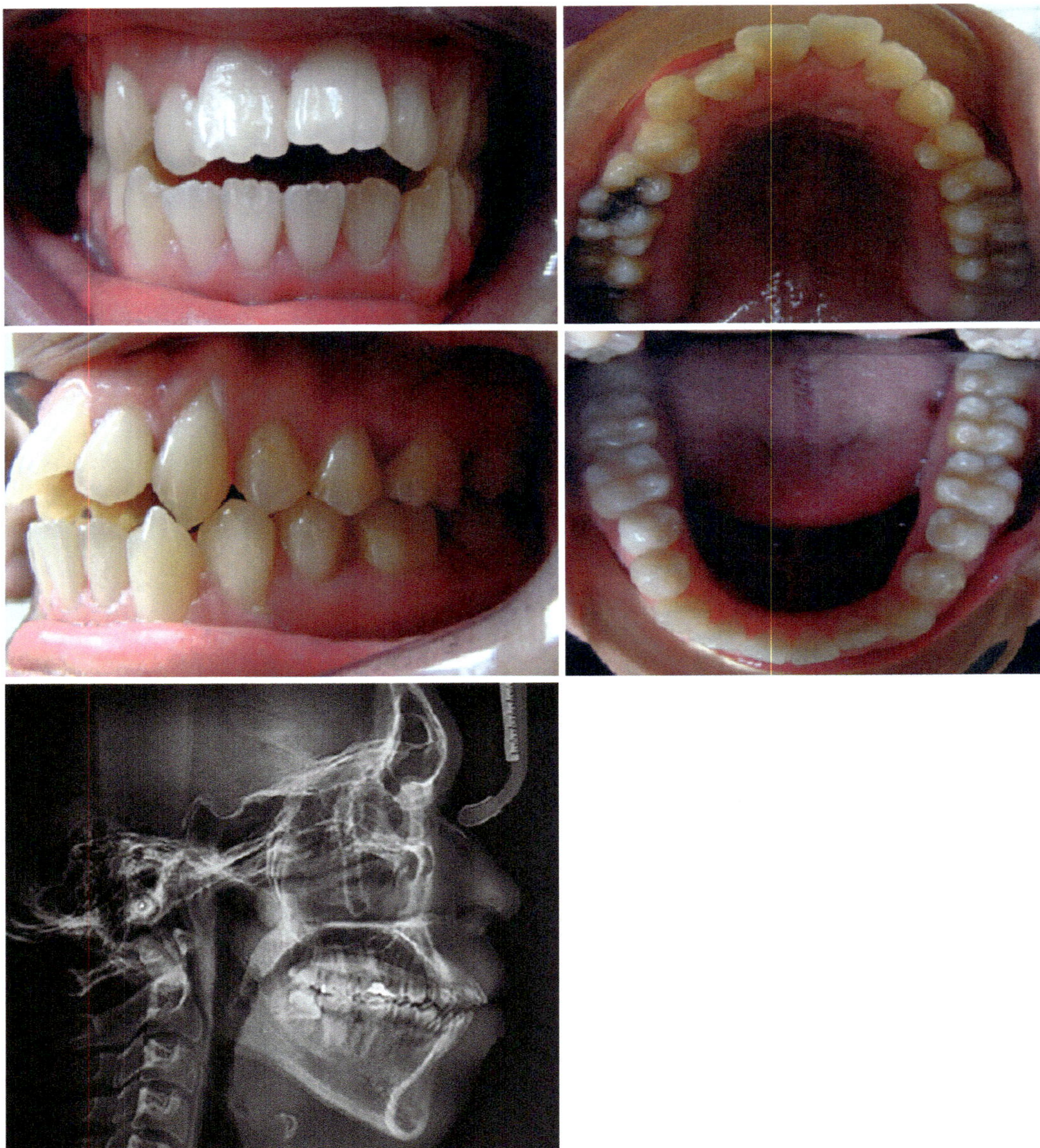

Fig. 7.2 For the treatment of this Class I malocclusion with moderate maxillary and mandibular crowding, moderate anterior open bite, and bimaxillary protrusion, we extracted four first premolars. The retraction of the maxillary and mandibular incisors allowed for their relative extrusion, which was essential for this patient's anterior open bite closure

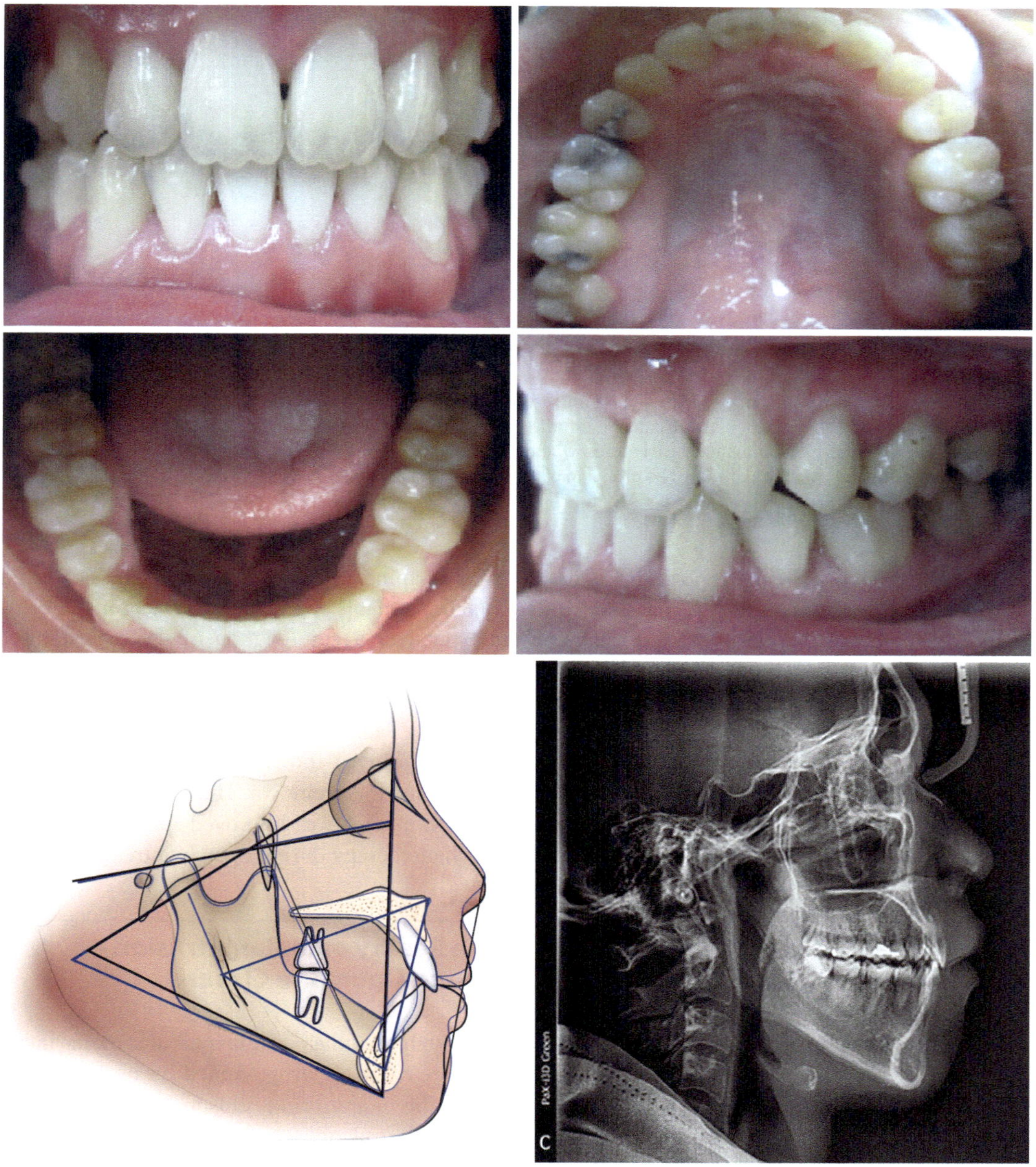

Fig. 7.2 (continued)

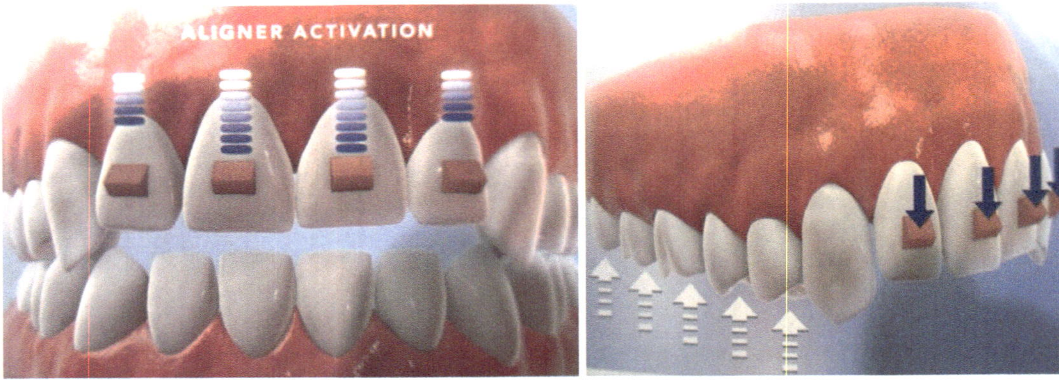

Fig. 7.3 One of the G4 modifications included optimized extrusion attachments to enhance the extrusion of the maxillary incisors. These attachments are triggered when programmed extrusion exceeds 0.5 mm. The clinician can consider omitting these attachments when other predictable means of extrusion have been planned, such as relative extrusion through maxillary incisor retraction

intrusive forces on the posterior teeth. Nevertheless, the nature of the clear aligner, with its full coverage of the dentition, represents an advantage during intrusion because it limits undesired extrusive movements.

Finishing after Anterior Open Bite Closure

Following the closure of the anterior open bite, a lateral open bite frequently develops due to heavy anterior interferences (Fig. 7.5). In these cases, the buccal segments need to be extruded either through an additional course of aligners, vertical elastics, or a combination of the two methods. The clinician should also consider alleviation of the heavy anterior contacts to facilitate closure of the lateral open bite.

Factors Affecting Bite Closure

As in fixed appliances, the success of open bite treatment largely depends on the removal of functional etiological factors prior to any mechanotherapy. These range from tongue disposition, digital habits, abnormal swallowing pattern, to mouth breathing. These can be addressed either through myofunctional therapy, forms of behavioral shaping to cease oral habits or abnormal functions, habit appliances such as tongue cribs or spurs, or a combination of these modalities [17]. When indicated, more invasive intervention may be required, such as in the case of mouth breathing, which may warrant a referral to the otolaryngologist for evaluation of the lymphatic tissues and their removal. The addressing of these factors allows for improved predictability of mechanotherapy during open bite treatment.

The Reality of Molar Intrusion during Open Bite Closure

Although maxillary and mandibular molar intrusion are routinely programmed for open bite closure, the majority of closure occurs through anterior extrusion, whether absolute or relative, as opposed to molar intrusion and mandibular autorotation. An early study of open bite treatment without the use of auxiliaries such as TADs concluded that the primary mechanism for bite closure occurred through extrusion of the anterior teeth [18]. This is also supported by recent studies which have observed there were more dental than skeletal changes contributing to open bite closure with clear aligner therapy [10].

It is difficult to achieve molar intrusion greater than 1 mm in a single arch without skeletal

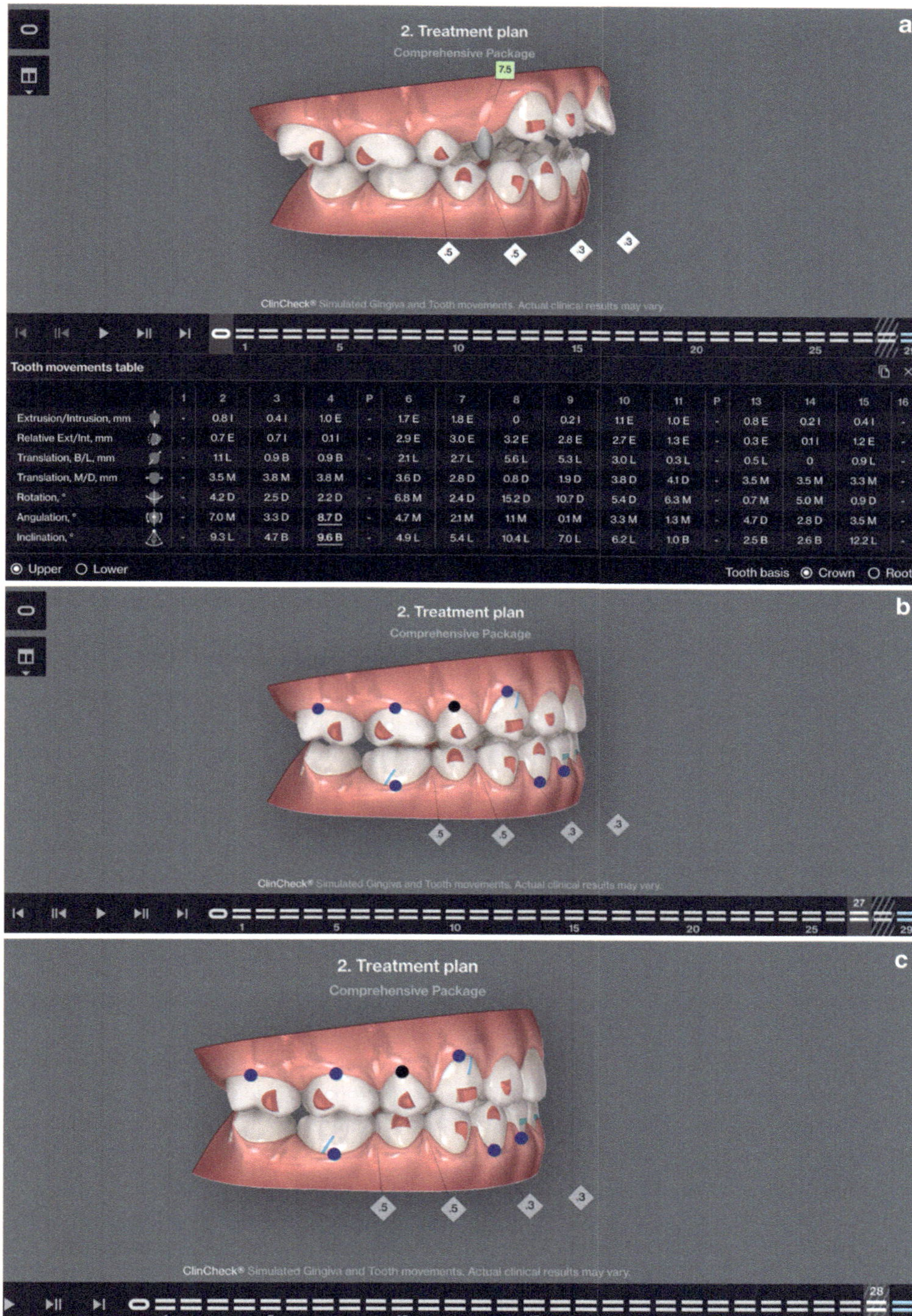

	1	2	3	4	P	6	7	8	9	10	11	P	13	14	15	16
Extrusion/Intrusion, mm	-	0.8 I	0.4 I	1.0 E	-	1.7 E	1.8 E	0	0.2 I	1.1 E	1.0 E	-	0.8 E	0.2 I	0.4 I	-
Relative Ext/Int, mm	-	0.7 E	0.7 I	0.1 I	-	2.9 E	3.0 E	3.2 E	2.8 E	2.7 E	1.3 E	-	0.3 E	0.1 I	1.2 E	-
Translation, B/L, mm	-	1.1 L	0.9 B	0.9 B	-	2.1 L	2.7 L	5.6 L	5.3 L	3.0 L	0.3 L	-	0.5 L	0	0.9 L	-
Translation, M/D, mm	-	3.5 M	3.8 M	3.8 M	-	3.6 D	2.8 D	0.8 D	1.9 D	3.8 D	4.1 D	-	3.5 M	3.5 M	3.3 M	-
Rotation, °	-	4.2 D	2.5 D	2.2 D	-	6.8 M	2.4 D	15.2 D	10.7 D	5.4 D	6.3 M	-	0.7 M	5.0 M	0.9 D	-
Angulation, °	-	7.0 M	3.3 D	8.7 D	-	4.7 M	2.1 M	1.1 M	0.1 M	3.3 M	1.3 M	-	4.7 D	2.8 D	3.5 M	-
Inclination, °	-	9.3 L	4.7 B	9.6 B	-	4.9 L	5.4 L	10.4 L	7.0 L	6.2 L	1.0 B	-	2.5 B	2.6 B	12.2 L	-

Fig. 7.4 (**a**) For adult patient H.S., who presented with a severe anterior open bite, increased overjet, and Class II div I malocclusion, treatment included the extraction of maxillary first premolars and intrusion of the maxillary molars. A bite jump was programmed on stage 28 (**b**, **c**) for mandibular autorotation and complete closure of the anterior open bite. We planned for significant relative extrusion of the maxillary incisors through retraction, as shown in the tooth movement assessment table. Light Class II elastics (1/4", 2.7 oz) were worn to supplement retraction of the maxillary incisors

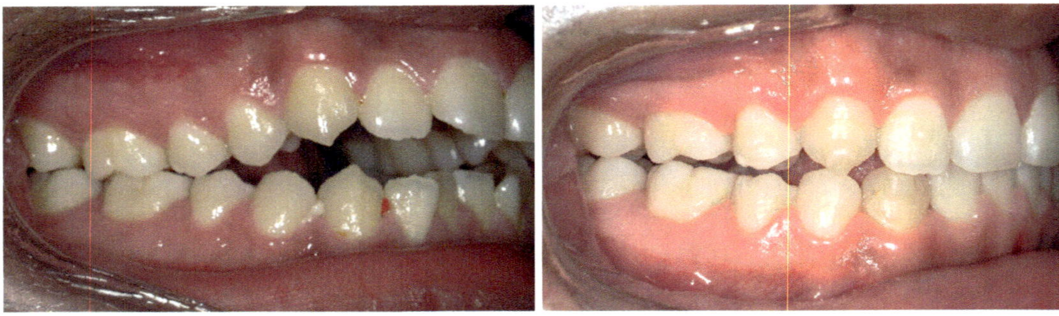

Fig. 7.5 Autorotation of the mandible for anterior open bite closure will often result in lateral open bites. Mild lateral open bites can be corrected by sectioning the maxillary aligner to allow for occlusal settling, while more severe lateral open bites may require vertical elastics or a refinement course for complete closure

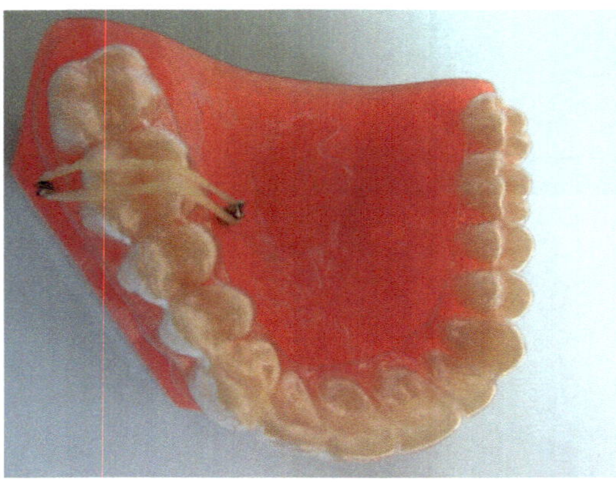

Fig. 7.6 A TAD can be placed on both the buccal and palatal sides of the molar to be intruded. The patient can wear an elastic (with a tension of ¼″, 4 oz. or 6 oz.) from the buccal to the palatal TAD to supplement intrusion to the molar

anchorage. Studies typically show both maxillary and mandibular molar intrusion of <1 mm during bite closure and <2 mm of intrusion additively from both arches. If >1 mm of intrusion is desired, then it is necessary to supplement intrusion with TADs. The miniscrews can be placed in the buccal and palatal bone respective to the tooth requiring intrusion. A power chain can be extended between the two TADs for the exertion of an intrusive force as bodily as possible (Fig. 7.6). Intrusion of <1 mm per maxillary and mandibular molars has been shown to result in the autorotation of the mandible and closure of the mandibular plane [8]. However, it is still difficult to achieve molar intrusion of greater than 2 mm per tooth, and therefore greater than 4 mm collectively for both arches.

The Incorporation of Bite Jumps

In the Clincheck plan of open bite closure, the bite jump simulates the closure of the anterior open bite (Fig. 7.7). It is important to program the bite jump into the Clincheck to accurately model the course of treatment. However, though the bite jump will simulate an autorotation of the mandible, it is unlikely significant autorotation is achieved in nonsurgical treatment without skeletal anchorage and more likely that the bite closure occurred through dental movements.

The bite jump is typically prescribed within the final aligner, though bite closure will often occur earlier. It is difficult to predict when anterior open bite closure or the bite jump will actually occur during treatment, but it is usually observed in the middle of a course of aligners or occasionally, as early as the first third of treatment (Fig. 7.8).

TAD-Assisted Molar Intrusion for Bite Closure

Ideally, when indicated, skeletal anchorage should be incorporated for bite closure so that miniscrews can supplement both maxillary and mandibular molar intrusion. However, clinicians have shown success with either exclusively

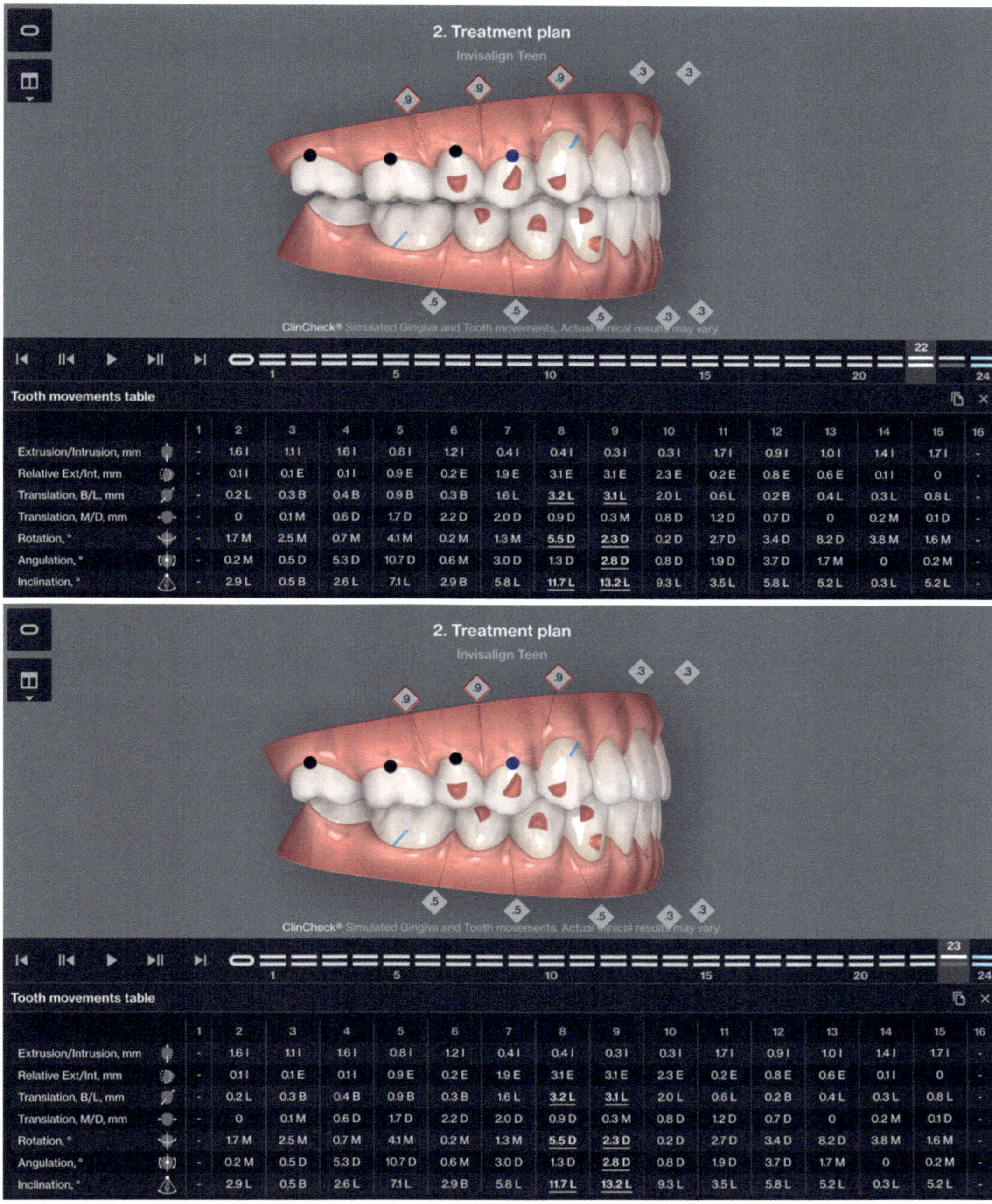

Fig. 7.7 Stage 23 represents a bite jump, portraying mandibular autorotation for anterior open bite closure. Significant intrusion was programmed for the maxillary premolars and molars, while significant relative extrusion was programmed for the maxillary and mandibular incisors

intruding the maxillary molars or exclusively intruding the mandibular molars in fixed appliances [19]. Recent reports have shown similar success with clear aligners by supplementing intrusion of the mandibular molars with skeletal anchorage [20]. Therefore, the clinician may consider a therapeutic diagnosis by incorporating skeletal anchorage for the intrusion of molars in one arch and then reevaluating during treatment the need for skeletal anchorage for molar intrusion in the opposing arch. This approach is less invasive than placing skeletal anchors in both arches at the outset, especially as the literature has demonstrated efficacy with bite closure using skeletal anchorage in a single arch.

The incorporation of skeletal anchorage for open bite treatment has been shown to decrease treatment time compared to treatments without skeletal anchorage, either with or without extractions. In fixed appliances, open bite treatments supported by skeletal anchorage have also been observed to achieve stability similar to that of surgical approaches, though relapse ranging from 10 to 30% has been observed for maxillary and mandibular molars that have been intruded with skeletal anchorage [21].

The Reality of Open Bite Closure with Clear Aligner Therapy

Whether in fixed appliances or clear aligner therapy, the successful treatment of open bites requires the accurate diagnosis of its etiology and the removal or management of any functional contributory factors, such as mouth breathing and tongue disposition. The principal therapeutic modalities of bite closure to target the dental and skeletal components of the malocclusion are extrusion of the anterior segments and intrusion of the posterior segments, both of which are often combined during therapy. In clear aligner therapy, the predictability of anterior extrusion can be enhanced by combining true extrusion with more predictable movements, such as lingual crown tip, while the predictability of significant poste-

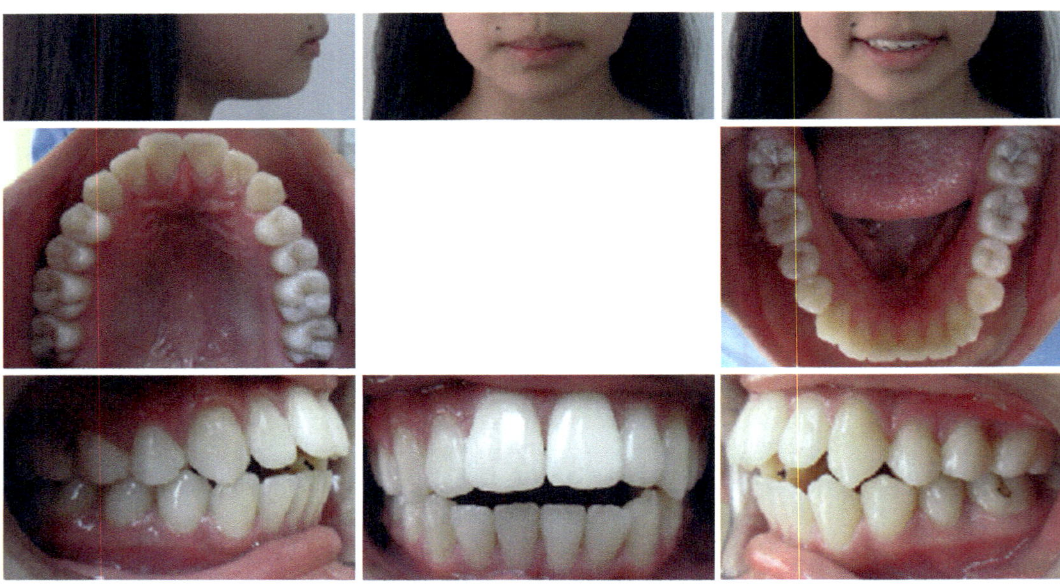

Fig. 7.8 For patient T. S., the anterior open bite was treated with both extrusion of the maxillary and mandibular incisors and maxillary and mandibular molar intrusion. The bite jump or anterior open bite closure occurred after 5 months of treatment, or within the first third of the total treatment duration

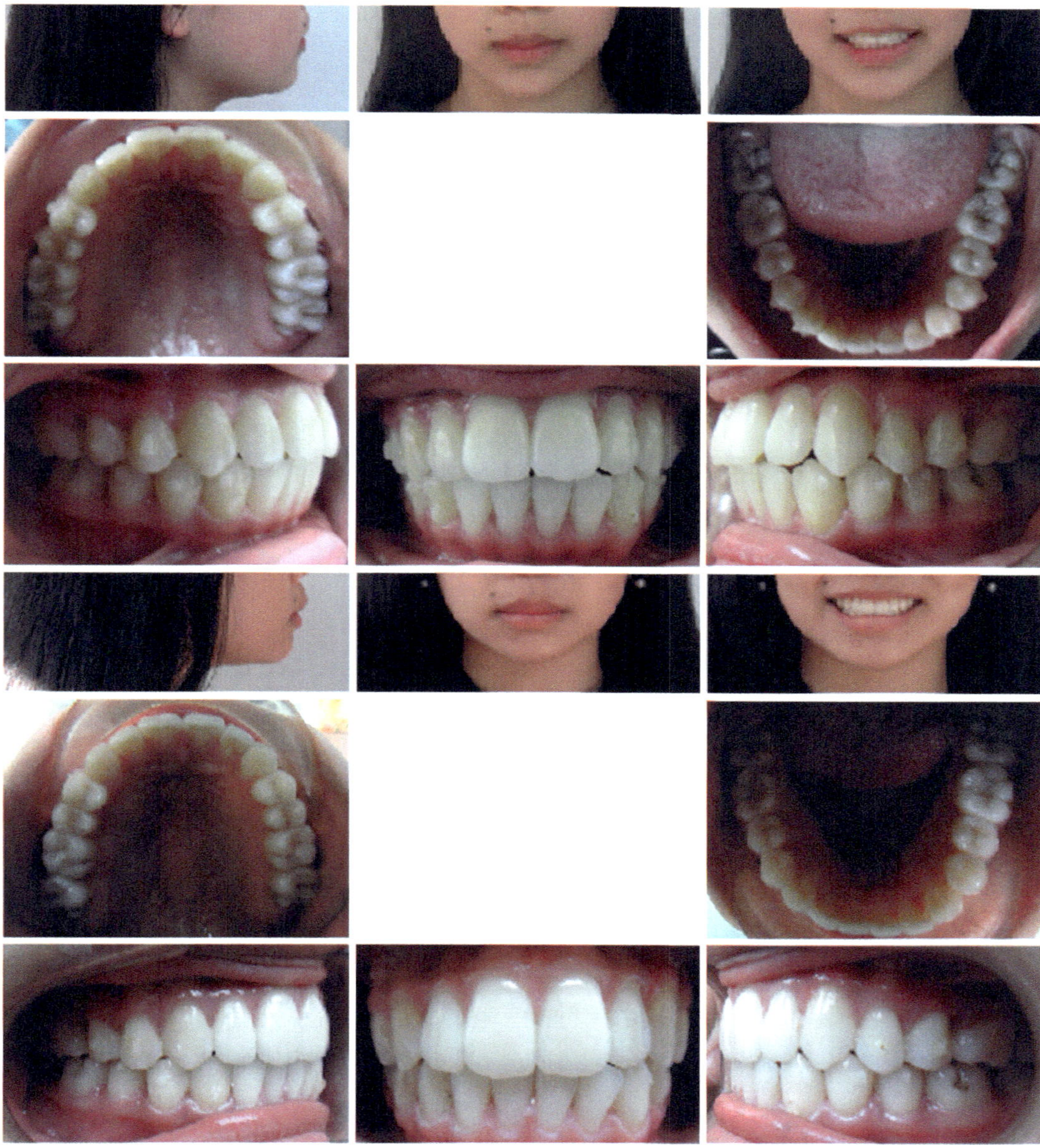

Fig. 7.8 (continued)

rior intrusion can be enhanced with the judicious use of skeletal anchorage.

It has been shown that anterior open bites with nonsurgical clear aligner therapy are closed through a combination of incisor extrusion, molar intrusion, and mandibular autorotation. However, the evidence also demonstrates bite closure occurs more through dental than skeletal changes and that only slight mandibular autorotation occurs during treatment.

References

1. Sandler PJ, Madahar AK, Murray A. Anterior open bite: aetiology and management. Dent Update. 2011;38(8).:522–4, 527–8, 531–2.
2. Reichert I, Figel P, Winchester L. Orthodontic treatment of anterior open bite: a review article--is surgery always necessary? Oral Maxillofac Surg. 2014;18(3):271–77.
3. Almeida RR, Ursi WJ. Anterior open bite etiology and treatment. Oral Health. 1990;80(1):27–31.
4. Matsumoto MA, Romano FL, Ferreira JT, Valério RA. Open bite: diagnosis, treatment and stability. Braz Dent J. 2012;23(6):768–78.
5. Greenlee GM, Huang GJ, Chen SS, Chen J, Koepsell T, Hujoel P. Stability of treatment for anterior open-bite malocclusion: a meta-analysis. Am J Orthod Dentofac Orthop. 2011;139(2):154–69.
6. Sherwood K. Correction of skeletal open bite with implant anchored molar/bicuspid intrusion. Oral Maxillofac Surg Clin North Am. 2007;19(3).:339–50, vi.
7. Schupp W, Haubrich J, Neumann I. Treatment of anterior open bite with the Invisalign system. J Clin Orthod. 2010;44(8):501–7.
8. Moshiri S, Araújo EA, McCray JF, Thiesen G, Kim KB. Cephalometric evaluation of adult anterior open bite non-extraction treatment with Invisalign. Dental Press J Orthod. 2017;22(5):30–8.
9. Align Technology. Align Technology Introduces Invisalign G4. 2011. https://investor.aligntech.com/news-releases/news-release-details/align-technology-introduces-invisalign-g4. Accessed 18 Apr 2021.
10. Harris K, Ojima K, Dan C, Upadhyay M, Alshehri A, Kuo CL, Mu J, Uribe F, Nanda R. Evaluation of open bite closure using clear aligners: a retrospective study. Prog Orthod. 2020;21(1):23.
11. Giancotti A, Germano F, Muzzi F, Greco M. A miniscrew-supported intrusion auxiliary for open-bite treatment with Invisalign. J Clin Orthod. 2014;48(6):348–58.
12. Haouili N, Kravitz ND, Vaid NR, Ferguson DJ, Makki L. Has Invisalign improved? A prospective follow-up study on the efficacy of tooth movement with Invisalign. Am J Orthod Dentofac Orthop. 2020;158(3):420–5.
13. Kravitz ND, Kusnoto B, BeGole E, Obrez A, Agran B. How well does Invisalign work? A prospective clinical study evaluating the efficacy of tooth movement with Invisalign. Am J Orthod Dentofac Orthop. 2009;135(1):27–35.
14. Proffit WR. Contemporary orthodontics. Toronto: Elsevier; 2013.
15. Boyd RL. Esthetic orthodontic treatment using the invisalign appliance for moderate to complex malocclusions. J Dent Educ. 2008;72(8):948–67.
16. Dai FF, Xu TM, Shu G. Comparison of achieved and predicted tooth movement of maxillary first molars and central incisors: first premolar extraction treatment with Invisalign. Angle Orthod. 2019;89(5):679–87.
17. Tanny L, Huang B, Naung NY, Currie G. Non-orthodontic intervention and non-nutritive sucking behaviours: a literature review. Kaohsiung J Med Sci. 2018;34(4):215–22.
18. Khosravi R, Cohanim B, Hujoel P, Daher S, Neal M, Liu W, et al. Management of overbite with the Invisalign appliance. Am J Orthod Dentofac Orthop. 2017;151(4):691–9.
19. Erverdi N, Keles A, Nanda R. The use of skeletal anchorage in open bite treatment: a cephalometric evaluation. Angle Orthod. 2004;74(3):381–90.
20. Pinho T, Santos M. Skeletal open bite treated with clear aligners and miniscrews. Am J Orthod Dentofac Orthop. 2021;159(2):224–33.
21. González Espinosa D, de Oliveira Moreira PE, da Sousa AS, Flores-Mir C, Normando D. Stability of anterior open bite treatment with molar intrusion using skeletal anchorage: a systematic review and meta-analysis. Prog Orthod. 2020;21(1):35.

8 Power Ridges: How Powerful Are They?

Contents

Torquing with Clear Aligners

Torque expression is one of the most important elements of orthodontic treatment. The faciolingual inclination of the crown is considered the third key of occlusion. Torque control in both the anterior and posterior segments is critical for achieving ideal overjet and overbite, adequate anterior guidance, balanced occlusal contacts, and optimal distribution of spaces [1]. Torque is also critical for smile esthetics and a harmonious soft tissue profile. Inadequate torque can result in poor lip support, reduced buccal corridors, and occlusal interferences.

The efficacy of torque expression in clear aligner therapy has been studied in clinical trials and in vitro biomechanical simulations. Studies have shown that buccal-lingual crown tip is one of the most accurate movements with clear aligners, when compared to movements in the other dimensions, such as rotation and intrusion [2]. However, recent studies have also demonstrated that clear aligners are more than twice as predictable at performing pure crown tipping than torque in incisors [3]. It has also been shown that labial root movement is significantly more accurate than lingual root movement with clear aligners [3]. This result has been partly explained by the greater prevalence of root fenestrations in the labial side compared to that in the lingual side [4]. In clear aligners, the inadequate expression of torque commonly results in excessive crown tipping during translation. For example, during the retraction of the maxillary incisors, loss of incisor torque can occur due to excessive lingual crown tip and inadequate expression of lingual root torque.

The primary adjunct for torquing movements in clear aligners is the alteration of aligner geometry in the form of a pressure line located at the cervical region on the facial surface of the crown. In the Invisalign system, this feature is known as the power ridge. It has been shown that the incorporation of a power ridge allows for the generation

A. T. Huang, D. Huang, *Controversies in Clear Aligner Therapy*,
https://doi.org/10.1007/978-3-030-92810-0_8

of a greater moment for the desired torquing movement [5]. The true effect of power ridges on torquing efficacy has not been determined, though they have been demonstrated to improve the accuracy of incisor torquing [6].

The use of power ridges is not limited to controlling maxillary incisor torque during incisor retraction, but also extends to a wide range of applications, including maintaining incisor inclination during posterior protraction, dental decompensation for orthognathic surgery, treatment of Class II and Class III malocclusions, and the detailing of lingually displaced teeth. In this chapter, we discuss the efficacy of power ridges, the indications and mechanotherapy for their use, and modifications in design to address their current limitations.

The Indications of Power Ridges

Incisor Retraction

The most common indication for the use of power ridges is to control incisor torque during retraction (Fig. 8.1). The incorporation of power ridges is important to prevent over-retraction of either the maxillary or mandibular incisors (Fig. 8.2). Supplementation with power ridges should be considered for incisors planned for significant retraction in extraction therapy and non-extraction therapy, especially in Class II division 1 cases requiring maxillary incisor retraction and Class I bimaxillary protrusion cases requiring both maxillary and mandibular incisor retraction (Fig. 8.3). A study on the efficacy of extraction therapy with clear aligners observed greater lingual crown torque and extrusion than predicted [7]. The clinicians neglected to place power ridges or attachments to supplement lingual root torque. They recommended the use of power ridges, attachments, or overcorrection with greater facial crown inclination for torque control in extraction therapy [7]. In extraction cases with significant retraction of the maxillary or mandibular incisors, power ridges can often be combined with intrusion to control both the inclination and vertical position of the incisors. Frequently, the amount of anterior intrusion has to be exaggerated to compensate for bite deepening during retraction, so the Clincheck simulation may show an edge-to-edge overbite at the end of treatment (Fig. 8.4).

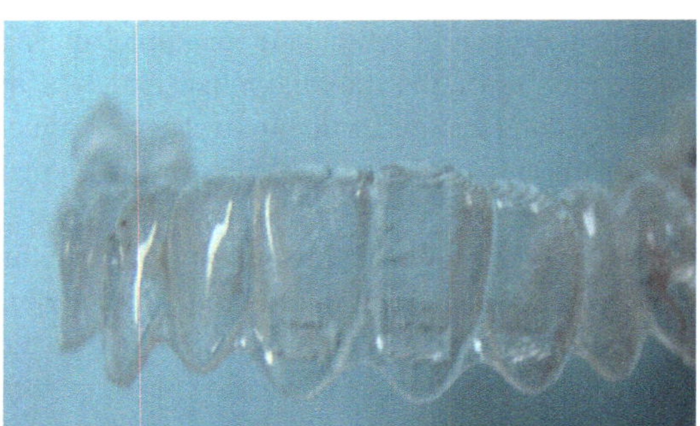

Fig. 8.1 Power ridges or pressure lines have been incorporated into the aligner on the facial surfaces near the gingival margins for the mandibular incisors. The power ridges are employed for supplementing lingual root torque

Posterior Protraction

The incorporation of power ridges is also important for controlling incisor torque when protracting posterior teeth during space closure. In the arch where posterior protraction is desired, the power ridges will function as anterior anchorage to supplement either the maintaining or labialization of the incisors (Fig. 8.5). This use of power ridges is indicated in cases with significant existing spaces, posterior protraction in the maxillary arch in Class III treatment, or posterior protraction in the mandibular arch in Class II treatment. For example, in Class II therapy with four premolar extractions, power ridges should be considered on the mandibular incisors to maintain torque during protraction of the mandibular posterior teeth.

Lingually Displaced Maxillary Lateral Incisors

Lingually displaced maxillary lateral incisors are typically inclined with their roots excessively

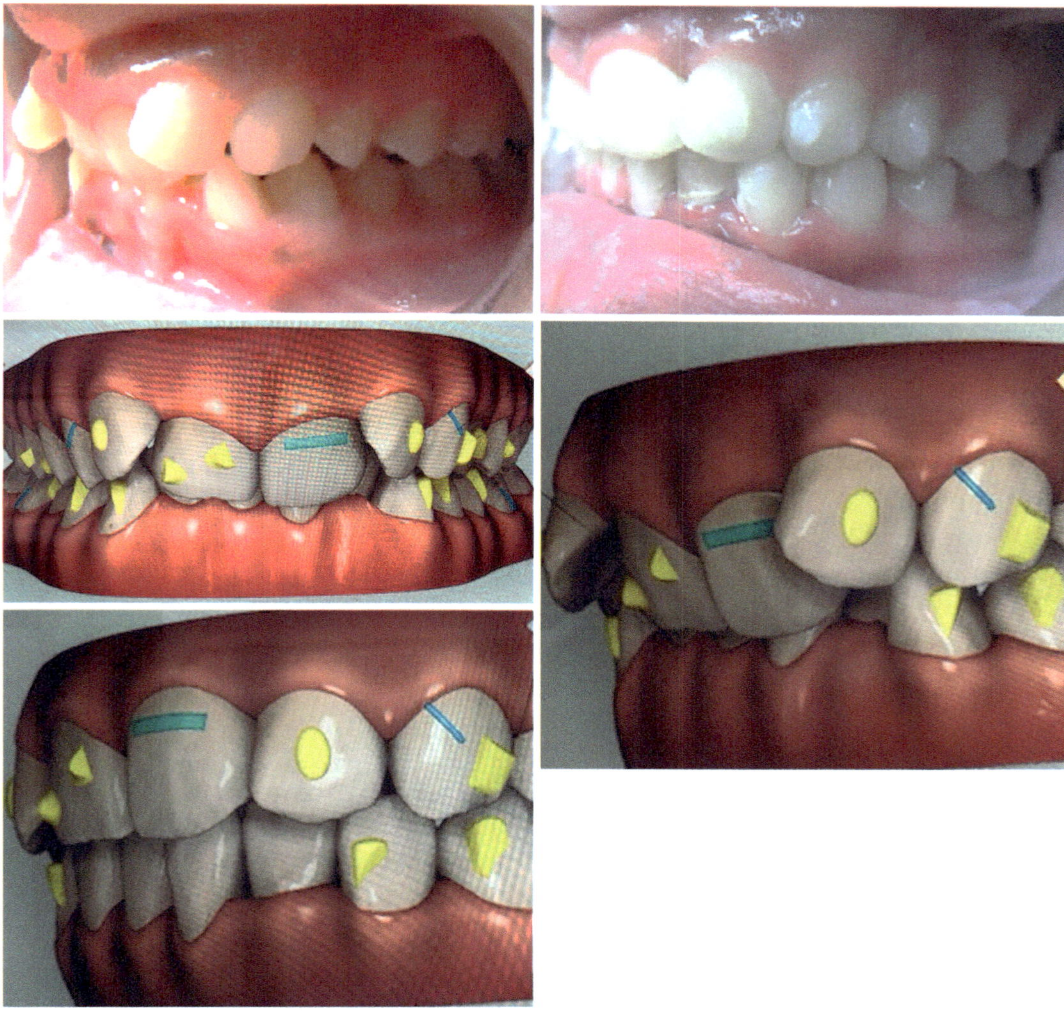

Fig. 8.2 The incorporation of power ridges can be beneficial in correcting excessively lingualized incisors. They are also important in preventing over-retraction of incisors when lingualization is planned

lingual. Therefore, these lateral incisors require significant facial root torque for ideal positioning. Though it has been shown that incisor labial root torque is more accurate than lingual root torque with clear aligners, it is likely significant labial root torque will require the use of adjuncts to achieve the desired movement [3]. In the Invisalign system, supplementing facial root torque is problematic because power ridges can only be placed on the facial surfaces of either maxillary or mandibular incisors. An alternative solution can be to manually alter aligner geometry. Specifically, the clinician can create a pressure line in the linguocervical area of the displaced maxillary lateral incisor with a 3 mm horizontal dimple plier. This pressure line can be incorporated for a series of aligners until the desired amount of facial root torque has been achieved.

However, in the uLab aligner system, pressure lines and pressure points are freely manipulated by the clinician. In this case, for a lingually displaced maxillary lateral incisor, the clinician can prescribe a pressure line on the linguocervical area and a pressure point on the facial surface near the incisal edge. This arrangement will allow

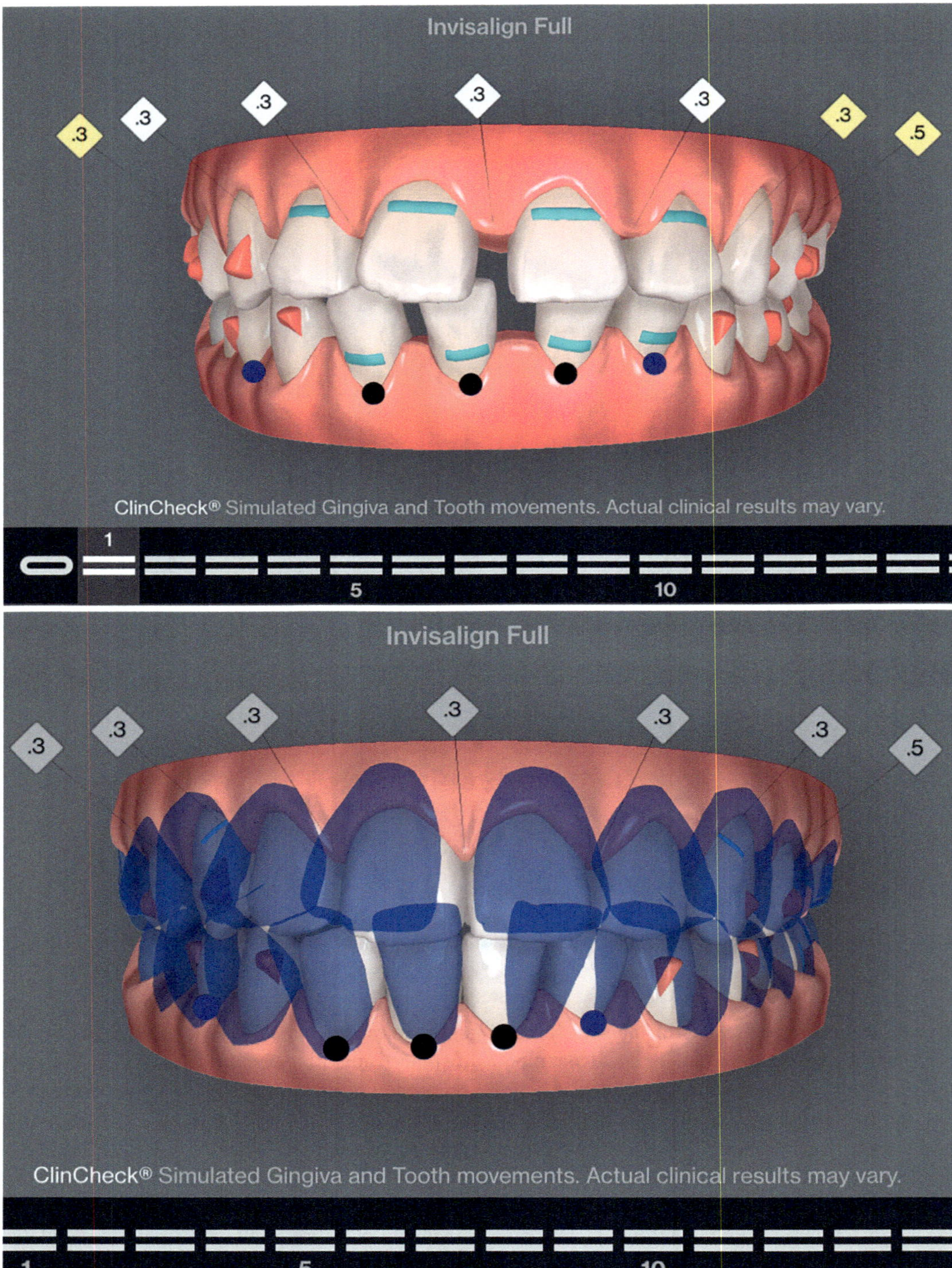

Fig. 8.3 The incorporation of power ridges is essential for maintaining torque during significant incisor retraction. For patient K.C., power ridges were placed on the maxillary and mandibular incisors throughout the course of treatment to maintain torque during incisor retraction for space closure and achievement of ideal overjet. Superimpositions of initial and final tooth positions show significant maxillary and mandibular incisor retraction

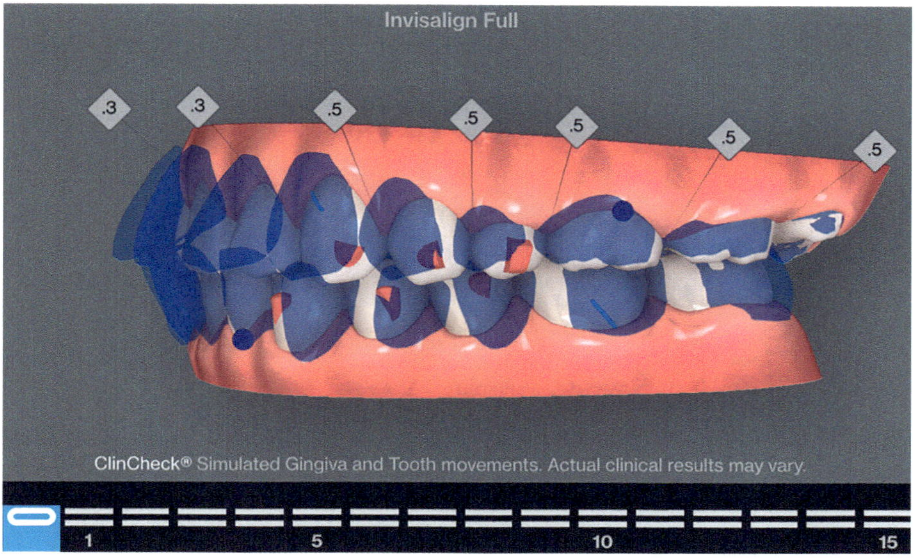

Fig. 8.3 (continued)

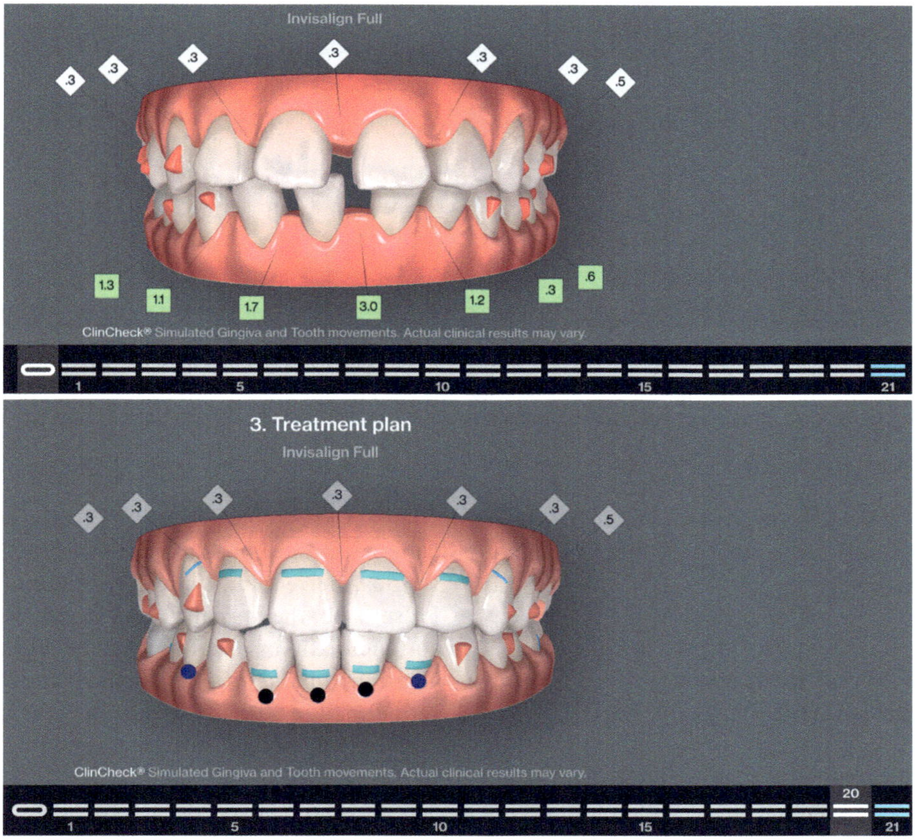

Fig. 8.4 In deep bite cases with significant incisor retraction, requiring control of incisor torque, anterior intrusion may be programmed with power ridges for bite opening and control of incisor inclination. In the treatment of deep bite cases, overbite is routinely overcorrected for more predictable overbite reduction

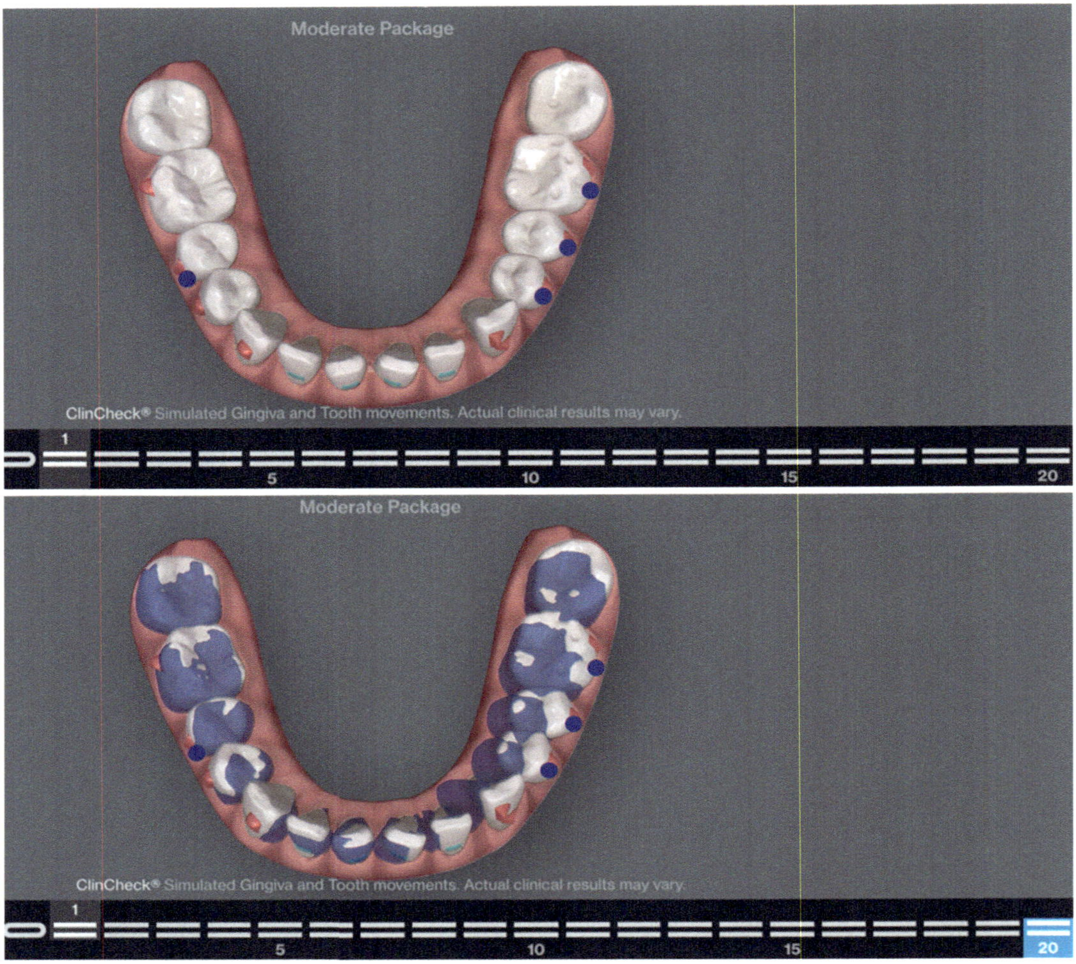

Fig. 8.5 The placement of power ridges assists in maintaining anterior torque during protraction of posterior teeth. For patient X.W., placement of power ridges on the mandibular incisors allowed for torque control during significant mandibular posterior protraction

for the generation of greater coupling moments and improve the accuracy of the facial root torquing movement.

Dental Decompensation for Orthognathic Surgery

Dental decompensation is frequently needed prior to orthognathic surgery in combined surgical and orthodontic treatment. One of the significant components of decompensation is the calibration of incisor inclination to undo compensatory changes and to facilitate surgical correction. For example, prior to Class III surgical correction, typically with a mandibular setback, the maxillary and mandibular incisor inclinations usually must be normalized. The mandibular incisors, which are typically retroclined in Class III malocclusions, must be significantly advanced into normal inclination. In these cases, the incorporation of power ridges would be beneficial for achieving the planned lingual root torque of the mandibular incisors during presurgical dental decompensation (Fig. 8.6).

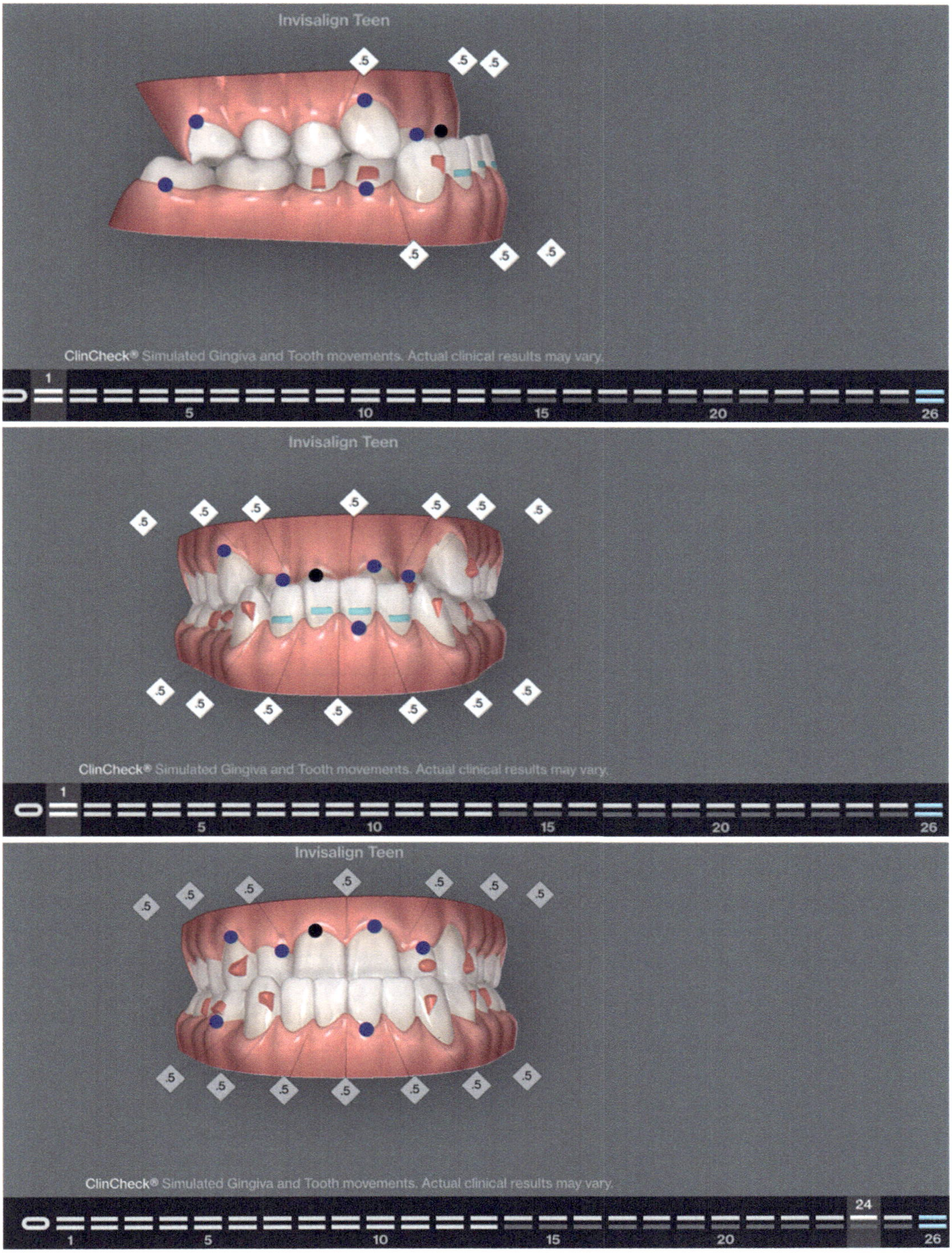

Fig. 8.6 Power ridges can be incorporated for controlling torque during surgical decompensation. For patient L.M., power ridges were placed on the mandibular incisors for enhancing lingual root torque to normalize incisor inclinations prior to a BSSO mandibular setback

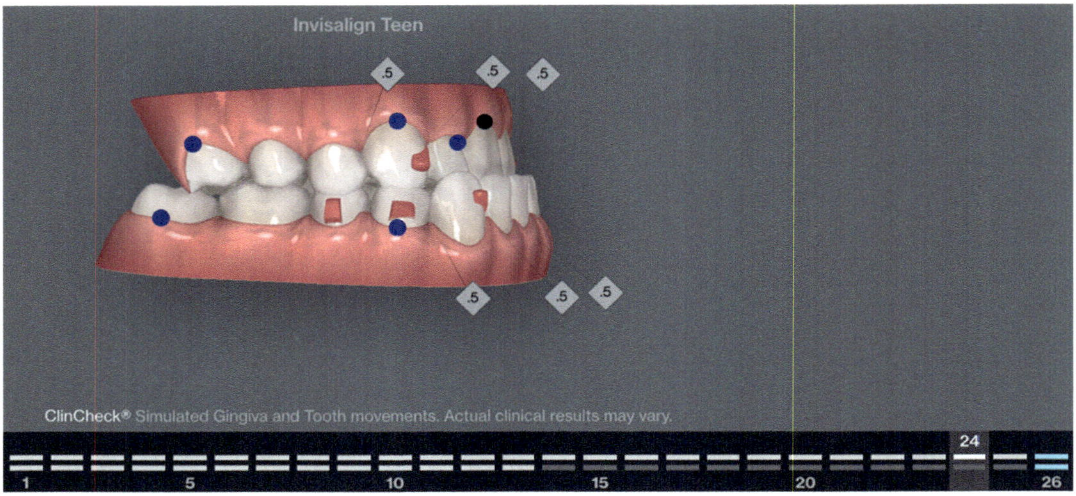

Fig. 8.6 (continued)

Intermaxillary Forces

Power ridges and pressure lines can also be useful in controlling the adverse effects of intermaxillary elastics on incisors. For example, the heavy use of Class III elastics can result in unfavorable lingualizing forces on the mandibular incisors. In these circumstances, to counter this effect, the clinician should consider the incorporation of power ridges on the mandibular incisors to supplement lingual root torque. Conversely, in cases involving the heavy use of Class II elastics, the clinician should consider supplementing labial root torque on the mandibular incisors, either with pressure lines when available or the manual alteration of aligner geometry.

Distalization in Class II Treatment

Power ridges are also important in controlling maxillary incisor torque with Class II division 1 cases treated non-extraction with significant maxillary arch distalization. The power ridges should be considered because of the significant retraction involved (Fig. 8.7a, b). It is important to note that during Clincheck design, the clinician should be mindful in only prescribing the number of stages of power ridges necessary, rather than indiscriminately prescribing power ridges throughout the entire treatment to avoid undesired tooth movements, such as excessive incisor proclination (Fig. 8.7c).

The Efficacy of Power Ridges

Certain in vitro studies have argued that the efficacy of power ridges may be compromised by the nature of the clear aligner appliance [8]. In particular, Hahn et al. showed that because aligners tend to "lift up" during torquing movements, the incisor edge will not remain in close contact with the aligner surface [8]. This biomechanical phenomenon limits the production of an effective force couple for root movement and supports the need for overcorrection. It has also been postulated that the distortion of the aligner during the torquing movement causes an undesired intrusive effect [9]. Nevertheless, these in vitro studies have also concluded that improved root control might be achievable for incisors with the use of attachments and alterations in aligner geometry [10].

Although no clinical trials have rigorously evaluated the efficacy of power ridges for producing root torque, case studies have shown an average of 55–70% of requested lingual root

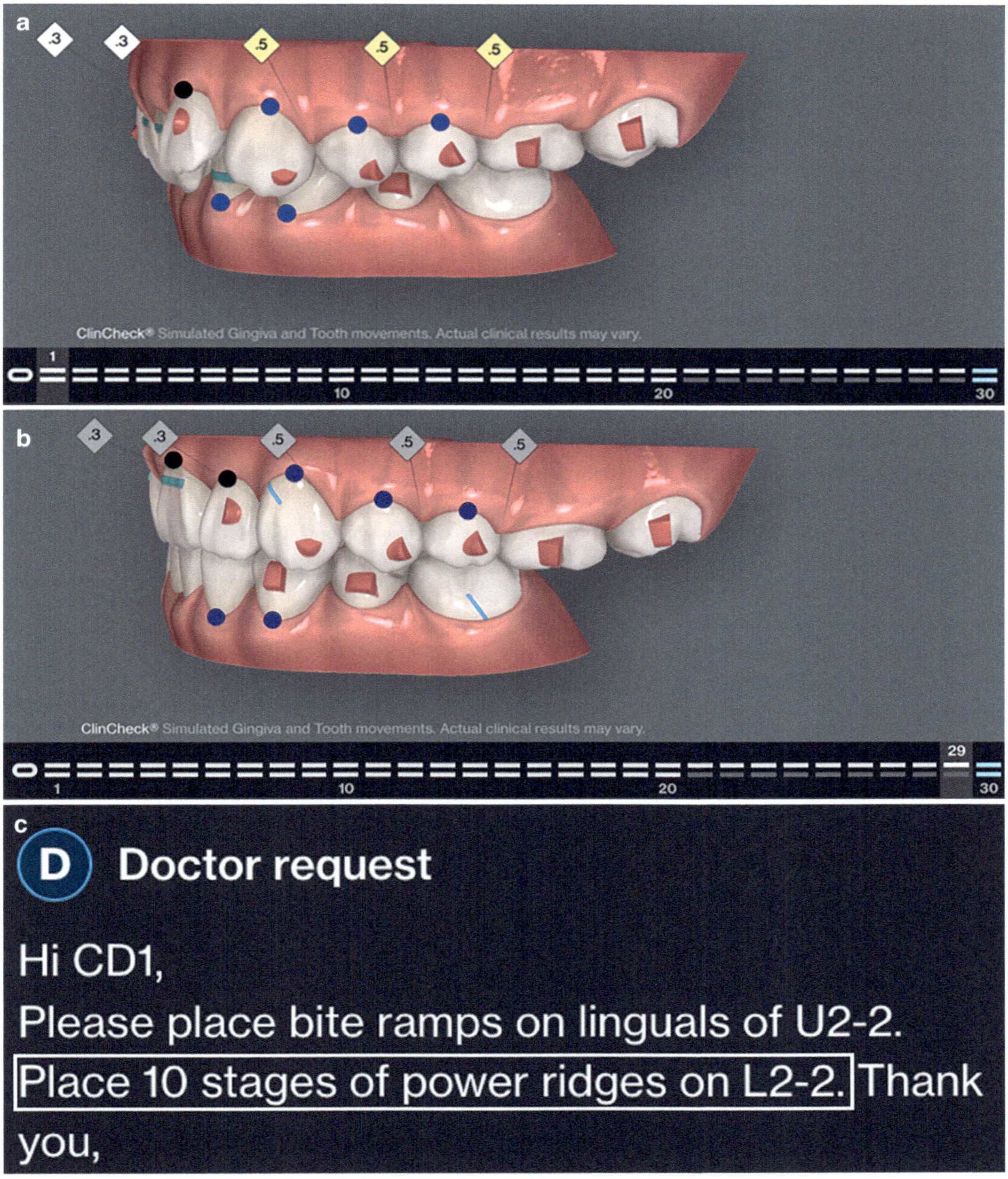

Fig. 8.7 (**a**, **b**) Power ridges should be incorporated for maxillary incisors within normal inclination or that are lingualized during significant retraction. For patient K.W., who presented with a Class II div II malocclusion and severe deep bite, power ridges were placed on the maxillary central incisors during retraction for lingual root torque during the entire duration of the first course of aligners. (**c**) Power ridges can be requested for a specific number of stages rather than the entire treatment to control the amount of lingual root torque and prevent excessive incisor proclination

torque achieved with the incorporation of power ridges [11]. Our clinical findings have shown comparable results of approximately 1° of proclination achieved with 2–3 stages of power ridges. Clinicians should be mindful of this margin of error and consider overcorrection when prescribing power ridges, especially in cases requiring significant root torque.

Torque control can be enhanced by combining pressure lines and pressure points on the incisal region of the opposing surface (as discussed in Chap. 1). For example, lingual root torque can be enhanced by placing the power ridge on the labial surface near the gingival margin of a mandibular incisor in addition to a pressure point on the lingual surface near the incisal edge. Currently, unlike the uLab software which allows for the free manipulation of pressure lines and pressure points, the Invisalign system does not allow the clinician placement of either power ridges or pressure points. Pressure points would have to be manually incorporated with dimple pliers when not automatically placed by the software.

Controlling Torque with Clear Aligners

The incorporation of power ridges is essential for improving torque control during clear aligner treatment. Clinical and in vitro trials have shown the adjunct's efficacy in enhancing the accuracy of root movement. Planned torque is frequently not achieved, likely due to the nature of the clear aligner appliance and the difficulty of root movement. Because of this margin of error, torque control remains a major liability in clear aligner therapy. Consequently, the clinician should consider the judicious use of adjunctive strategies for significant torquing movements and torque control, including pressure lines, pressure points, manual alteration of aligner geometry, and overcorrection.

References

1. Sfondrini MF, Gandini P, Castroflorio T, et al. Buccolingual inclination control of upper central incisors of aligners: a comparison with conventional and self-ligating brackets. Biomed Res Int. 2018;2018:9341821.
2. Haouili N, Kravitz ND, Vaid NR, Ferguson DJ, Makki L. Has Invisalign improved? A prospective follow-up study on the efficacy of tooth movement with Invisalign. Am J Orthod Dentofac Orthop. 2020;158(3):420–5.
3. Jiang T, Jiang YN, Chu FT, Lu PJ, Tang GH. A cone-beam computed tomographic study evaluating the efficacy of incisor movement with clear aligners: assessment of incisor pure tipping, controlled tipping, translation, and torque. Am J Orthod Dentofac Orthop. 2021;159(5):635–43.
4. Pan HY, Yang H, Zhang R, Yang YM, Wang H, Hu T, et al. Use of cone-beam computed tomography to evaluate the prevalence of root fenestration in a Chinese subpopulation. Int Endod J. 2014;47:10–9.
5. Simon M, Keilig L, Schwarze J, Jung BA, Bourauel C. Forces and moments generated by removable thermoplastic aligners: incisor torque, premolar derotation, and molar distalization. Am J Orthod Dentofac Orthop. 2014;145(6):728–36.
6. Simon M, Keilig L, Schwarze J, Jung BA, Bourauel C. Treatment outcome and efficacy of an aligner technique--regarding incisor torque, premolar derotation and molar distalization. BMC Oral Health. 2014;14:68.
7. Dai FF, Xu TM, Shu G. Comparison of achieved and predicted tooth movement of maxillary first molars and central incisors: first premolar extraction treatment with Invisalign. Angle Orthod. 2019;89(5):679–87.
8. Hahn W, Zapf A, Dathe H, Fialka-Fricke J, Fricke-Zech S, Gruber R, Kubein-Meesenburg D, Sadat-Khonsari R. Torquing an upper central incisor with aligners--acting forces and biomechanical principles. Eur J Orthod. 2010;32(6):607–13.
9. Brezniak N. The clear plastic appliance: a biomechanical point of view. Angle Orthod. 2008;78(2):381–2.
10. Bollen AM, Huang G, King G, Hujoel P, Ma T. Activation time and material stiffness of sequential removable orthodontic appliances. Part 1: ability to complete treatment. Am J Orthod Dentofac Orthop. 2003;124(5):496–501.
11. Boyd R. How successful is Invisalign for treatment of anterior open bite and deep overbite? American Association of Orthodontics. 2013. https://www.aaoinfo.org/system/files/media/documents/Boyd,Robert%2D%2DTreatmentofDeepandOpenbitewithClearAligners.pdf. Accessed 13 Jun 2021.

Overcoming Limitations in Extraction Therapy

9

Contents

How Predictable Is Extraction Therapy with Clear Aligners?

Extraction therapy remains one of the most formidable challenges for clear aligners. Clinical trials and case reports have shown that extraction cases with clear aligners often do not achieve predicted outcomes [1]. Notably, teeth adjacent to premolar extraction spaces tend to tip significantly during space closure. Also, in first premolar extraction cases, clear aligners have demonstrated poor incisor torque control, characterized by greater lingual tipping than programmed for the maxillary incisors [2]. Anchorage loss and poor incisor torque control constitute two of the major limitations of extraction therapy with clear aligners.

In 2015, Invisalign introduced the G6 protocol to improve the efficacy of extraction therapy (Fig. 9.1). Specifically, the protocol incorporated optimized attachments on premolars and molars adjacent to extraction spaces for supplementing posterior anchorage and optimized attachments on canines to improve the bodily retraction of canines. Also, the protocol introduced aligner activations or specific force systems to reduce undesired tipping and incisor extrusion during retraction. Early clinical trials have shown greater accuracy with G6-optimized attachments in controlling the mesial translation of first molars when compared to conventional vertical attachments [2]. Other clinical trials have also suggested similar effectiveness as measured by ABO scores between clear aligners and fixed appliances in four premolar extraction cases after the G6 modifications, though the clear aligner cases typically required longer treatment times with courses of refinement [3].

For extraction therapy with clear aligners, strategic treatment planning and Clincheck development and the judicious use of adjuncts and auxiliaries such as power ridges and partial fixed

A. T. Huang, D. Huang, *Controversies in Clear Aligner Therapy*,
https://doi.org/10.1007/978-3-030-92810-0_9

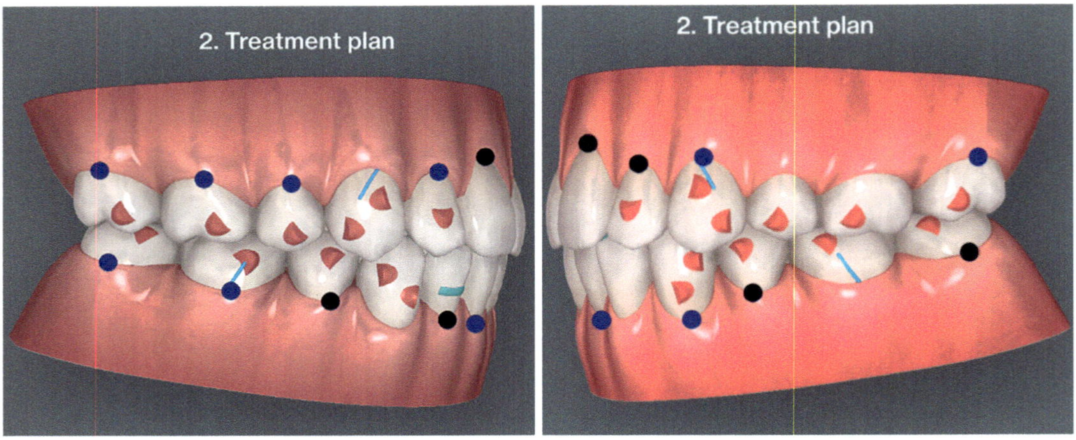

Fig. 9.1 For patient Z. L., we designed a four premolar extraction pattern to decrowd the maxillary and mandibular arches and to reduce the significant overjet. Invisalign's G6 attachments were placed in all four quadrants for space closure with moderate anchorage. The optimized retraction attachments on all four canines allegedly supplement bodily movement during retraction, while the optimized moderate anchorage attachments on the premolars and molars supposedly enhance posterior anchorage during space closure

appliances are essential for ideal outcomes. The careful planning of incisor retraction and space closure with adjunctive measures such as virtual gable bends can minimize undesired tooth movements. The incorporation of auxiliaries such as a course of partial fixed appliances can be applied either during or after clear aligner therapy to assist in achieving planned movements by uprighting tipped teeth adjacent to extraction sites [4]. Anchorage management can also be supplemented with intermaxillary elastics and auxiliary miniscrews.

In this chapter, we describe the current limitations of extraction therapy with clear aligners. We then discuss both current and prospective approaches in treatment planning and mechanotherapy for their management.

Treatment Planning Considerations for Predictable Extraction Therapy

Premolar extractions in the mandible are usually more challenging than those in the maxilla, most likely due to resistance to bodily movement from the greater density of the mandible [5]. As a result, significant undesired tipping can occur in the teeth adjacent to extraction sites in both arches, often with greater severity in the mandible (Fig. 9.2) [6]. Studies have shown a trend for greater tipping of mandibular teeth into extraction spaces when compared to that of maxillary teeth [1]. Therefore, it would be prudent for the clinician to consider atypical extraction patterns instead of four premolar extractions. Commonly, an atypical pattern of extraction such as the extraction of maxillary premolars and IPR or the extraction of a mandibular incisor can be a viable alternative for the treatment of crowding in the mandibular arch. An atypical extraction pattern can often minimize the adverse effects of conventional four premolar extractions, including excessive tipping of teeth adjacent to extraction sites, lateral open bites, and loss of torque in the mandibular incisors (Fig. 9.3). Therefore, the clinician should plan for two premolar extractions in the mandibular arch, along with extractions of two maxillary premolars, only when truly necessary.

Clincheck Development for Extraction Therapy

Tipping During Space Closure

In Clincheck development for extraction therapy, it is important to judiciously plan space closure to minimize adverse effects, especially

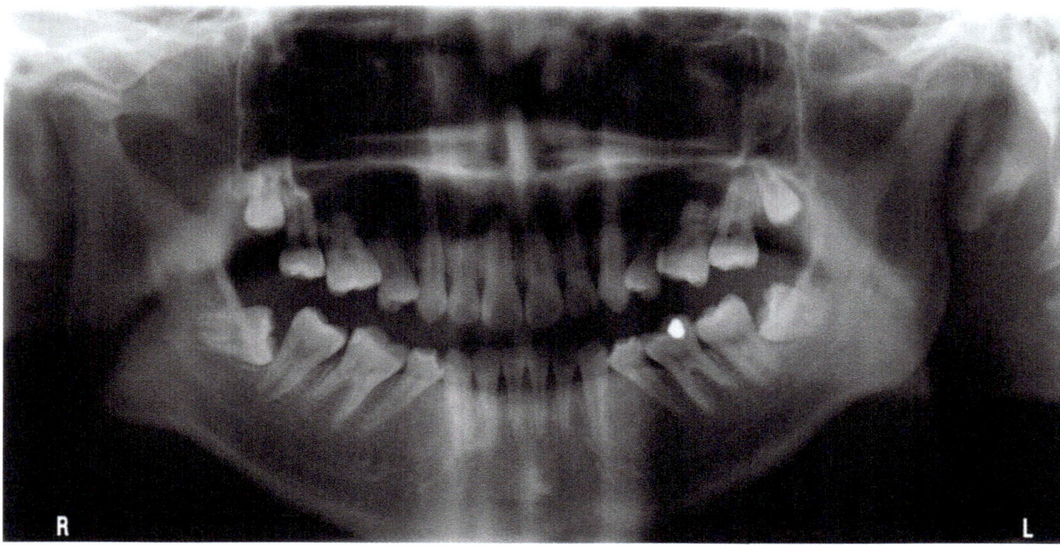

Fig. 9.2 Excessive tipping tends to occur with more severity in teeth adjacent to mandibular extraction sites compared to those adjacent to maxillary extraction sites. Excessive tipping in the mandible can be avoided or minimized with treatment planning for atypical extractions and careful virtual setups of extraction space closure

excessive tipping in the teeth adjacent to the extraction space. One of the current limitations of available clear aligner software is that they do not allow the clinician to visualize the movements produced by virtual gable bends (VGB). As a result, the clinician can only approximate the predicted effects of the VGB. Ideally, clear aligner software should display the precise movements created by the VGB so the clinician can adjust its staging. At present, the clinician can only request a certain number of stages of VGB, with an arbitrary amount of movement produced in each stage. Nevertheless, the clinician should ensure that the VGB has been incorporated during extraction space closure to prevent excessive tipping and to achieve root parallelism.

In addition to the VGB, the clinician should consider overcorrection of root movement to prevent excessive crown tipping (Fig. 9.4). The overcorrection can be requested along with the VGB. Overcorrection during extraction therapy has been advocated for movements challenging for aligners, such as body movement during space closure and lingual root torque for incisors during retraction [2]. The clinician should be mindful that the application of anterior lingual root torque will result in a reciprocal mesial tipping force for the first molar [7]. As a result, the clinician should consider overcorrecting distal crown tip, analogous to a tip-back bend in fixed appliances. Studies have suggested that overcorrecting the distal tip of first molars in addition to attachment use during space closure might help counteract a mesial tipping force and maintain tooth angulation for more bodily tooth movement.

Ideally, excessive tipping and associated adverse effects including lateral open bite could be controlled through the incorporation of pressure points or power ridges on the lingual surfaces of posterior teeth. Early studies have demonstrated that the G6 optimized attachment showed improved resistance to mesial tipping of maxillary molars compared to conventional attachments [2]. Opposing pressure points could enhance G6 optimized attachments to produce a coupling effect and more bodily translation (Fig. 9.5).

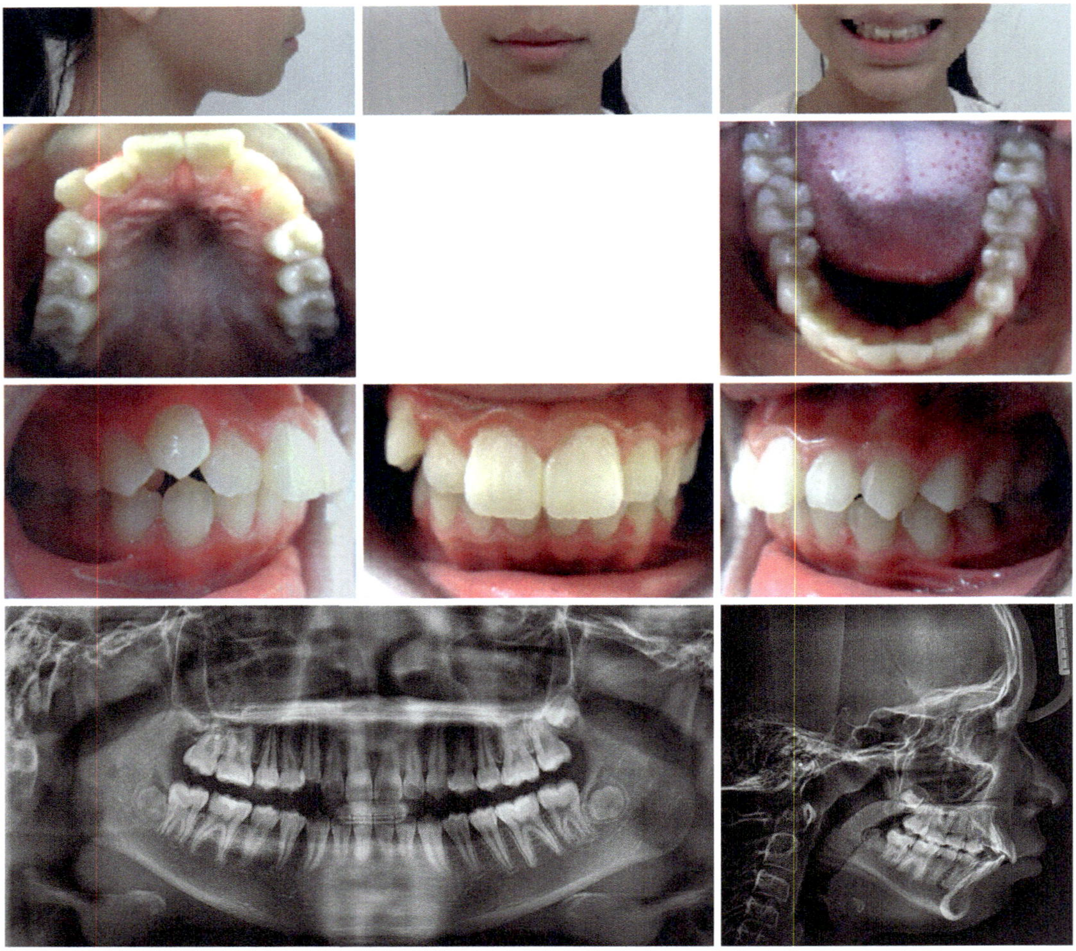

Fig. 9.3 In patient K.J., an atypical extraction pattern of two maxillary first premolars and IPR in the lower arch allowed for avoiding adverse effects, such as lateral open bite, excessive tipping of mandibular posterior teeth, and loss of torque in the mandibular incisors. Nearly ideal root parallelism was achieved, as shown by the final panoramic radiograph

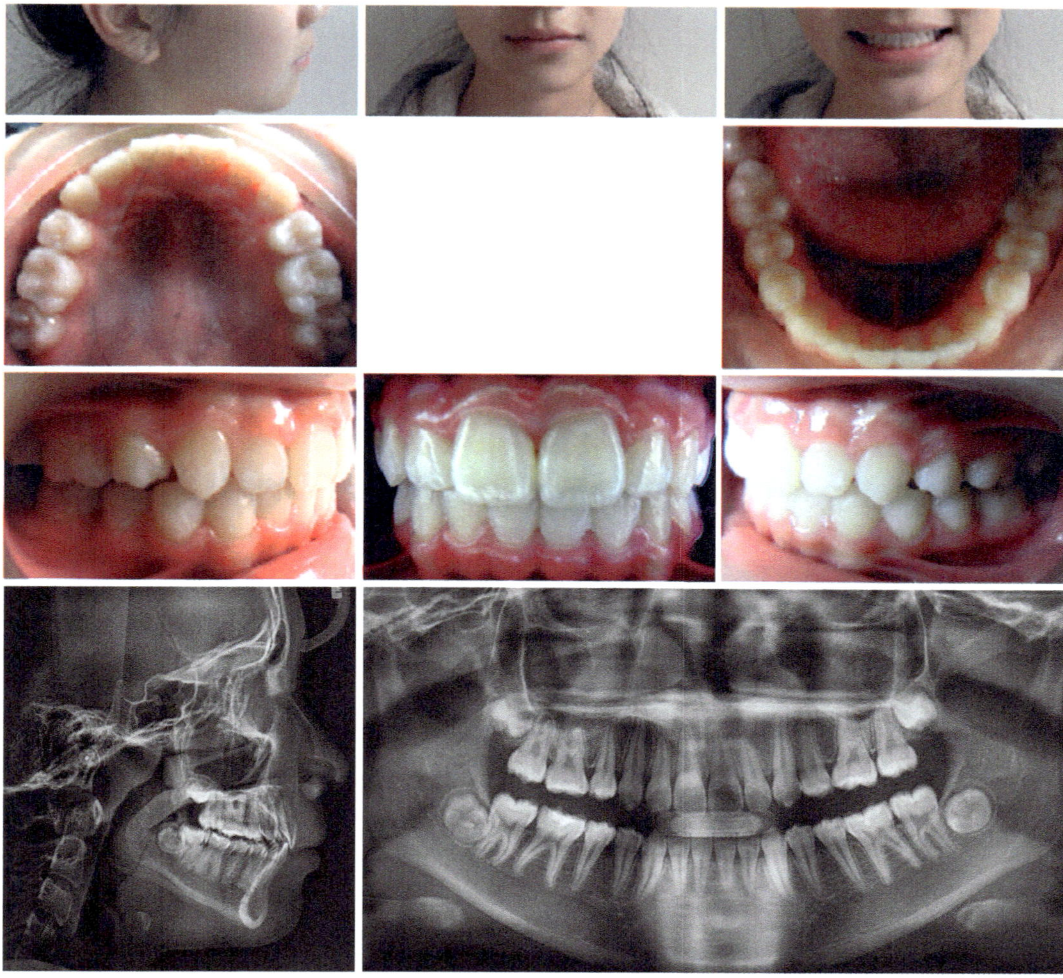

Fig. 9.3 (continued)

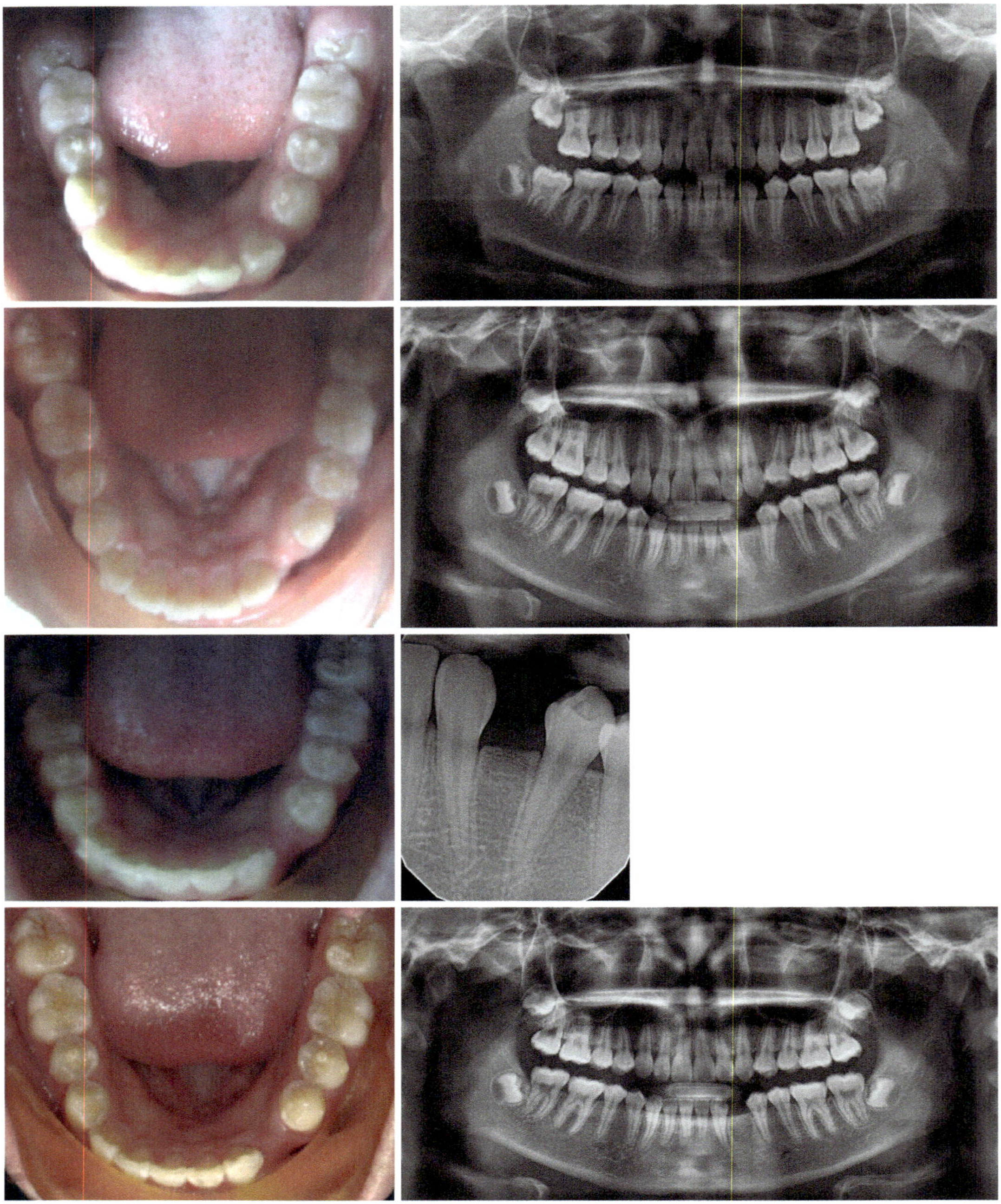

Fig. 9.4 For patient N.P., an implant space for the mandibular left canine was required, as the mandibular left canine was planned to substitute the congenitally missing left mandibular lateral incisor. In the first course of aligners, which lasted 10 months, the mandibular left canine was mesialized, while the mandibular left first premolar was distalized to create an implant space between the two teeth. However, a VGB was not incorporated in the first course, leading to excessive tipping of both teeth and poor root parallelism. In a 12-month refinement course, a VGB in addition to overcorrection of root movement was incorporated to separate the roots. The addition of the VGB and overcorrection of root movement allowed for full separation of the canine and premolar roots

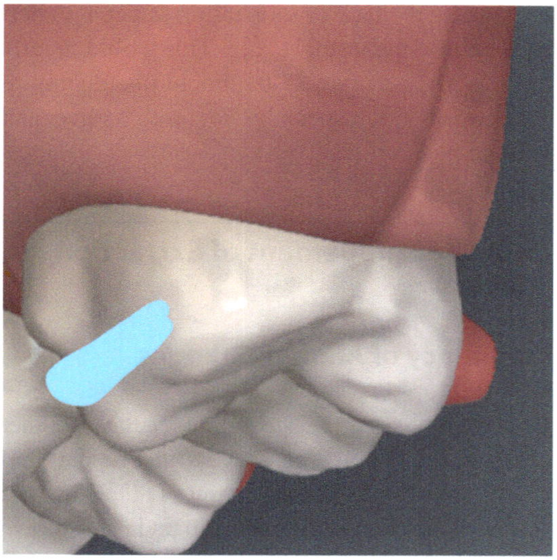

Fig. 9.5 Ideally, a pressure point could be incorporated on the lingual surfaces of the posterior teeth near their occlusal tables. The pressure point's buccal force can oppose the lingual force created by the G6 attachment to produce a couple. This couple would allow for more bodily translation of posterior teeth during space closure

Considerations for Posterior Protraction

One of the most important considerations during Clincheck development is the amount of posterior protraction during space closure. If the posterior teeth are planned for significant protraction, such as >3 mm, then the clinician should anticipate excessive crown tipping, lateral open bite, and loss of incisor torque. During extraction therapy, the greater the amount of planned translation, the greater the likelihood for crown tipping. This is supported by clinical trials which have shown that extraction therapy in cases with greater crowding showed less translation and less mesial tipping of first molars [2]. It has also been demonstrated that less anchorage loss is correlated with greater severity of initial crowding [8]. In crowded arches, the extraction space is predominately used for relieving crowding and anterior retraction instead of posterior protraction. The clinician should be cautious in planning for extraction therapy involving significant posterior protraction and consider a non-extraction approach to avoid adverse effects.

Controlling Posterior Torque

Controlling buccolingual inclination of the posterior teeth is essential for achieving proper posterior interdigitation, ideal buccal overjet, and preventing occlusal interferences. Commonly, the posterior teeth exhibit inadequate buccal root torque, resulting in plunging palatal cusps, occlusal interferences, and lateral open bites. To achieve proper posterior buccolingual inclination, the clinician should ensure in the virtual setup that the arches are sufficiently expanded and the posterior maxillary molars have adequate buccal root torque [4].

Invisalign's G8 modifications have supposedly improved the application of buccal root torque during posterior expansion through optimized expansion attachments and specific contouring in aligner surfaces [9]. However, the efficacy of the G8 modifications has not been rigorously evaluated and they are frequently not triggered in extraction cases (G8 activation is only triggered when a specific amount of expansion has been programmed). Ideally, aligner activation should be default whenever significant buccal root torque is programmed. Likewise, power ridges or pressure points should be made available for posterior teeth to supplement buccal root torque in the Invisalign software, although they can be currently incorporated in the uLab software (Fig. 9.6).

Controlling Incisors During Retraction

One of the primary challenges of extraction therapy is controlling incisor torque and vertical position during retraction. Incisors tend to demonstrate greater lingual tipping than programmed leading to over-retraction and deep overbites [2]. Often, the clinician will have to overcorrect the planned intrusion of the maxillary incisors to prevent excessive bite deepening (Fig. 9.7). This is in accordance with recommendations from studies which have suggested overcorrection to improve the efficacy of anterior intrusive movements [10]. As discussed in Chap. 6, overcorrec-

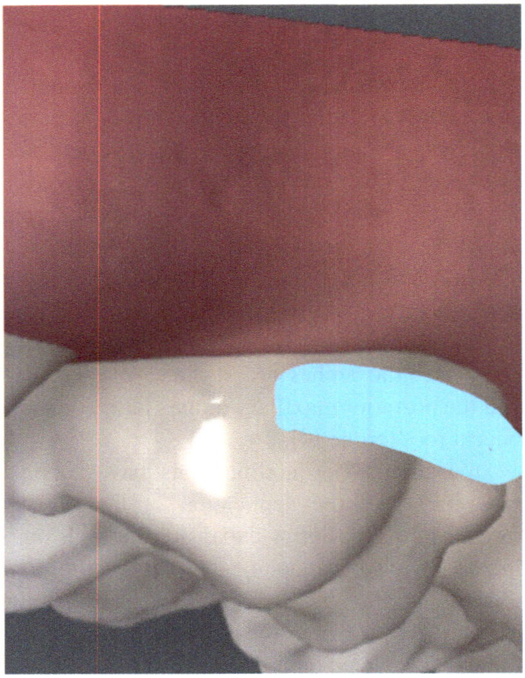

Fig. 9.6 Ideally, the incorporation of a power ridge or pressure point on the lingual surfaces of posterior teeth near their cervical areas can supplement buccal root torque during extraction therapy. However, at present, the Invisalign software does not allow a power ridge or pressure point placement on lingual surfaces or on posterior teeth (though the uLab software does offer these options). It is important to confirm in the software that posterior teeth have adequate buccal root torque to prevent plunging palatal cusps, occlusal interferences, and lateral open bites

tion of intrusion for the incisors will often result in a final simulated overbite that appears shallow. The incorporation of power ridges in extraction arches should also be considered, especially if initial incisor inclinations are within normal range or retroclined. Studies have also advocated overcorrecting lingual root torque for incisors during the virtual setup for torque control.

In patients who initially present with excessively deep overbites and vertical maxillary excess, the use of anterior TADs should be considered to supplement maxillary incisor intrusion and to avoid bite deepening during incisor retraction (Fig. 9.7).

One of the limitations in controlling incisors during extraction therapy with the various current software is the lack of integration of cephalometric data into the virtual setup. This would greatly improve the accuracy of treatment planning incisor movements, especially for both torque and vertical position (Fig. 9.8).

Clinical Management of Extraction Therapy

Frequency of Aligner Changes

Invisalign has suggested that 7-day aligner changes are viable for successful clinical outcomes and shorter treatment times [11]. However, studies have contested this claim and have shown that complex movements such as distal crown tipping, buccal-crown torque, and mandibular posterior intrusion were more accurate with 14-day aligner changes when compared to both 7 and 10-day aligner changes [12]. Early studies also demonstrated that patients with 14-day aligner changes were more likely to complete a course of aligners compared to those changing aligners weekly [13]. Considering the complexity of the movements involved in extraction therapy, which include significant posterior crown tipping and torquing, 14-day aligner changes are recommended for accurate tooth movement. This 14-day regimen would be especially recommended for adults, whose velocity of orthodontic tooth movement has been shown to be slower than that of children [14].

Tipping During Therapy

Commonly, the teeth adjacent to the extraction site will excessively tip during the course of therapy and manifest as poor tracking with the aligner. In these cases, the clinician can consider extending wear time for the patient on the poorly tracking aligner to allow for more movement on the tipped teeth toward their programmed positions. The clinician can also incorporate pressure points with hand instruments onto the aligner in problematic areas for improved tracking and

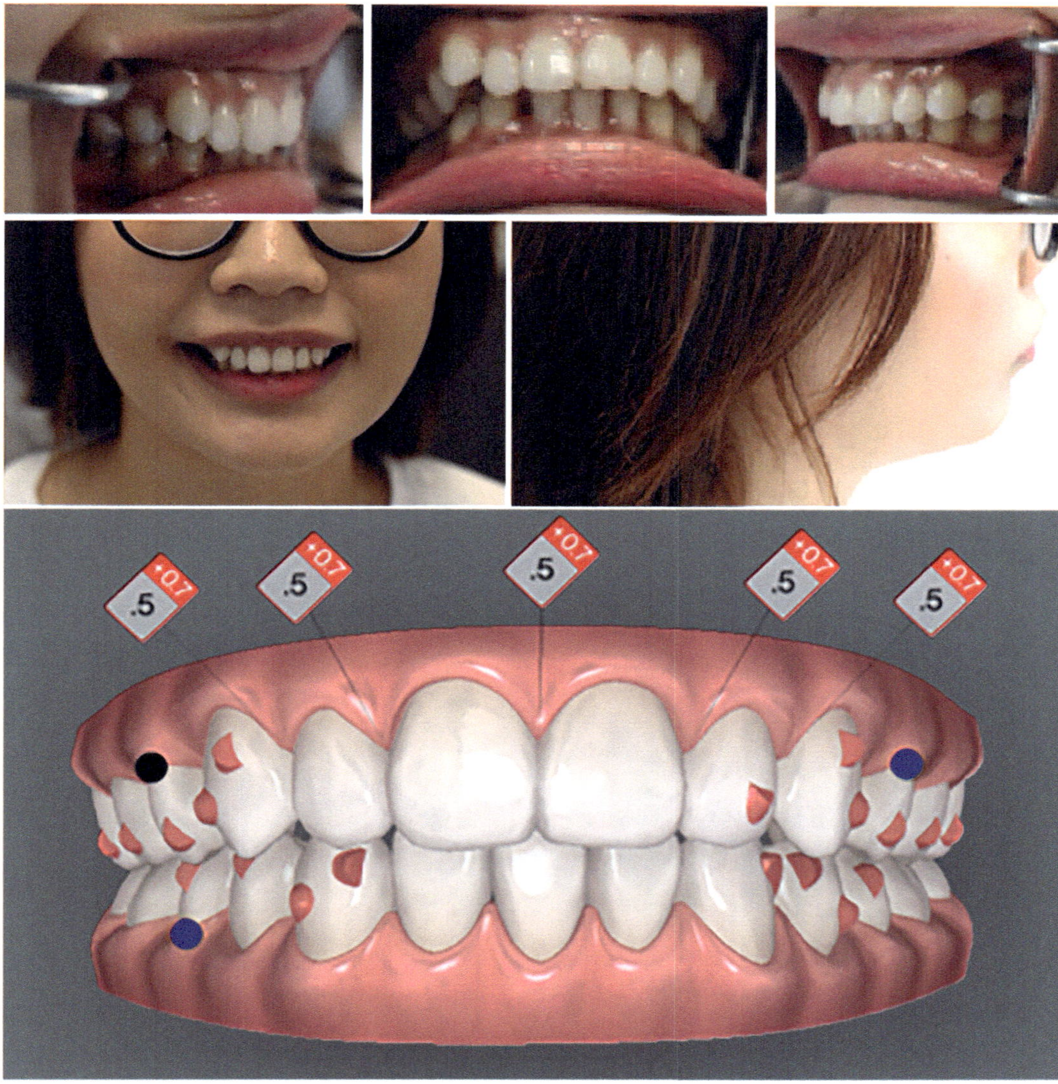

Fig. 9.7 In patient W.W., a clinician extracted maxillary first premolars with poor torque control of the maxillary incisors during retraction. As a result, there was a significant loss of incisor torque, as shown by the progress cephalometric radiograph. The loss of torque also led to incisor extrusion, bite deepening, and an unesthetic increase of gingival display. The clinician planned for inadequate intrusion and lingual root torque on the maxillary incisors. The clinician also planned for a final bite that was excessively deep. To minimize the gingival display, TADs will be placed distal to the maxillary lateral incisors for an intrusive force. The incisors will have to be torqued and significantly intruded to aid in bite opening

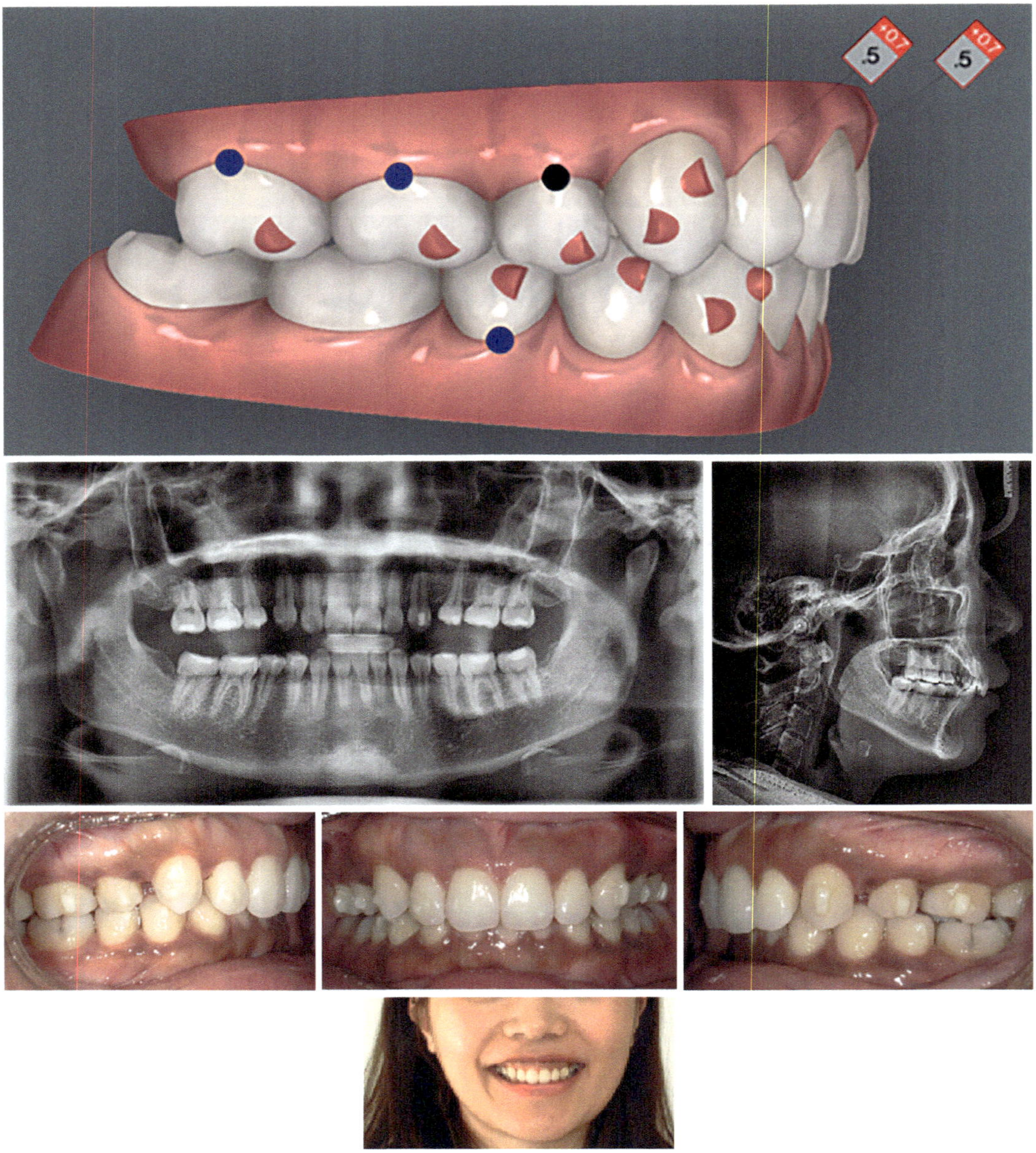

Fig. 9.7 (continued)

encapsulation. For example, dimples can be placed in the cervical area of the aligner to improve retention for an excessively tipped molar. Importantly, addressing poor tracking during the course of aligners can minimize the duration of refinement and the need for auxiliaries, including partial fixed appliances.

Combination Treatment

The timely intervention with combination treatment is essential for successful outcomes and minimizing treatment times in clear aligner extraction therapy. Frequently, excessively tipped teeth adjacent to extraction sites will require aux-

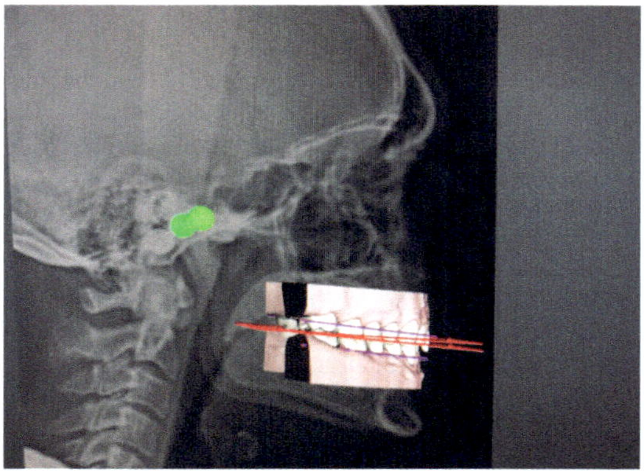

Fig. 9.8 At present, no software has fully integrated cephalometric data with teeth movement. Ideally, clear aligner software should allow for projections of cephalometric changes over the course of treatment. This integration would allow for more precise planning of incisor movements in all dimensions

iliary methods for uprighting. The clinician should consider either partial braces or metal buttons for vertical elastics prior to a course of refinement (Fig. 9.9) [6]. After the posterior crowns have been significantly uprighted, a refinement course can be employed for additional detailing and finishing. A comparison between fixed appliances and clear aligners in the treatment of first premolar extraction cases showed comparable efficacy but as much as 7 months of refinement for cases treated with clear aligners [3]. This method of timely combination treatment can more predictably upright tipped crowns and lessen the duration of the refinement course and overall treatment time.

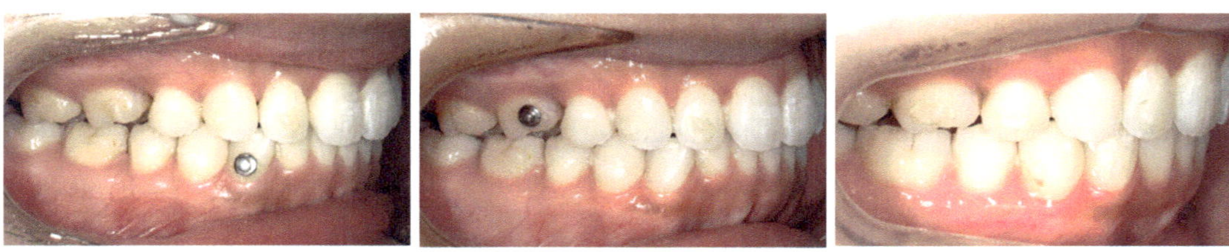

Fig. 9.9 The addition of an auxiliary at the end of the first course of aligners during extraction therapy can correct tipped posterior teeth in an efficient manner. For this patient, a button was bonded on the maxillary right molar for vertical elastics to the opposite arch (usually a precision cut on the right mandibular second premolar). After 3 months of vertical elastic wear, the molar was extruded into ideal inclination and proper interdigitation prior to a refinement for detailing and finishing

Improving the Efficacy of Clear Aligner Extraction Therapy

Recent studies have suggested improved efficacy for extraction therapy with clear aligners due to the G6 protocol and the use of auxiliaries [15]. However, the method is still limited by major liabilities during space closure and anterior teeth retraction, which can result in loss of anterior torque, deepening of overbite, excessive tipping of teeth adjacent to extraction sites, and poor posterior interdigitation. These sequelae can be minimized or avoided through treatment planning in view of the appliance's typical behavior with extraction therapy, judicious planning of incisal and molar movements during the virtual setup, and timely treatment modification, with auxiliaries as necessary, during the course of therapy. These methods aim at improving the predictability of movements during extraction therapy and therefore minimizing adverse effects. It is evident the future of clear aligner extraction therapy lies in innovating its biomechanical features, whether within the aligner material or its auxiliaries, for producing more ideal force systems for more accurate movements.

References

1. Baldwin DK, King G, Ramsay DS, Huang G, Bollen AM. Activation time and material stiffness of sequential removable orthodontic appliances. Part 3: premolar extraction patients. Am J Orthod Dentofac Orthop. 2008;133(6):837–45.
2. Dai FF, Xu TM, Shu G. Comparison of achieved and predicted tooth movement of maxillary first molars and central incisors: first premolar extraction treatment with Invisalign. Angle Orthod. 2019;89(5):679–87.
3. Gaffuri F, Cossellu G, Lanteri V, Brotto E, Farronato M. Comparative effectiveness of Invisalign and fixed appliances in first-premolar extraction cases. J Clin Orthod. 2020;52(5):294–301.
4. Bowman SJ, Celenza F, Sparaga J, Papadopoulos MA, Ojima K, Lin JC. Creative adjuncts for clear aligners, part 3: extraction and interdisciplinary treatment. J Clin Orthod. 2015;49(4):249–62.
5. Devlin H, Horner K, Ledgerton D. A comparison of maxillary and mandibular bone mineral densities. J Prosthet Dent. 1998;79(3):323–7.
6. Zhu Y, Li X, Lai W. Treatment of severe anterior crowding with the Invisalign G6 first-premolar extraction solution. J Clin Orthod. 2019;53(8):459–69.
7. Tuncay O, Bowman SJ, Amy B, Nicozisis J. Aligner treatment in the teenage patient. J Clin Orthod. 2013;47:115–9.
8. Geron S, Shpack N, Kandos S, Davidovitch M, Vardimon AD. Anchorage loss--a multifactorial response. Angle Orthod 2003;73(6):730–37.
9. Align Technology. Align Technology announces Invisalign G8 with new Smartforce aligner activation features. 2020. https://investor.aligntech.com/news-releases/news-release-details/align-technology-announces-invisalign-g8-new-smartforce. Accessed 25 Jul 2021.
10. Haouili N, Kravitz ND, Vaid NR, Ferguson DJ, Makki L. Has Invisalign improved? A prospective follow-up study on the efficacy of tooth movement with Invisalign. Am J Orthod Dentofac Orthop. 2020;158(3):420–5.
11. Fry R. Weekly aligner changes to improve Invisalign treatment efficiency. J Clin Orthod. 2017;51(12):786–91.
12. Al-Nadawi M, Kravitz ND, Hansa I, Makki L, Ferguson DJ, Vaid NR. Effect of clear aligner wear protocol on the efficacy of tooth movement. Angle Orthod. 2021;91(2):157–63.
13. Bollen AM, Huang G, King G, Hujoel P, Ma T. Activation time and material stiffness of sequential removable orthodontic appliances. Part 1: ability to complete treatment. Am J Orthod Dentofac Orthop. 2003;124(5):496–501.
14. Dudic A, Giannopoulou C, Kiliaridis S. Factors related to the rate of orthodontically induced tooth movement. Am J Orthod Dentofac Orthop. 2013;143(5):616–21.
15. Gaffuri F, Cossellu G, Lanteri V, Brotto E, Farronato M. Comparative effectiveness of Invisalign and fixed appliances in firstpremolar extraction cases. J Clin Orthod. 2020;52(5):294–301.

The Predictability of Bite Jumps 10

Contents

What Are Bite Jumps?

Bite jumps constitute a significant feature of virtual setups for the treatment of complex malocclusions. The bite jumps simulate extensive movements in the maxilla, mandible, or a combination, resulting in changes in maxillomandibular relationships. These include large anteroposterior movements, rotation of the maxilla or mandible for anterior open bite closure, and rotation of the maxilla or mandible about a vertical axis for the correction of asymmetries. Currently, the Invisalign software possesses the most developed bite jump feature among available software for anteroposterior, vertical, and transverse movements in either the maxilla or mandible. The clinician can select the bite jump in the prescription form for the virtual setup or request a bite jump during the development of the setup.

The most common issues associated with bite jumps are its proper indications and its timing for use during therapy. During the virtual setup, the bite jump should be considered as a projected change in skeletal relationships in the anteroposterior, vertical, or transverse dimensions. The primary indications for the bite jump include growing patients in which the clinician anticipates significant jaw growth, open bite closure involving mandibular autorotation, and cases involving orthognathic surgical correction. The use of the bite jump to project unrealistic movements such as extensive space closure or significant Class II correction in the absence of a functional regulator or growth can result in the planning of unachievable dental and jaw movements and an inaccurate virtual setup.

A. T. Huang, D. Huang, *Controversies in Clear Aligner Therapy*,
https://doi.org/10.1007/978-3-030-92810-0_10

The bite jump can be incorporated as a single stage or as a series of stages for incremental skeletal movements. Typically, a single stage is employed to simulate open bite closure or surgical correction, though the precise timing of open bite closure in nonsurgical treatments can be difficult to predict. Multiple incremental stages would be applicable for treatment with a functional regulator, such as the MA appliance. This setup would simulate the effects of traditional functional appliances, which have shown greater short-term gains in Class II correction with incremental mandibular advancement when compared to maximal mandibular advancement [1]. A shorter series of stages can also be incorporated to simulate maxillary arch distalization with a distalizing appliance.

In this chapter, we describe the major indications, contraindications, and principles for the use of the bite jump in virtual setups for accurate treatment planning and predictable outcomes. We will also consider their application in both growing and nongrowing patients, as well as in cases involving functional regulators, orthopedic appliances, distalizing appliances, and orthognathic surgery.

Indications for Bite Jumps

Growing Patients

One of the most essential indications for bite jumps is the realistic simulation of skeletal growth in growing children and adolescents (Table 10.1). The bite jump is frequently indicated for Phase I treatment with clear aligners, or Invisalign First, as these patients are certain to experience significant jaw growth during treatment. In particular, the bite jump should be prescribed for growing Class II or Class III patients to predict anteroposterior orthopedic changes. For example, as discussed in Chap. 2, a Class III patient can be treated with a combination approach consisting of clear aligners and RPFM for maxillary protraction. The incorporation of a bite jump would be necessary to simulate both the significant forward movement of the maxilla and the jumping of the anterior crossbite (Fig. 10.1).

Table 10.1 The common indications and contraindications for the use of the bite jump

Indications	Contraindications
Growing patients	Correction of excessive overjet without adequate mechanotherapy
Mandibular autorotation during open bite closure	Extraction space closure
Orthognathic surgery	TAD-assisted movements
Dental functional shift	Extensive space closure

Similarly, a Class II patient can be treated with a combination approach consisting of clear aligners and a Class II orthopedic appliance, such as the cervical headgear. This form of therapy would also require a bite jump to simulate the forward growth of the mandible during treatment. The incorporation of the bite jump would allow for a more realistic representation of the Class II correction (Fig. 10.2). When planning for a bite jump, the clinician should also consider the amount of growth remaining with growth indicators frequently used for the treatment of Class II malocclusions, such as the hand and wrist maturation method, standing height, and the cervical vertebrae maturation method (CVM) [2]. For Class II patients with little to no growth remaining, a bite jump simulating significant forward movement of the mandible would be contraindicated (unless the clinician were planning for a surgical correction).

Importantly, in Phase I treatment with growing patients, the bite jump would also be indicated for Class II and Class III patients treated with clear aligners and intermaxillary elastics (without an orthopedic appliance). Though it has been shown that the effects of intermaxillary elastics are primarily dentoalveolar, a bite jump would still be indicated because the growing patient will predictably experience significant mandibular growth [3]. The clinician can program the bite jump to simulate jaw growth during therapy (Fig. 10.3).

In patients treated with clear aligners and the mandibular advancement feature, the bite jump

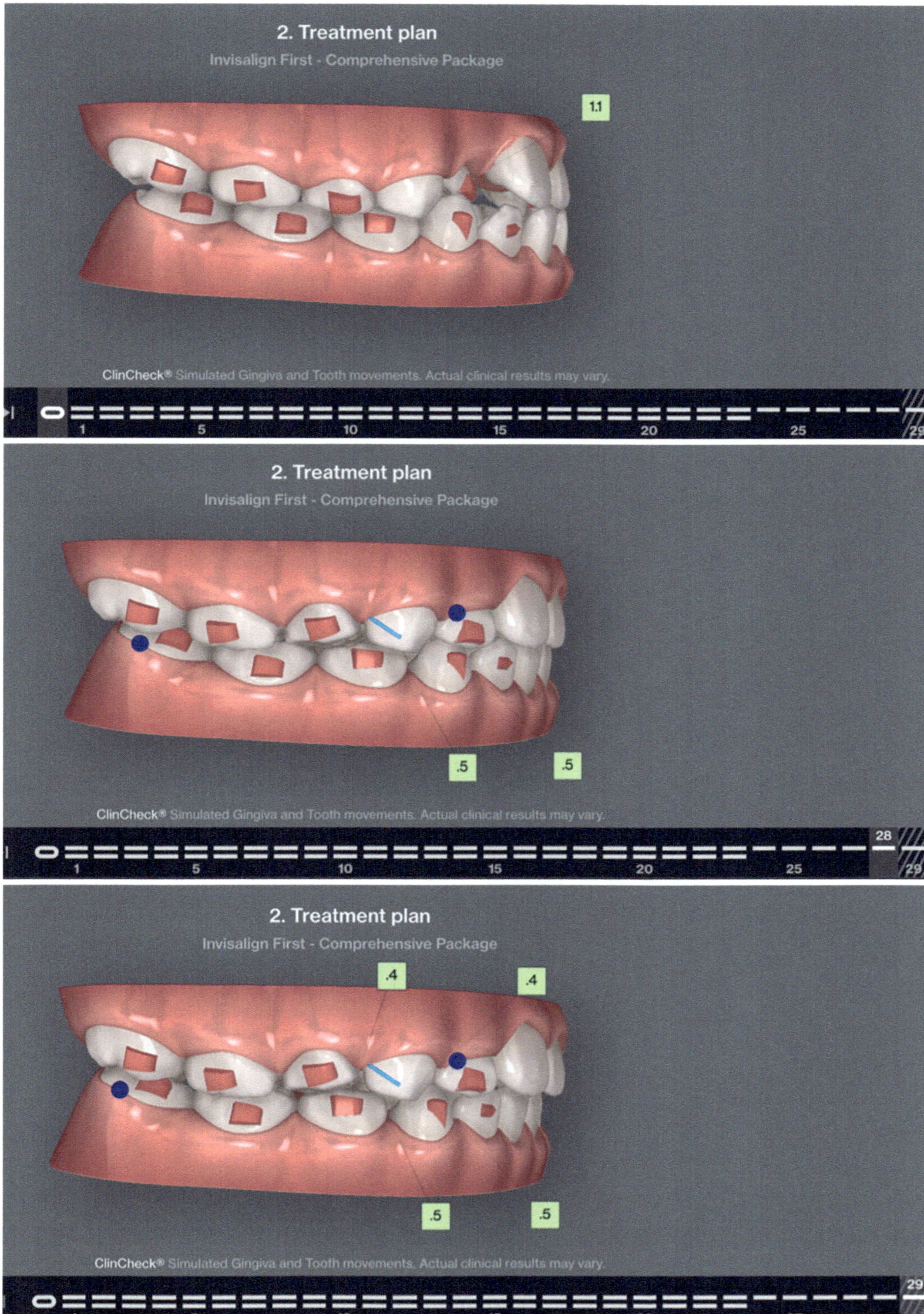

Fig. 10.1 For patient A.P., a bite jump was planned for stage 29 to represent forward movement of the maxilla through growth and orthopedic maxillary protraction with RPFM

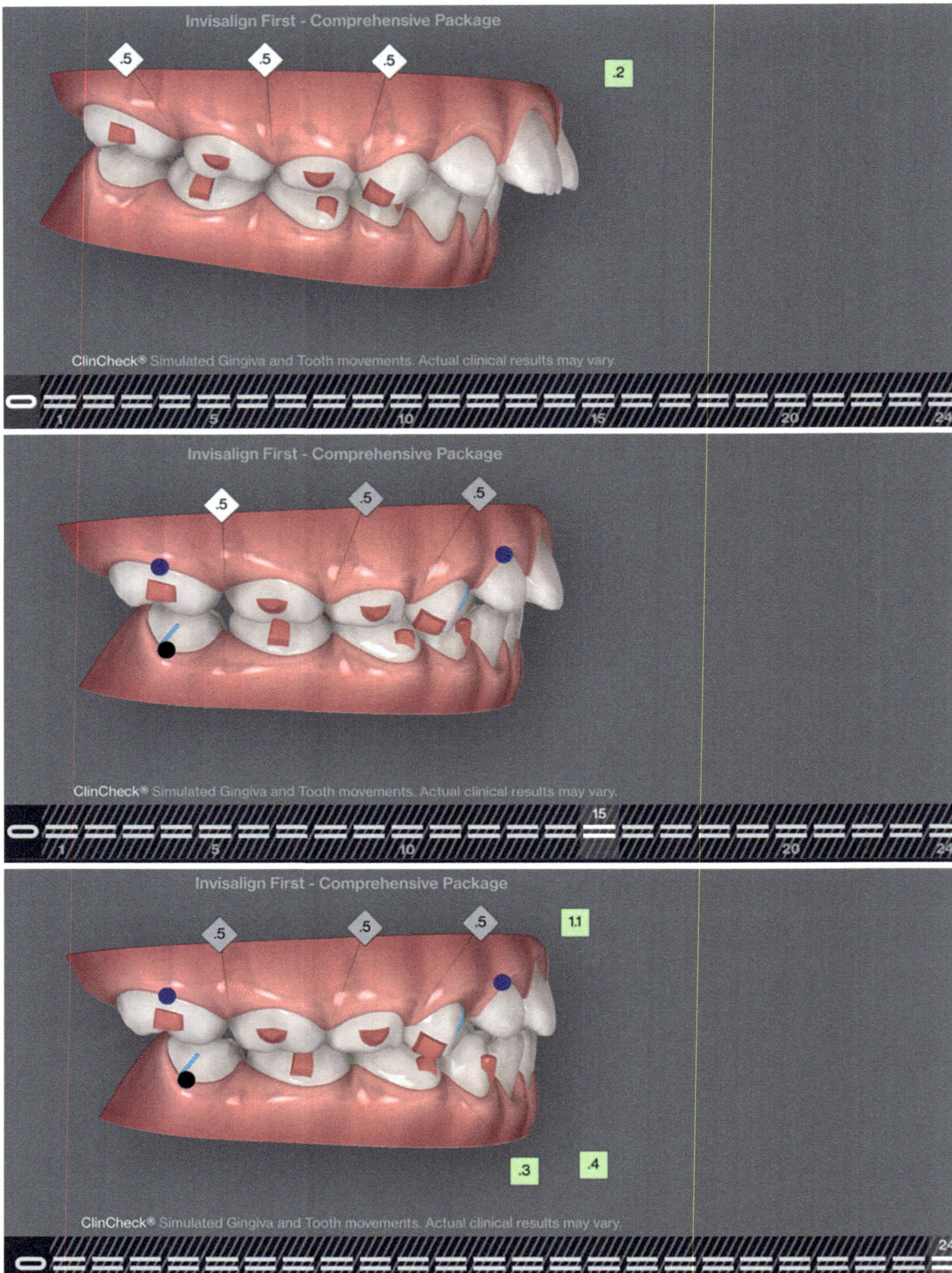

Fig. 10.2 The orthopedic treatment of Class II malocclusion in a growing patient can be simulated using continuous bite jumps to represent the forward growth of the mandible. In patient M.S., cervical headgear supplemented a distalizing force to the maxillary arch for Class II correction

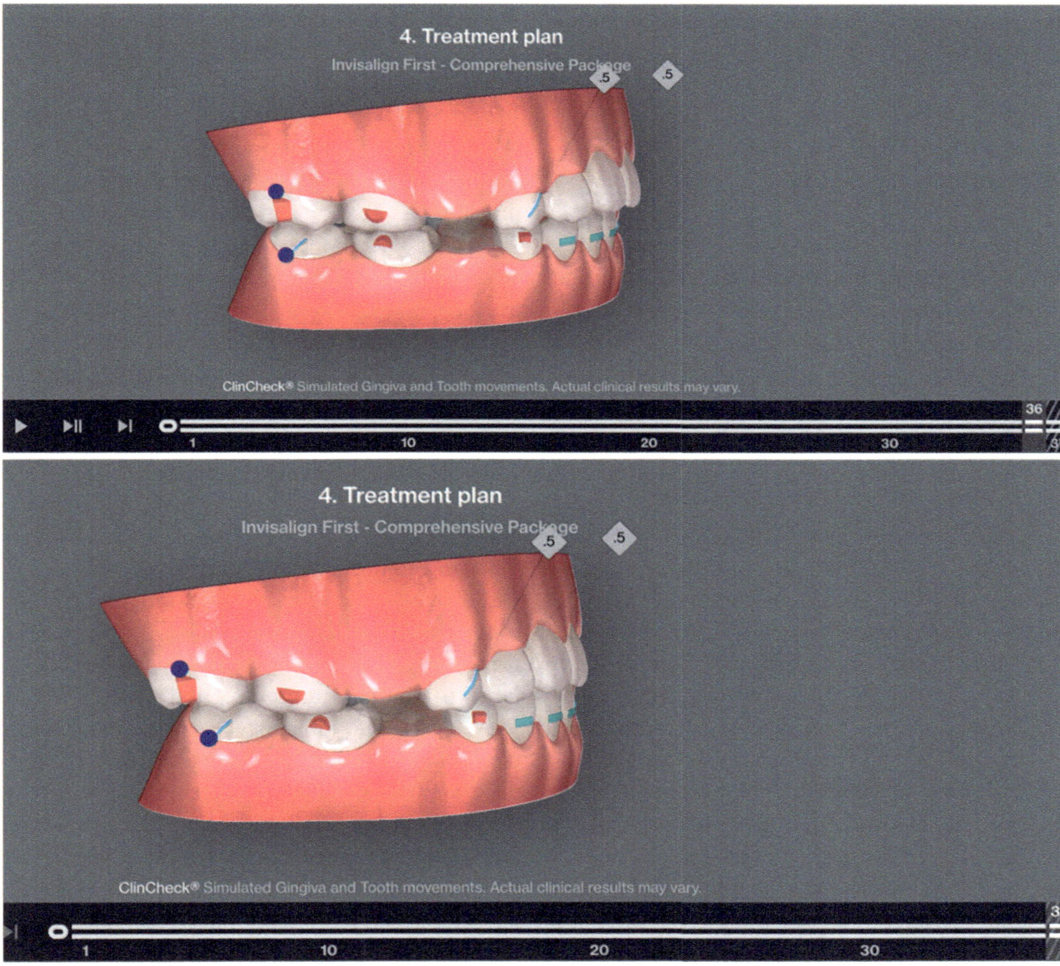

Fig. 10.3 For patient O.S., the incorporation of a bite jump on stage 37 simulates Class II correction from predicted mandibular growth during the initial course of aligners. Class II correction was also supplemented with Class II elastics

is necessary to set up the mandibular forward position. As discussed in Chap. 3, the MA appliance is more likely to produce skeletal effects in patients during the pubertal peak as compared to those in a prepubertal stage [4]. The bite jump must be incorporated in the virtual setup for the MA appliance, usually in 2 mm advancements of the mandible until an edge-to-edge position (or an overcorrected position), though the exact amount of advancement can be adjusted by the clinician.

Open Bite Closure

Studies on open bite treatment with clear aligners have demonstrated that bite closure occurs through a combination of incisor extrusion, molar intrusion, and counterclockwise rotation of the mandible [5]. A bite jump would be indicated to realistically model the autorotation of the mandible. In most cases of open bite treatment, the virtual setup will show intrusion of the posterior teeth, extrusion of the maxillary and mandibular incisors, and a bite jump simulating autorotation and anterior open bite closure toward the end of therapy.

Orthognathic Surgery

The significant jaw movements in orthognathic surgery should be modeled with a bite jump at the end of the presurgical course of therapy. It is recommended that the clinician coordinate the design of the bite jump with the attending surgeon for a definitive treatment plan and the planning of presurgical movements that will optimize the effectiveness of the surgery [6]. For example, the bite jump and the presurgical movements will differ significantly for a Class III patient treated with a mandibular setback and maxillary advancement compared to those for the same patient treated with only a mandibular setback. In either case, presurgical movements would include incisor decompensation to increase the negative overjet but exact movements in all dimensions would differ depending on the type of surgery planned. If the patient has a transverse discrepancy severe enough to warrant a segmental maxillary surgery, then a posterior crossbite and midline discrepancy would be left untreated in the presurgical phase. In contrast, for a single-jaw surgery, a midline discrepancy can be corrected in the nonsurgical arch during the presurgical phase [6].

Dental Functional Shift

In certain cases, occlusal interferences can result in functional shifts that manifest in midline deviations, posterior crossbites, and other transverse discrepancies. The bite jump would be indicated for such dental functional shifts. Typically, the bite jump would be planned at the end of the course of aligners on the virtual setup after the interference has been relieved through dental movements.

Principles of Bite Jump Use

Predictability of the Bite Jump

When prescribing bite jumps, the clinician should confirm that the planned dental and skeletal movements are likely to occur. If there is a high degree of uncertainty regarding the movements represented by a bite jump, then it should be avoided in the virtual setup. Conceptually, the bite jump should be considered as a simulation of skeletal movements of either the maxilla, mandible, or a combination. An exception would be the correction of a functional shift, whose bite jump would represent dental movements.

It is essential to note that the bite jump should not be employed as an alternative for movements that are biomechanically unrealistic. For example, if there is excessive overjet remaining at the end of a virtual setup for a nongrowing patient, then it would be impractical to prescribe a bite jump to simulate the correction of the overjet. This sort of bite jump would not be indicated if mechanics were not applied to realistically produce significant Class II correction (Fig. 10.4). Recent studies have shown that no anteroposterior improvement was achieved in clear aligner treatments of Class II malocclusion with Class II elastics [7]. Therefore, it is questionable whether Class II elastics alone would be able to produce the significant overjet correction predicted by a bite jump.

Timing

For open bite closure, the bite jump is usually prescribed at the end of the course of aligners in the virtual setup. The bite jump can be represented as the final stage following the virtual maxillary and mandibular first molar-to-first molar power chains (known as maxillary and mandibular virtual C-chains for Invisalign clear aligners). It is difficult to predict when precisely open bite closure will occur, so it would be more judicious to place the bite jump toward the end

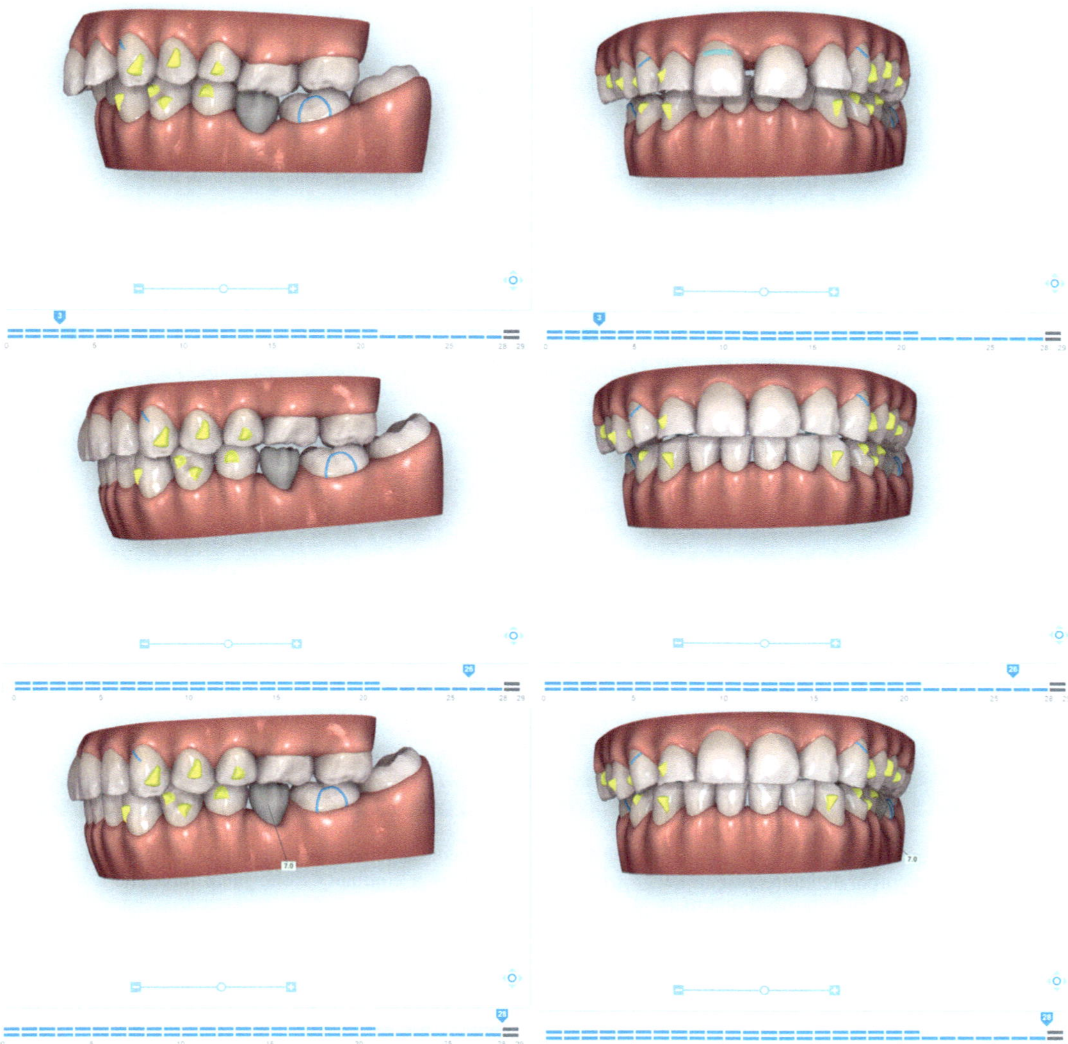

Fig. 10.4 Bite jumps should not be used to simulate the corrections of large overjet without the application of adequate Class II mechanotherapy. In this virtual setup, the clinician programmed a highly unrealistic bite jump in stage 28, in which they simulated both significant midline correction and overjet reduction without applying mechanotherapy to predictably produce these effects. This approach would result in discrepancies between predicted and achieved occlusal outcomes

of therapy (rather than at the middle or near the beginning of the course of aligners). Nevertheless, we have observed that bite closure usually occurs in the middle of the course of aligners. The bite jump would also be placed at the end of the virtual setup for a presurgical phase of clear aligner therapy to represent the surgical correction after all presurgical movements have been completed.

In growing patients, the bite jump may need to be incorporated throughout the entire treatment to accurately simulate continuous jaw growth (Fig. 10.5). In this case, the bite jump would appear in every aligner stage. This continuous mode of bite jumps is indicated for Class II orthopedic treatment, Class II and Class III mechanics in actively growing patients, and Class III orthopedic treatment, typically with RPFM.

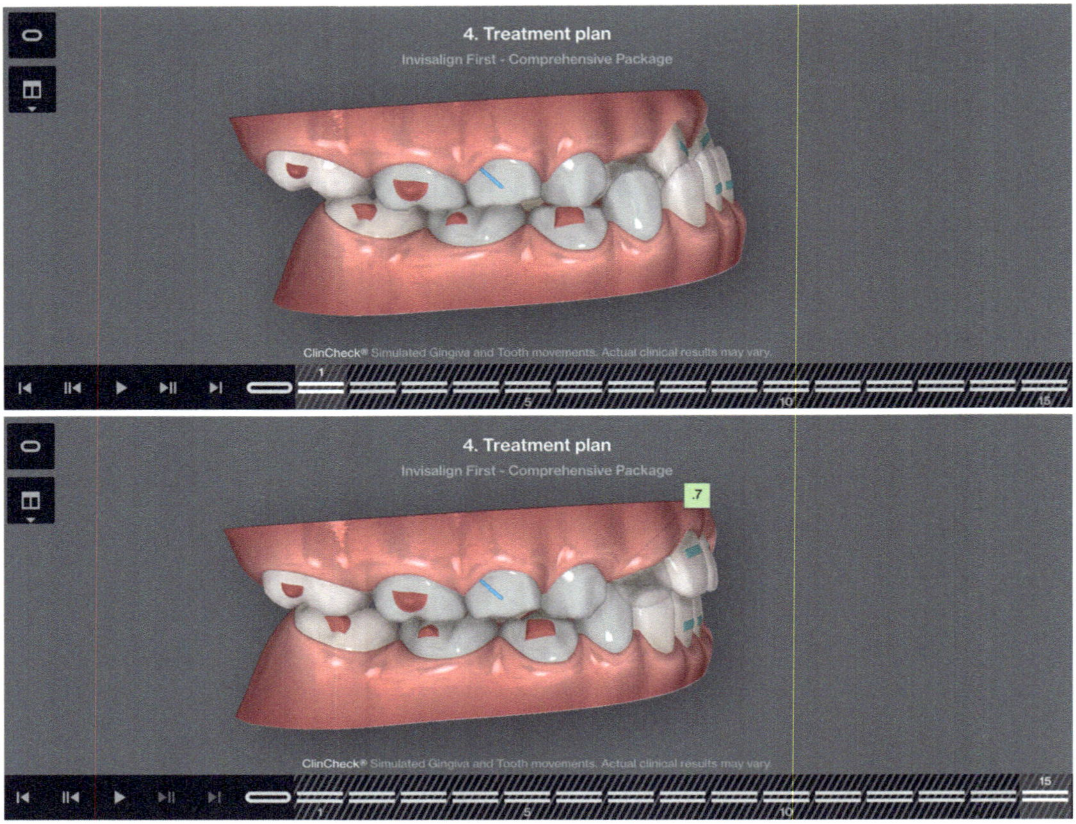

Fig. 10.5 For growing patients, a continuous bite jump may have to be incorporated to represent jaw growth. For patient W. W., the patient's forward maxillary growth and orthopedic maxillary protraction through RPFM was simulated by a continuous bite jump throughout the initial course of aligners

For the mandibular advancement appliance, the bite jump can also be prescribed as incremental changes for gradual forward movement of the mandible. This mode of activation agrees with recent studies that have observed a stepwise mandibular advancement in either fixed or removable functional appliances allowed for a greater reduction of ANB and greater control of incisor proclination compared to single-step maximum bite jumping [8]. Typically, each bite jump advances the mandible about 2 mm. But the clinician can calibrate the precise amount of mandibular advancement for each bite jump until an edge-to-edge position.

Another less common but viable timing pattern for the bite jump would be a short sequence of stages in the middle of a course of aligners. This pattern would be indicated for significant distalization of maxillary or mandibular posterior teeth (Fig. 10.6), in ranges of 2–2.5 mm [9]. The bite jump would represent the stages of Class II correction (or Class III correction) during distalization, showing retraction of the maxillary arch. This scenario would likely require an auxiliary device, such as a distalizer, to predictably achieve the planned amount of distalization.

Controversial Uses of the Bite Jump

Excessive Overjet in Nongrowing Class II Patients

One of the most common misuses of the bite jump is its prescription for significant overjet correction in nongrowing Class II patients in the

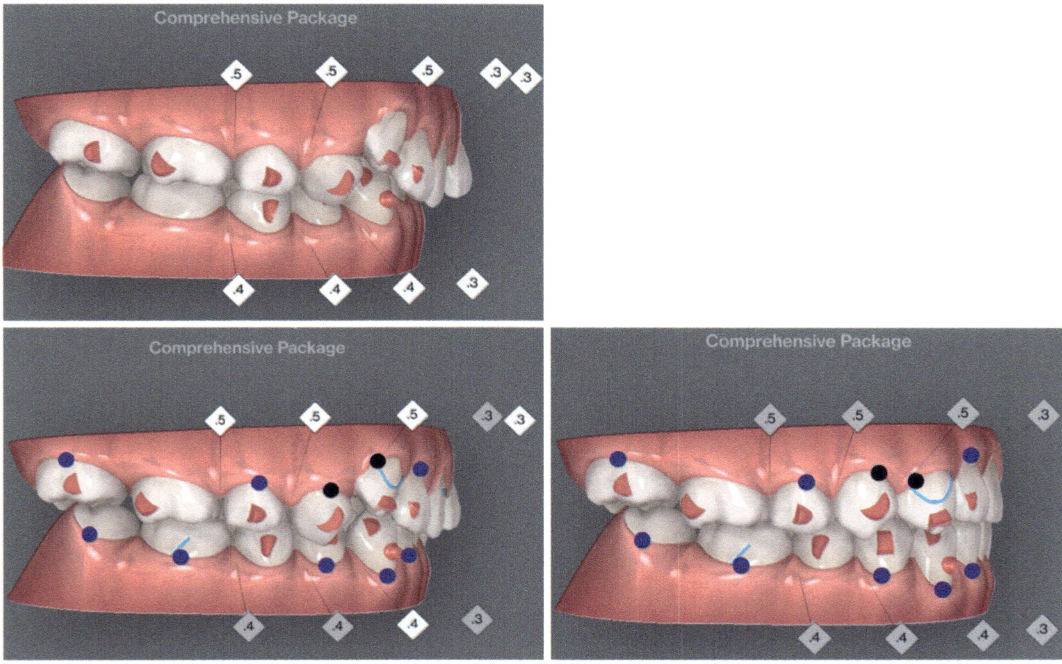

Fig. 10.6 A bite jump can be used to simulate the effects of distalization. For patient A.C., the bite jump distalizes the right maxillary posterior segment by about 1.5 mm

absence of adequate mechanics, such as a functional regulator or a distalizer. This application of the bite jump is impractical because it represents an unrealistic movement. As a result, the overjet correction will likely not be achieved, so that the clinical outcome will significantly deviate from the outcome rendered on the virtual setup.

This misuse is also commonly observed in compromised treatments for adults with severe Class II or Class III discrepancies. In these cases, without a surgical correction or auxiliaries for Class II correction, it is recommended to avoid prescription of the bite jump and to develop a more realistic virtual setup.

TAD-Assisted Cases

For movements that are supplemented with TADs, it is more predictable to incorporate overcorrection for the movement rather than a bite jump (Fig. 10.7). For example, as discussed in Chap. 6, in patients with deep bites and vertical maxillary excess, an additional 2–3 mm of intrusion of the maxillary anterior teeth can be achieved with supplementary forces from TADs. The clinician should program overcorrection of the maxillary anterior teeth rather than a bite jump to realistically portray the intrusive movements. An exception would be TAD-supplemented intrusion of maxillary and mandibular posterior teeth for open bite closure (Chap. 7). A bite jump would be indicated to represent the mandibular autorotation, as it is a realistic movement [10].

Extraction Cases

In extraction cases, the bite jump is usually not indicated, as it may mispresent dental movements and changes in jaw relationships in all dimensions. As discussed in Chap. 9, the clinician should plan extraction cases with measures such as the G6 protocol to ensure predictable extraction space closure and incisor movements [11]. The extensive jaw movements of the bite jump would typically not occur in extraction cases (except in cases involving mandibular autorotation).

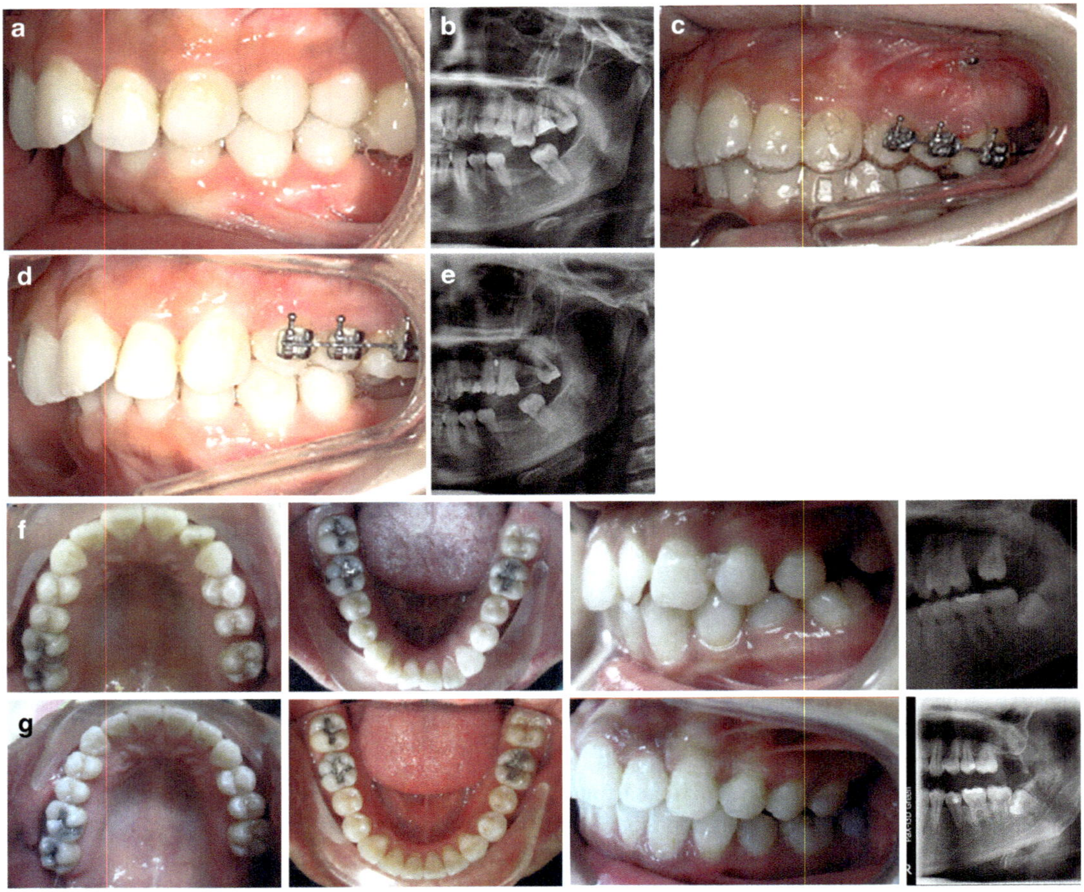

Fig. 10.7 (**a, b**) For patient O.L., the left maxillary first molar required significant intrusion to create space for an opposing implant restoration. A bite jump was not programmed for left maxillary first molar intrusion, as this would reflect unrealistic tooth movements. (**c**) Combination therapy with partial fixed appliances and a TAD was employed to supplement intrusion, while controlling the buccolingual inclination of the molar. (**d, e**) Significant intrusion of the left maxillary first molar was achieved after six months of treatment. Additional intrusion will be necessary to create adequate clearance for the opposing molar restoration. (**f, g**) A bite jump should not be employed to simulate extensive space closure. Instead, closure of large spaces should be programmed in a stepwise fashion for predictability. For patient J.Y., the residual space between the left maxillary second premolar and left maxillary second molar was closed with an initial course of aligners without the use of a bite jump followed by a short course of partial fixed appliances in the left maxillary posterior segment to upright the maxillary second molar

Extensive Space Closure

The bite jump is rarely indicated for representing the movements involved in extensive space closure. Instead, the clinician should realistically stage the dental movements, such as the mesialization of a second molar into a first molar space. Significant space closure may require combination treatment with fixed appliances. For example, the mesialization of a second molar into a first molar space can be supplemented with braces and a mesializing force from an anterior anchoring segment of the mandibular first and second premolars (Fig. 10.7).

Mandibular Shifts

The bite jump is sometimes indicated for mandibular shifts in cases where the resolution of the

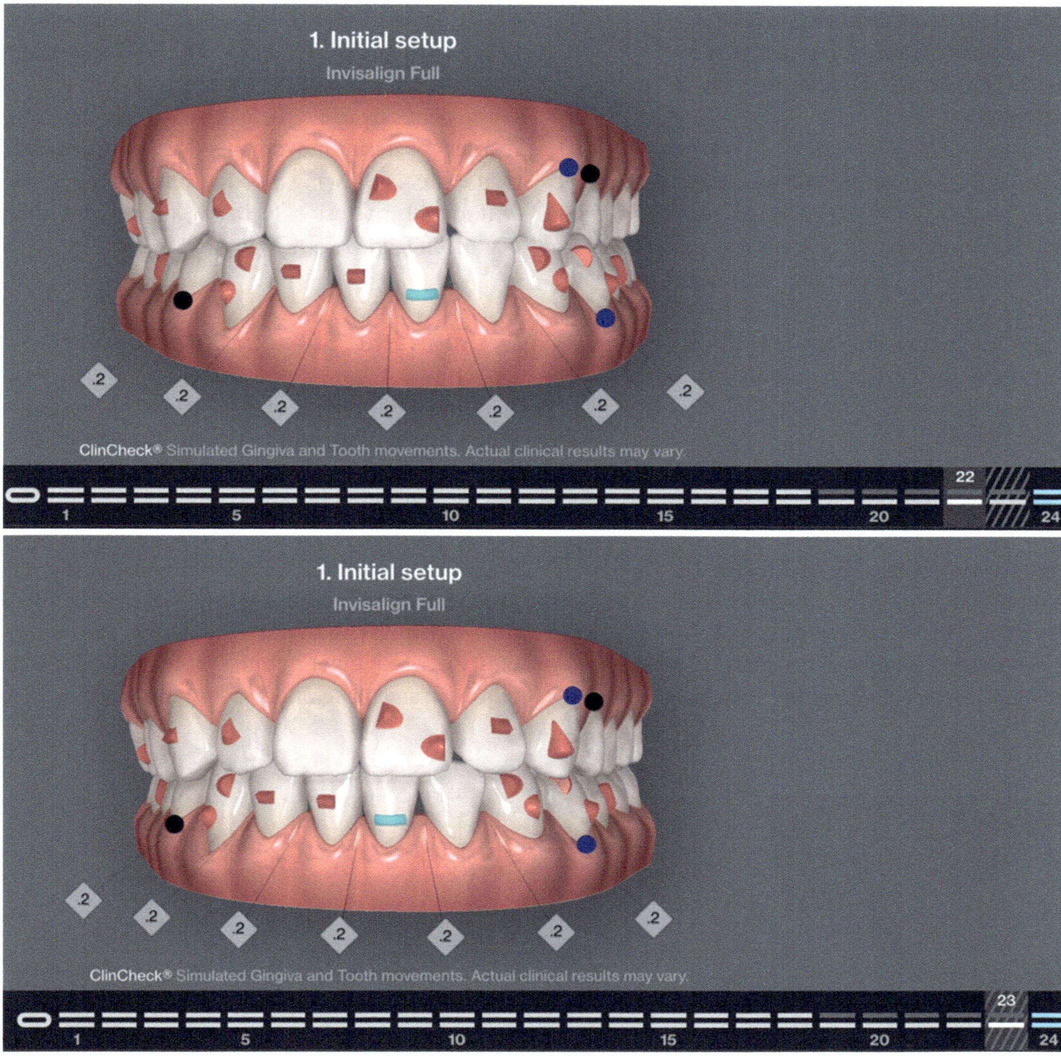

Fig. 10.8 For patient F. C., a bite jump was programmed for stage 23 to represent the differential BSSO. The bite jump portrays the translation of the mandible to the patient's right, the coordination of maxillary and mandibular midlines, and the correction of the left posterior crossbite

shift can be predictably achieved. For a patient with a mandibular asymmetry treated with a differential BSSO orthognathic surgery, a bite jump would be indicated to represent the surgical correction (Fig. 10.8). Another viable use of the bite jump would be for patients with dental-related shifts, in which one is certain orthodontic treatment would address the etiology. For example, a bite jump would be indicated if the dental functional shift was caused by a single-tooth anterior crossbite, as the crossbite would likely be alleviated in the course of aligners.

However, for a patient with skeletal mandibular asymmetry treated without skeletal correction in a compromised fashion through methods such as asymmetrical elastics, a bite jump would be contraindicated, as significant skeletal correction of the asymmetry would not occur.

Solutions for Discrepancies Between Clinical Outcomes and Outcomes Predicted by Bite Jumps

Frequently, even with judicious application of the bite jump, clear aligner treatments will not achieve clinical outcomes as programmed. In these cases, it is necessary to further adjust the occlusion toward the outcome simulated by the bite jump, either through refinements or alternative methods, such as combination therapy with fixed appliances.

Growing Patients

For growing Class II and Class III patients, a comprehensive course of additional aligners is usually required for detailing and finishing. This is especially common for patients receiving mandibular advancement, as the forward positioning of the mandible will almost always result in heavy anterior interferences and a bilateral posterior open bite, which must be closed with a refinement course. The MA appliance also restricts posterior movements due to the presence of the precision wings, so the refinement course will detail posterior teeth positions and their occlusion (Fig. 10.9).

Orthognathic Surgery Cases

A refinement course usually cannot be avoided for ideal detailing and finishing in cases involving orthognathic surgery [12]. An intraoral scan can be performed during the fourth week following the surgery and a course of refinement developed. For more complicated orthognathic surgical procedures, such as triple jaw surgery (LeFort I osteotomy, sagittal split osteotomy, and genioplasty), a refinement course will most likely be required and last longer compared to that of a

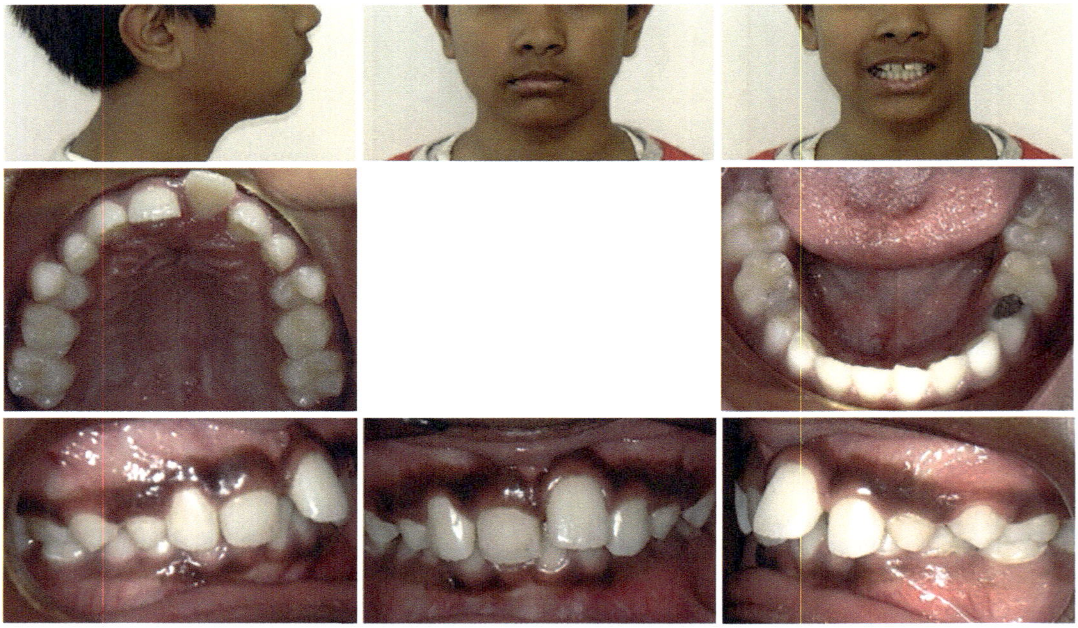

Fig. 10.9 In patient A.A, after an initial course of mandibular advancement, an additional course of refinement was necessary to detail the positions of the posterior segments. The MA appliance restricts the movements of posterior teeth and commonly results in heavy anterior interferences. The refinement included the closure of the bilateral posterior open bites and minimization of heavy anterior contacts

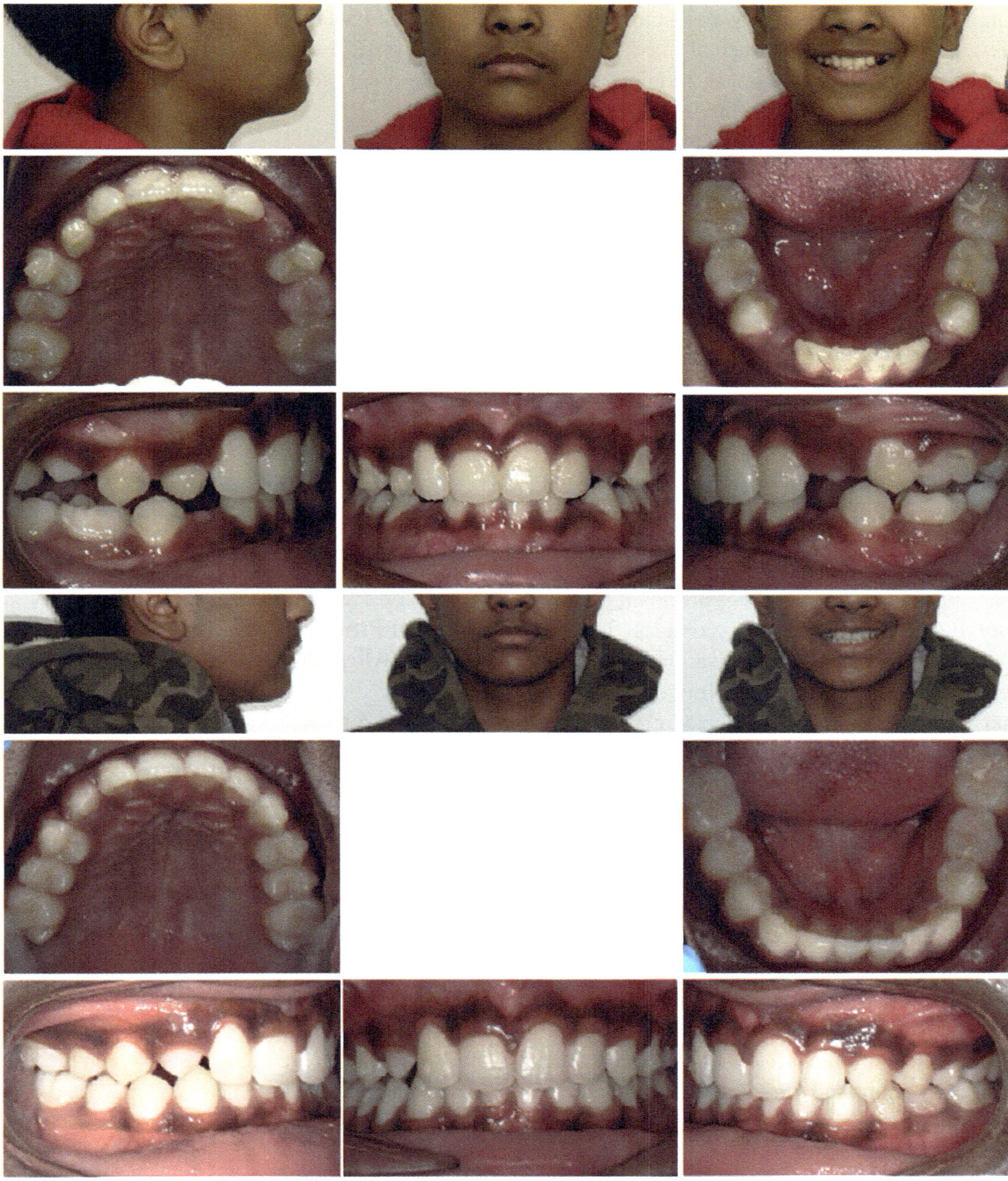

Fig. 10.9 (continued)

simpler orthognathic surgery. For example, a surgery involving both a segmental maxillary osteotomy and BSSO would require further adjustments to the maxillary arch form and transverse relationships between the maxilla and mandible, such as the correction of posterior crossbites [6].

Open Bite Closure

Further detailing and finishing will frequently be required after an initial course of aligners treating open bite closure [10]. Clinical outcomes often do not coincide with the ideal bite closure projected by the bite jump, although the treatment of mild anterior open bites may result in outcomes closer to the projected occlusion, only requiring minor adjustments. A bilateral posterior open bite often manifests after anterior open bite closure due to heavy anterior contacts, intrusive forces in the maxillary and mandibular posterior segments, and the unpredictability of the skeletal and dental movements involved in mandibular autorotation [5]. In these cases, the clinician should consider a course of refinement to extrude the maxillary and mandibular posterior segments. Alternatively, the clinician can employ auxiliaries, such as buttons on the posterior teeth for vertical elastics wear to achieve proper interdigitation.

Conversely, the initial course of aligners may result in an anterior open bite that has not been fully closed. As a result, the clinician will have to incorporate additional bite closure mechanics. These can be applied through a refinement course with additional extrusion of the anterior teeth and intrusion of the posterior teeth. For cases with a residual mild anterior open bite, a short course of anterior vertical elastics can be considered to achieve proper bite closure.

Dental Functional Shifts

Though dental functional shifts are usually resolved once the etiology is addressed, the occlusion may require further adjustments after the initial course of aligners to achieve outcomes projected by the bite jump. Specifically, a midline discrepancy may persist despite the alleviation of the shift and the removal of the etiological factor. Minor midline discrepancies can be corrected with an additional course of aligners incorporating unilateral IPR and a short course of asymmetric elastics (Fig. 10.10).

Optimal Planning of Bite Jumps in Clear Aligner Treatment

Bite jumps represent one of the most misused features in the virtual setups for clear aligner treatment. The misapplication of the bite jump can result in planning for impractical changes in maxillomandibular relationships and significant discrepancies between projected and clinical outcomes. The guiding principle when considering the incorporation of the bite jump should be a determination of its predictability—that is, the likelihood of the planned jaw movements with respect to mechanotherapy and the patient's dentofacial growth. Nevertheless, even when the bite jump is applied in a realistic manner, clinical outcomes frequently require further adjustments to achieve its projections.

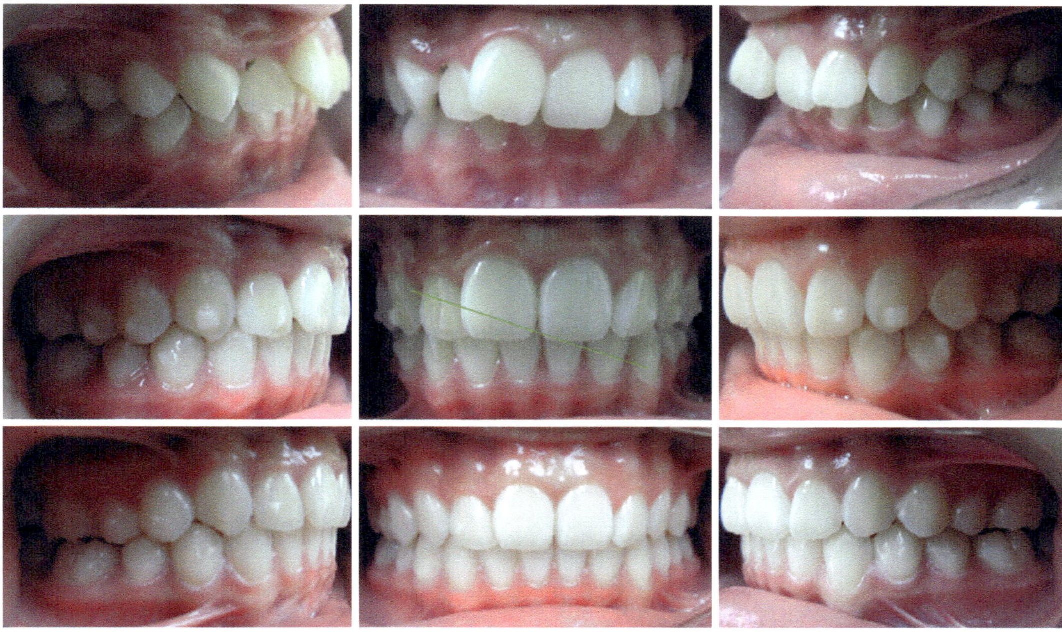

Fig. 10.10 After the correction of a functional shift through the relief of a heavy interference, a mild midline discrepancy may persist. This can be treated with a 3–4 month course of asymmetric elastics to ideally coordinate maxillary and mandibular midlines. For this patient, an initial course of aligners improved midline coordination through asymmetric mandibular IPR and relief of heavy anterior interferences. Afterward, a short course of asymmetric elastics (Class II on the left, Class III elastics on the right) were worn for 3 months to fully achieve maxillary and mandibular midline coordination

References

1. Santana LG, Avelar K, Flores-Mir C, Marques LS. Incremental or maximal mandibular advancement in the treatment of class II malocclusion through functional appliances: a systematic review with meta-analysis. Orthod Craniofac Res. 2020;23(4):371–84.
2. Perinetti G, Contardo L. Reliability of growth indicators and efficiency of functional treatment for skeletal class II malocclusion: current evidence and controversies. Biomed Res Int. 2017;2017:1367691.
3. Janson G, Sathler R, Fernandes TM, Branco NC, Freitas MR. Correction of class II malocclusion with class II elastics: a systematic review. Am J Orthod Dentofac Orthop. 2013;143(3):383–92.
4. Ravera S, Castroflorio T, Galati F, Cugliari G, Garino F, Deregibus A, Quinzi V. Short term dentoskeletal effects of mandibular advancement clear aligners in class II growing patients. A prospective controlled study according to STROBE guidelines. Eur J Paediatr Dent. 2021;22(2):119–24.
5. Moshiri S, Araújo EA, McCray JF, Thiesen G, Kim KB. Cephalometric evaluation of adult anterior open bite non-extraction treatment with Invisalign. Dental Press J Orthod. 2017;22(5):30–8.
6. Lou T, Caminiti M. Orthognathic surgery combined with clear aligner therapy. J Clin Orthod. 2021;55(1):44–58.
7. Patterson BD, Foley PF, Ueno H, Mason SA, Schneider PP, Kim KB. Class II malocclusion correction with Invisalign: is it possible? Am J Orthod Dentofac Orthop. 2021;159(1):e41–8.
8. Knösel M, Espinoza-Espinoza GE, Sandoval-Vidal P, Zaror C. Angle class II correction: stepwise mandibular advancement or bite jumping?: a systematic review and meta-analysis of skeletal, dental and condylar effects. J Orofac Orthop. 2020;81(4):286–300.
9. Ravera S, Castroflorio T, Garino F, Daher S, Cugliari G, Deregibus A. Maxillary molar distalization with aligners in adult patients: a multicenter retrospective study. Prog Orthod. 2016;17:12.
10. Harris K, Ojima K, Dan C, Upadhyay M, Alshehri A, Kuo CL, Mu J, Uribe F, Nanda R. Evaluation of open bite closure using clear aligners: a retrospective study. Prog Orthod. 2020;21(1):23.
11. Dai FF, Xu TM, Shu G. Comparison of achieved and predicted tooth movement of maxillary first molars and central incisors: first premolar extraction treatment with Invisalign. Angle Orthod. 2019;89(5):679–87.
12. Kankam H, Madari S, Sawh-Martinez R, Bruckman KC, Steinbacher DM. Comparing outcomes in orthognathic surgery using clear aligners versus conventional fixed appliances. J Craniofac Surg. 2019;30(5):1488–91.

Overcoming Limitations in Finishing

11

Contents

Detailing with Clear Aligner Therapy

Despite the significant advances to clear aligner therapy since its inception, it is still inhibited by a number of limitations in controlling orthodontic tooth movement, many of which manifest in the finishing stages [1]. Frequently, there is a mismatch between clinical and predicted treatment outcomes in clear aligner software models [2]. Research has shown that extrusion is the least accurate movement with clear aligner therapy, with one study reporting 30% predictability [3]. Rotation was the second least accurate movement with clear aligner therapy [1]. A prospective study analyzing the effects of attachments and interproximal reduction on canine movement showed a mean accuracy in rotation of 36% [4]. These inaccuracies in tooth movement often manifest as poor tracking for individual teeth during the course of therapy. Typically, these minor discrepancies, such as unrotated canines and lateral incisors and infraerupted lateral incisors, are resolved by an additional course of aligners. In such cases, the need to resolve minor occlusal discrepancies often results in a significant increase in treatment time, either in the form of interrupting a course of aligners or extended courses of refinement. However, there exist alternative methods of modifying aligner material with hand instruments or incorporating auxiliaries during a course of aligners to either resolve or improve minor occlusal discrepancies (Fig. 11.1, Table 11.1). In some cases, tooth movement through staging of the aligners and attachments may not be adequate to produce the desired tooth movements. Hand instruments, allowing for the alteration of aligner geometry, and auxiliaries like fixed appliances can both enhance movements difficult for clear aligners. As a result, the clinician can either avert or minimize an additional course of aligners. In this manner, the clinician can decrease overall treat-

A. T. Huang, D. Huang, *Controversies in Clear Aligner Therapy*,
https://doi.org/10.1007/978-3-030-92810-0_11

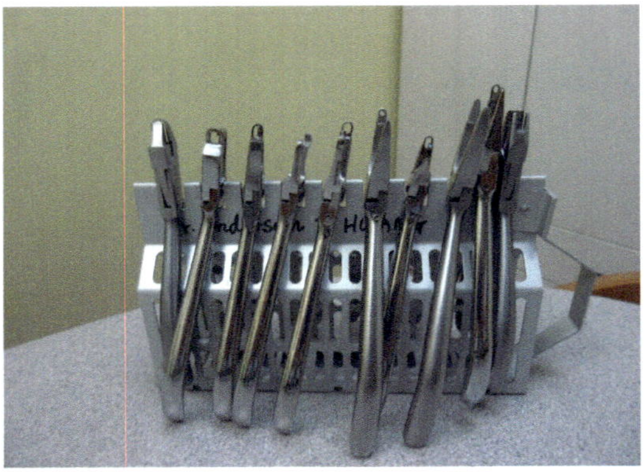

Fig. 11.1 Hand instruments can enhance the effectiveness of detailing and finishing by supplementing difficult movements or enhancing mechanotherapy. Their proper application can minimize or avoid courses of refinement and shorten overall treatment time

Table 11.1 Description of finishing instruments and their indications

Instrument	Indication
1 mm dimple plier	For labialization, derotation, lingualization and additional retention.
Spacer plier	To create space for labial or lingual tooth movement and derotation.
Eraser plier	To remove unwanted attachments or dimples.
3 mm dimple plier	To create power ridges and additional vertical or horizontal attachments.
Bite ramp plier	For the addition or modification of bite ramps.
Hole punch plier	To create precision cuts and button cutouts.
Precision cut plier	To create precision cuts.

ment time for more effective orthodontic treatment.

In the finishing stages, intervention with hand instruments or auxiliaries during the course of aligners can also be applied to inter-arch discrepancies in a variety of dimensions. During treatment, they can be used to enhance or modify mechanotherapy that did not achieve the desired effects or incorporate mechanotherapy in response to a need that was initially overlooked. The incorporation of hand instruments and auxiliaries expands the capabilities of the clear aligner to treat complex interocclusal problems and allows for increased adaptability of the appliance for problems that may arise during treatment.

In this chapter, we start by describing intra-arch occlusal discrepancies in a variety of dimensions that may arise during the finishing stages and their solutions. Then we discuss common inter-arch problems and their treatment with methods for enhancing the clear aligners through the incorporation or modification of mechanotherapy. Lastly, we outline the decision-making process and timing behind intervention for the management of discrepancies during the finishing stages.

Intra-arch Occlusal Discrepancies

Discrepancies in the First Order

Discrepancies in the buccolingual dimension most often manifest themselves in teeth that have not derotated as predicted and as a result, fail to track with the aligner. Research has shown that among the maxillary and mandibular anterior teeth, the maxillary and mandibular canines are the least accurate in regards to accuracy of rotation [4]. Inadequacies in premolar rotations have also been observed [5]. Though we have observed increased accuracy of derotation in the maxillary anterior region with recent innovations, including Invisalign's G7 optimized attachments for lateral incisor control, rotational discrepancies still persist and manifest themselves in the late stages of courses of clear aligners. We note that lateral incisors are often unforgiving with patient incompliance. Nevertheless, we still observe maxillary lateral incisors and maxillary canines that remain rotated despite satisfactory patient compliance (Fig. 11.2).

For teeth that have not been derotated and poorly track with their aligners, the respective aligner material can be modified with a hand instrument to supplement the rotational force supplied by the aligner. Firstly, the non-tracking tooth's adjacent contacts should be verified that adequate space has been created for derotation.

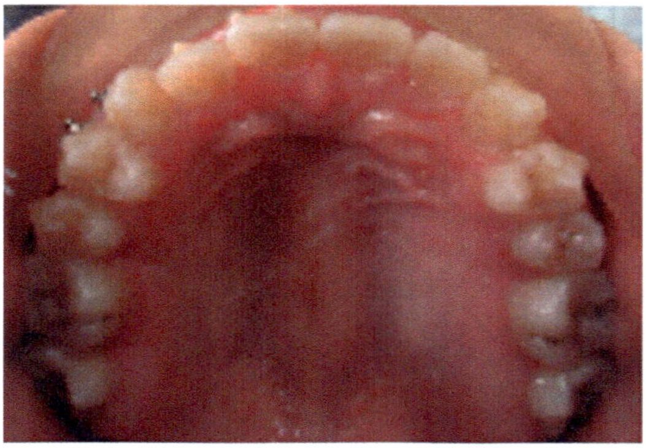

Fig. 11.2 For patient J. X., the right maxillary lateral incisor and right maxillary canine failed to derotate completely after an initial course of aligners

If the contacts are overly tight, the clinician should create sufficient interproximal space by stripping prior to modifying the aligner material. After, the aligner material can be modified with a dimple plier to create a coupled force to aid in derotation (Fig. 11.3). Dimples (indentations) should be placed on the mesiolingual and the distolabial surfaces to create a couple that rotates the tooth in a distolingual direction (Fig. 11.4a). Conversely, the dimples would be reversed for rotation in the opposite direction. The dimples should be about 1 mm in diameter so that the modified aligner can reseat onto the non-tracking tooth. Slightly larger dimples, such as 3 mm, can be used for additional force to address larger discrepancies. Thirdly, it should be noted greater force than usual will be needed for the patient to seat the aligner because it has been slightly deformed. Clinically, one can advise the patient to use a chewie (Fig. 11.4b) to secure the seating of aligners that have been modified with dimples.

There are limitations to this method of modifying the aligner to generate additional rotational forces. It seems to be more effective for anterior teeth as opposed to posterior teeth, most likely because of the latter's greater tooth mass. If the tooth is significantly off-track, such as greater than 15° from the predicted position, then it is unlikely the aligner can properly encapsulate the tooth to generate an appreciable rotational force. In such cases, it is

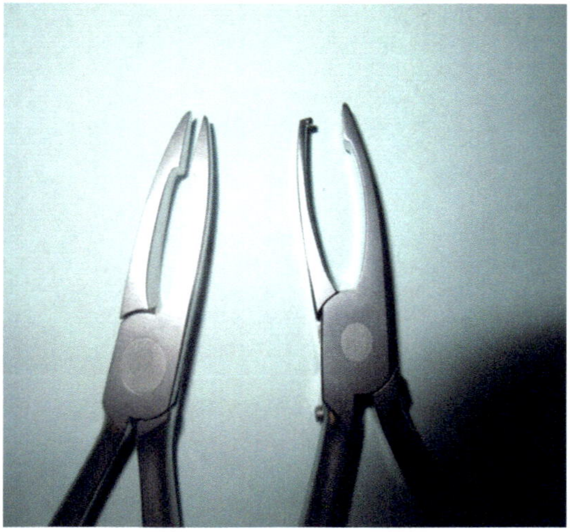

Fig. 11.3 The 1 mm dimple plier (right) can be used to alter aligner geometry and supplement forces for movements such as labialization, derotation, or lingualization

suggested that the clinician rescan the patient's occlusion and address the rotational discrepancy in a mid-course correction or refinement course. Alternatively, severely rotated teeth can also be treated with vertical elastics to bonded buttons or a combination of sectional brackets and archwires with clear aligners for a short period of time (Fig. 11.5a, b). In this method, the patient would be maintained on the same aligner, usually the final aligner, while the tooth is adjusted with fixed appliances. The aligner would be sectioned to allow for simultaneous wear of the aligner and the sectional brackets. We have observed that this combination type of treatment allows for the correction of rotated anterior teeth with greater efficiency than with forces produced solely by clear aligners.

Another discrepancy in the first order can also manifest in the form of a tooth that is labially or lingually tipped from its predicted position and failing to track with the aligner. In this case, the clinician should verify that the tooth's contact areas are not overly tight and perform light stripping as necessary for the tooth to move freely. Subsequently, the aligner can be modified with both a dimple plier and a spacer plier (Fig. 11.6). If an additional labializing force to the tooth is

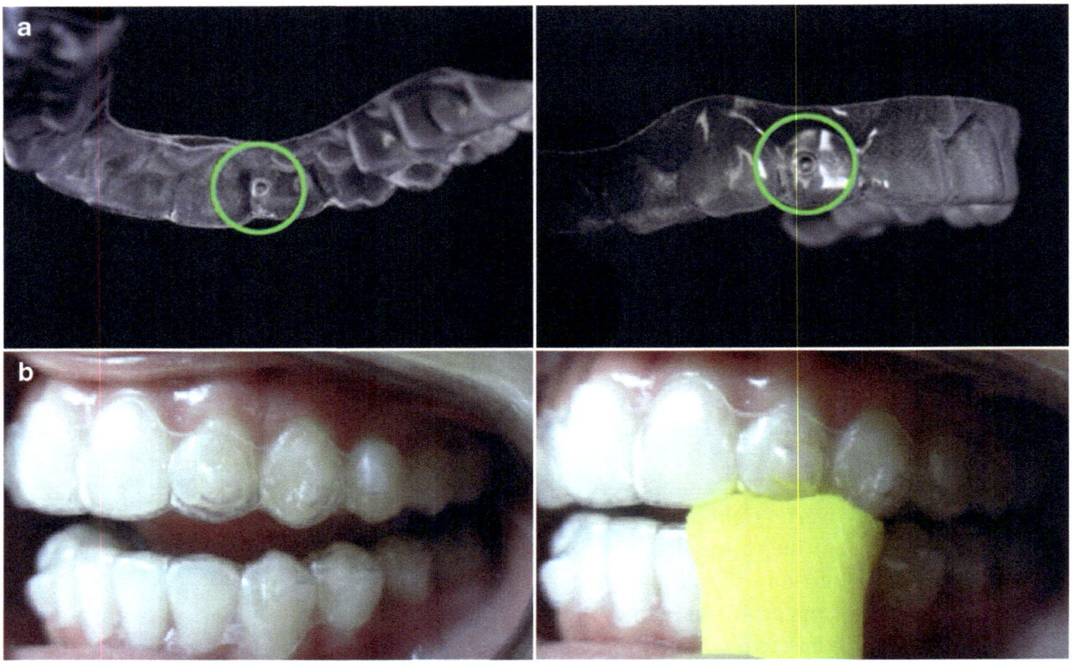

Fig. 11.4 (**a**) The placement of mesiolingual (left) and distolabial (right) dimples within the aligner can enhance the distolingual rotation of a maxillary lateral incisor. (**b**) After the placement of dimples, the distortion of the aligner may result in more difficulty for the patient in seating the aligner. The patient is recommended to use a chewie to improve fitting after alterations of aligner geometry

desired, then a 1 mm dimple should be placed on the lingual surface of the aligner, while additional space should be added to the labial surface with the spacer plier so that the tooth can move labially (Fig. 11.7a). For additional labial movement, two 1 mm dimples can be added on the lingual surface of the aligner material (Fig. 11.7b). For a lingualizing force, the placement of the dimple and the enlargement would be reversed. It should be noted that the dimple should be placed along the long axis of the tooth to produce a labializing or lingualizing force that is as bodily as possible.

There are cases when dimples are mistakenly placed in an area of the aligner that is not ideal for the optimal delivery of forces. The clinician can remove the dimple and restore the aligner material to its original state with an eraser plier (Fig. 11.8). In this way, the clinician can ensure optimal force delivery when intervening during a course of aligners and when modifying the aligner material.

Optimizing Tooth Movement

In certain cases, the aligner can be modified by other means to enhance orthodontic movements that are challenging for the appliance either because of the difficulty or the extent of tooth movement. Hand instruments can be used to incorporate new attachments or modify previously programmed attachments. We have discussed the significance of attachments in optimizing tooth movements [5, 6]. During treatment, the addition of attachments can serve as a means to increase retention of the aligners and facilitate the execution of planned tooth movements within the arch. For example, precision cuts on lower molars offer significant benefits for Class II elastics. However, one of the disadvantages of precision cuts as opposed to button cutouts is the possibility of the patient dislodging the mandibular aligner during elastic wear. Beveled attachments, including horizontal and vertical attachments, have been shown to increase reten-

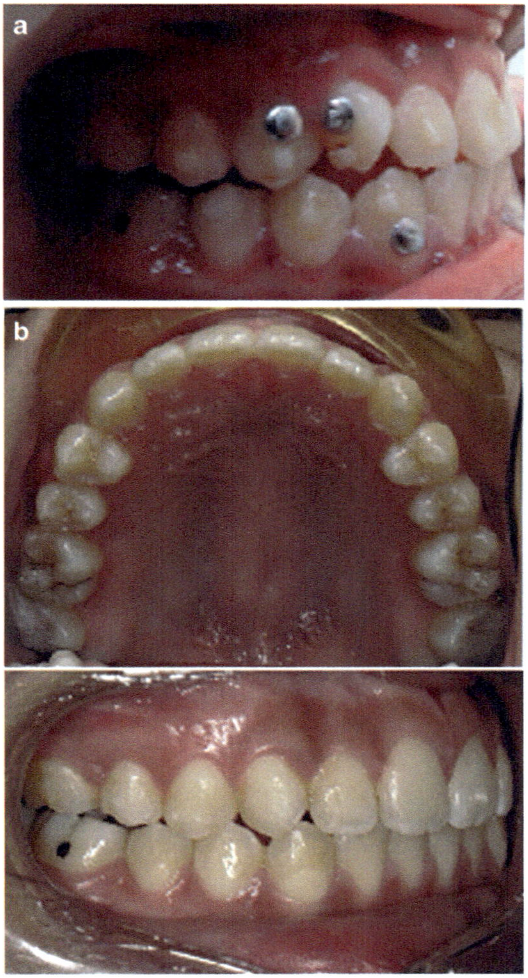

Fig. 11.5 (**a**, **b**) For patient J. X., the maxillary right canine remained rotated and infraerupted after the first course of aligners. A course of partial fixed appliances with metal buttons was employed to derotate and extrude the canine through a course of vertical elastics. The aligner was cut to allow vertical elastics wear. After 4 months, the canine rotation was completely corrected and the tooth extruded into ideal interdigitation

tion significantly, as compared with ellipsoid attachments and when no attachments are used [7]. To address the situation, a 3 mm horizontal dimple can be placed on either the mandibular first molar or the mandibular second molar with a 3 mm horizontal dimple plier (Fig. 11.9). The horizontal dimple will serve as the template for an additional attachment on the mandibular molar. Consequently, the aligner would be better

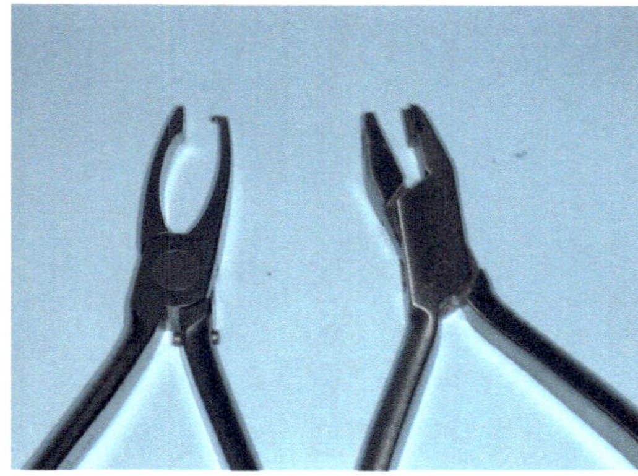

Fig. 11.6 The 1 mm dimple plier (left) can create a labializing or lingualizing force, while the spacer plier (right) can be concurrently used to create space into which the displaced tooth can be moved

retained with additional attachments on the mandibular molars and allow for both regular elastic wear and execution of the planned molar movements.

Discrepancies in the Third Order

It has been discussed that torque is difficult to achieve with clear aligners (Chap. 8). Studies have analyzed the efficacy of torque in clear aligner therapy and shown an improved movement accuracy with altered aligner geometry [5]. These geometric alterations can be applied during the course of treatment to enhance torquing movements in upright or proclined anterior teeth. For a tooth that is overly upright and not torqued in accordance with the software model, a horizontal dimple of 3 mm can be placed in the labiogingival region of the aligner material respective to the upright tooth with the horizontal dimple plier (Fig. 11.10a). The 3 mm horizontal dimple will serve as a power ridge and aid in tipping the crown labially and the root lingually (Fig. 11.10b). Another point of force or pressure point can be placed on the aligner material corresponding to the lingual surface of the incisor near the incisal edge. The two-point application of forces will create a couple to more effectively produce lingual root torque.

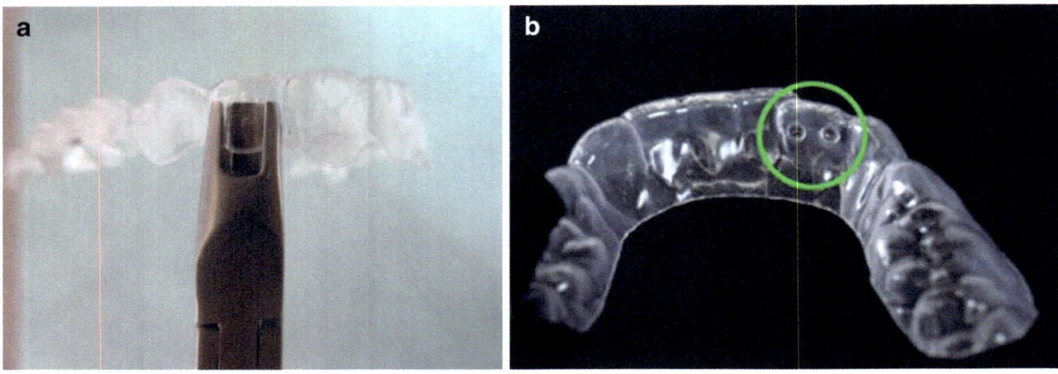

Fig. 11.7 (**a**) The enlargement on the labial surface of the aligner facilitates the labial movement of a lingually displaced tooth. (**b**) The placement of two dimples on the lingual surface of the aligner material can supplement the labializing force of the aligner

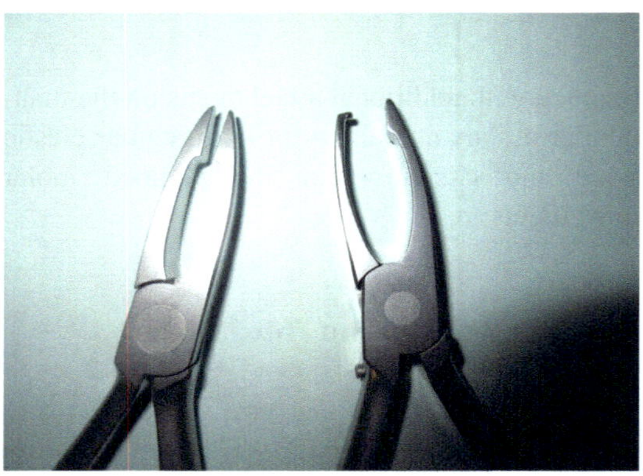

Fig. 11.8 The eraser plier (left) can remove attachments for the placement of dimples or remove dimples producing undesired forces

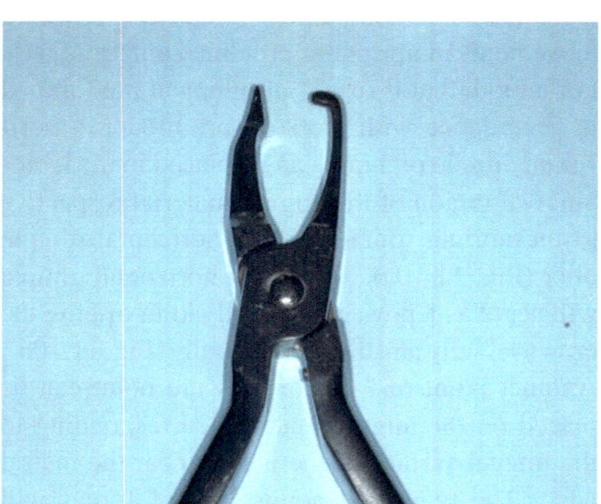

Fig. 11.9 The 3 mm horizontal dimple plier can create indentations for additional attachments or power ridges during the course of treatment

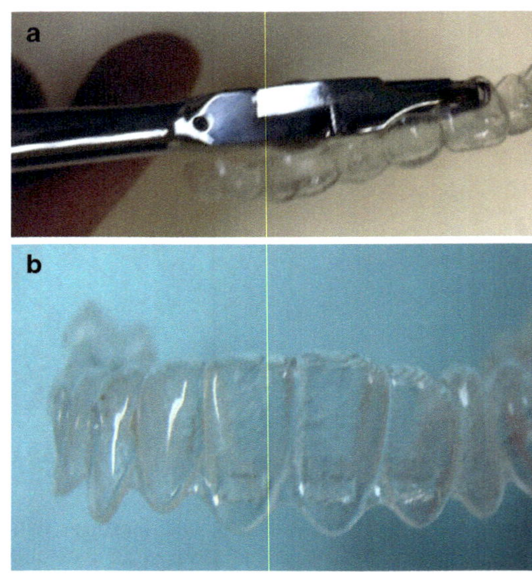

Fig. 11.10 (**a**) The 3 mm horizontal dimple plier can create an indent on either labial or lingual surfaces near cervical areas for lingual root torque or labial root torque, respectively. (**b**) A power ridge has been created with a 3 mm horizontal dimple plier for lingual root torque

Conversely, the horizontal dimple can also be placed in the lingual regions of the aligner material respective to maxillary and mandibular incisors for labial root torque. At present, power ridges for lingual regions of incisors cannot be programmed with most software, except for that of uLab. Therefore, in most software, the addition of power ridges with hand instruments is the only current method of altering aligner geometry to supplement labial root torque.

Inter-arch Discrepancies

During the course of a series of aligners, inter-arch discrepancies can arise that either were not anticipated, such as a midline discrepancy, or may persist due to inadequate biological response in the patient as a result of one's mechanics, such as a residual deep bite, open bite, or overjet. In these cases, the clinician can intervene with hand instruments and auxiliary measures to either shorten a refinement course or to aid in detailing and finishing to avoid an additional refinement course altogether.

Midline Discrepancies

Midline discrepancies may manifest during the course of treatment as a result of an inadequate biological response within the patient or as an unanticipated effect of tooth movement (Fig. 11.10). Practitioners have shown that cross midline elastics can be effective in the correction of dental asymmetries [8]. The cross midline elastic effect can be simulated in clear aligners by incorporating precision cuts on the aligner material respective to the mandibular left canine and the maxillary right canine to shift the mandibular midline to the right. Conversely, in order to shift the midline to the left, precision cuts would be incorporated on the aligner material respective to the mandibular right canine and the maxillary left canine. A minor midline discrepancy of 1–2 mm can be remedied in 6–8 weeks in a compliant patient (Fig. 11.11). These precision cuts can be programmed into the course of aligners during the initial Clincheck; however, they may have been initially omitted, often because of limitations in the clear aligner software. If a midline discrepancy manifests toward the end of a course of aligners, the clinician can modify the aligner material with either a hole punch plier (Fig. 11.12a) or a precision cut plier (Fig. 11.12b) to create the appropriate precision cuts and allow the patient to wear cross midline elastics (Fig. 11.13). In this way, the clinician can coordinate the maxillary and mandibular midlines in the final stages of a course of aligners.

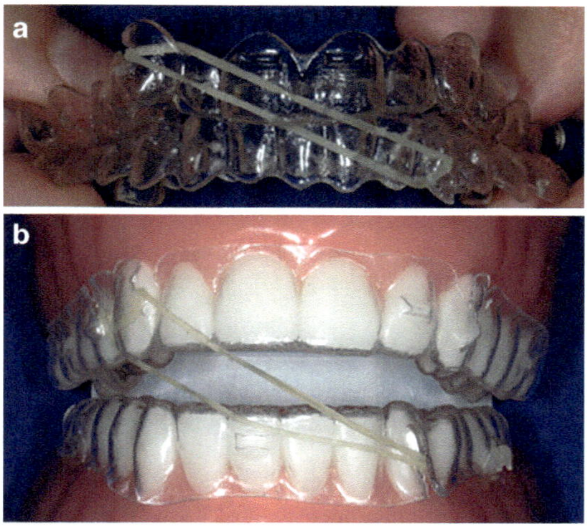

Fig. 11.11 (**a, b**) A midline discrepancy can occur during the course of treatment due to heavy occlusal interferences resulting in functional shifts, Bolton discrepancies, underlying skeletal asymmetries, or undesired tooth movements. A midline deviation of 1–2 mm can be corrected by creating precision cuts on opposite canines for cross midline elastics wear with 1/4", 2.7 oz. or 1.4", 4 oz. elastics

The clinician should also be conscious of the possibility that the aligners may dislodge with the use of cross elastics, especially with heavier elastics, like ¼", 4 oz. or 3/16", 4 oz. elastics. A solution to dislodging is the creation of button cutouts on the respective teeth, bonding metal or clear buttons, and instructing the patient to run the cross elastics between the buttons. The clinician should be cautious that the forces produced by the cross elastics do not cause unwanted rotations in the canines.

Deep Bites

Previously, we have discussed the difficulties in clear aligner therapy for the treatment of deep overbites (Chap. 6) [9]. Though the G5 protocol has allowed for increased effectiveness, it is still common for deep bites to persist toward the end of the first or even second course of aligners. In these cases, the clinician can modify the aligner material during the course of treatment to enhance bite opening mechanics. Often, the programmed placement of the bite ramps will be

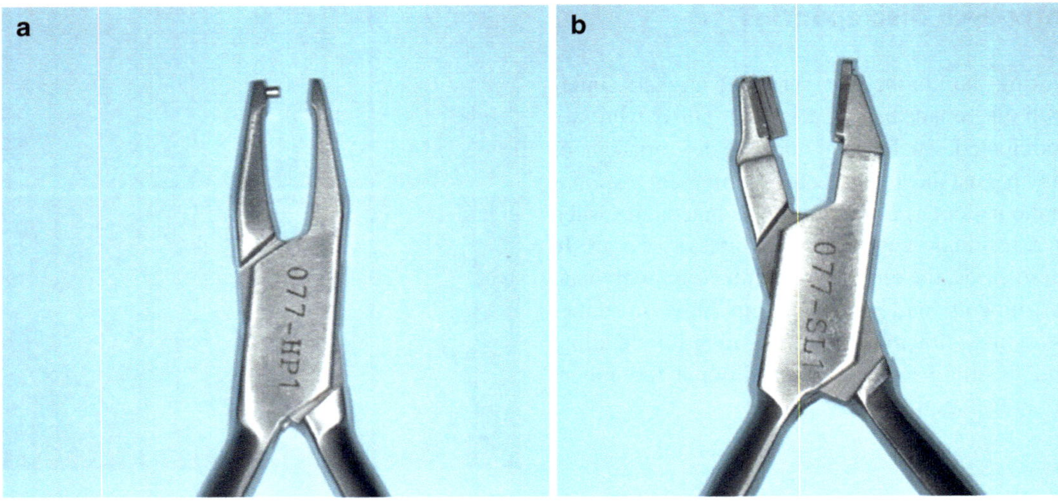

Fig. 11.12 (**a**) A hole punch plier can be useful in creating precision cuts for intermaxillary elastics or vertical elastics to opposing teeth. (**b**) The precision cut plier can create cuts for elastics wear

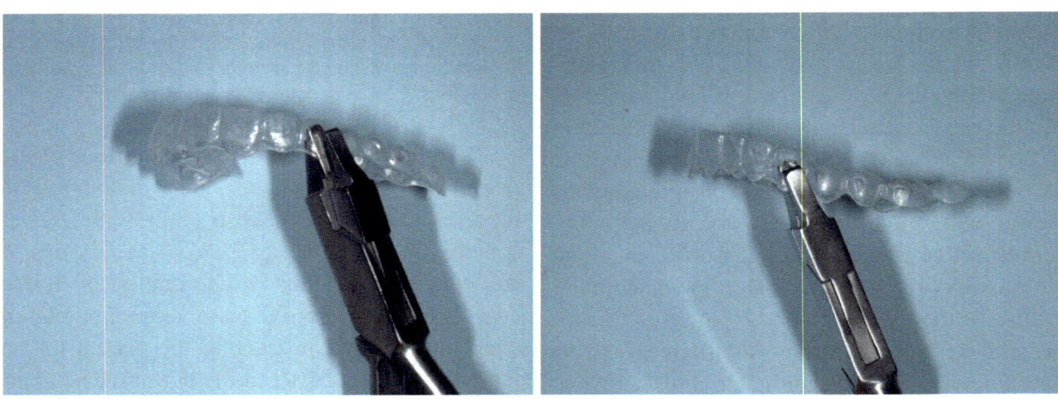

Fig. 11.13 The precision cut plier can be used for the addition of precision cuts for cross midline elastics

nonideal due to limitations in the software. For instance, in Class II patients with significant overjet, the bite ramps on the material respective to the lingual surfaces of the maxillary central and lateral incisors may not occlude with the opposing mandibular incisors. As a result, the bite ramps may not properly disocclude the posterior teeth and will therefore remain nonfunctional. The clinician can enlarge the bite ramps with the bite ramp plier so that they properly contact the opposing mandibular teeth (Fig. 11.14). Alternatively, the clinician can add bite ramps to the aligner material respective to the lingual surfaces of the maxillary canines for a greater disoccluding effect.

Anterior Open Bites

Clear aligners have been historically effective in the treatment of anterior open bites even when compared with fixed appliances (Chap. 7) [10]. However, situations may arise during a course of aligners in which the open bite has not been completely closed or more rarely, manifests for the first time during treatment. In these cases, the

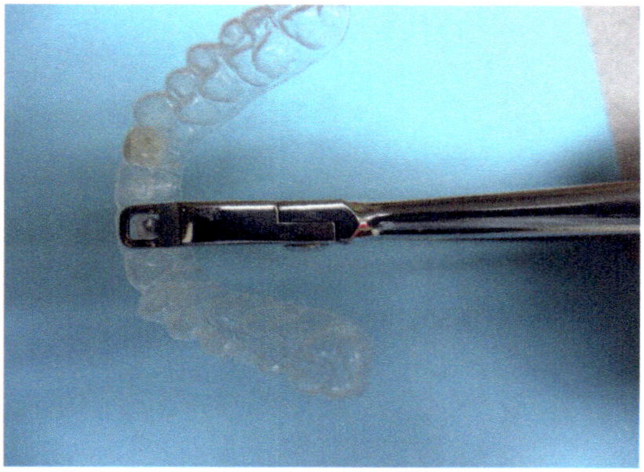

Fig. 11.14 The bite ramp plier allows the enlargement of bite ramps for contact with the mandibular incisors and proper disocclusion of the buccal segments to enhance bite opening in deep bite cases

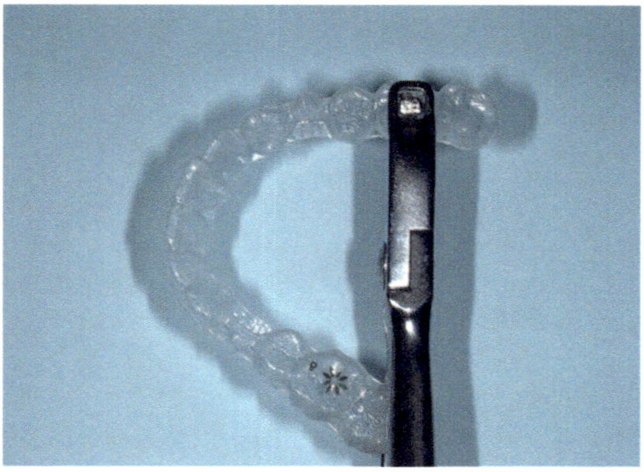

Fig. 11.15 In open bite cases, the addition of bite ramps onto maxillary molars can simulate a bite block effect and promote molar intrusion

patient will most likely require an additional course of refinement. However, the clinician can promote open bite closure by modifying aligner material to reduce total treatment time. In particular, bite ramps can be placed with a bite ramp plier on the occlusal surfaces of both maxillary or both mandibular molars to simulate the intrusive effects of a posterior bite block (Fig. 11.15). In this way, the clinician can enhance intrusive forces on maxillary or mandibular molars to promote open bite closure.

Posterior Open Bites

One of the most common criticisms leveled at clear aligner therapy is its clinical performance in finishing with solid posterior contacts and proper posterior interdigitation. In 2016, Invisalign introduced a number of enhancements in its G7 generation to improve finishing, including the minimization of posterior open bites. Specifically, heavy anterior contacts triggered the Invisalign software, which automatically created a 0.5 mm more than normal overjet to remove anterior interferences. This enhancement has lessened the frequency and severity of posterior open bites in the finishing stages of clear aligner therapy. The clinician should ensure that no heavy anterior interferences remain during Clincheck development as a means of preventing the development of posterior open bites later in treatment (we further discuss posterior open bite prevention in Chap. 12). However, despite these precautions and the incorporation of G7 innovations, posterior open bites still commonly manifest themselves. These discrepancies vary widely in severity and etiology and must be addressed with the appropriate strategy.

Minor posterior open bites which present with fewer than 1 mm interocclusal distance are most often due to the thickness of the aligner itself. These minor discrepancies can be resolved by switching the patient to nightly wear with Essix retainers to allow for occlusal settling. For a greater settling effect, the clinician can consider wraparound Hawley retainers for the maxilla and an Essix in the mandible (Fig. 11.16c–e).

Posterior open bites of moderate severity (1–2 mm interocclusal distance) are often attributed to residual heavy anterior interferences. One of the first solutions the clinician should consider is the sectioning of the maxillary aligner at the distal of the maxillary canines. The patient can then wear the sectioned canine-to-canine aligner for 4–6 weeks for extrusion of the posterior segments. If the posterior open bite persists, the cli-

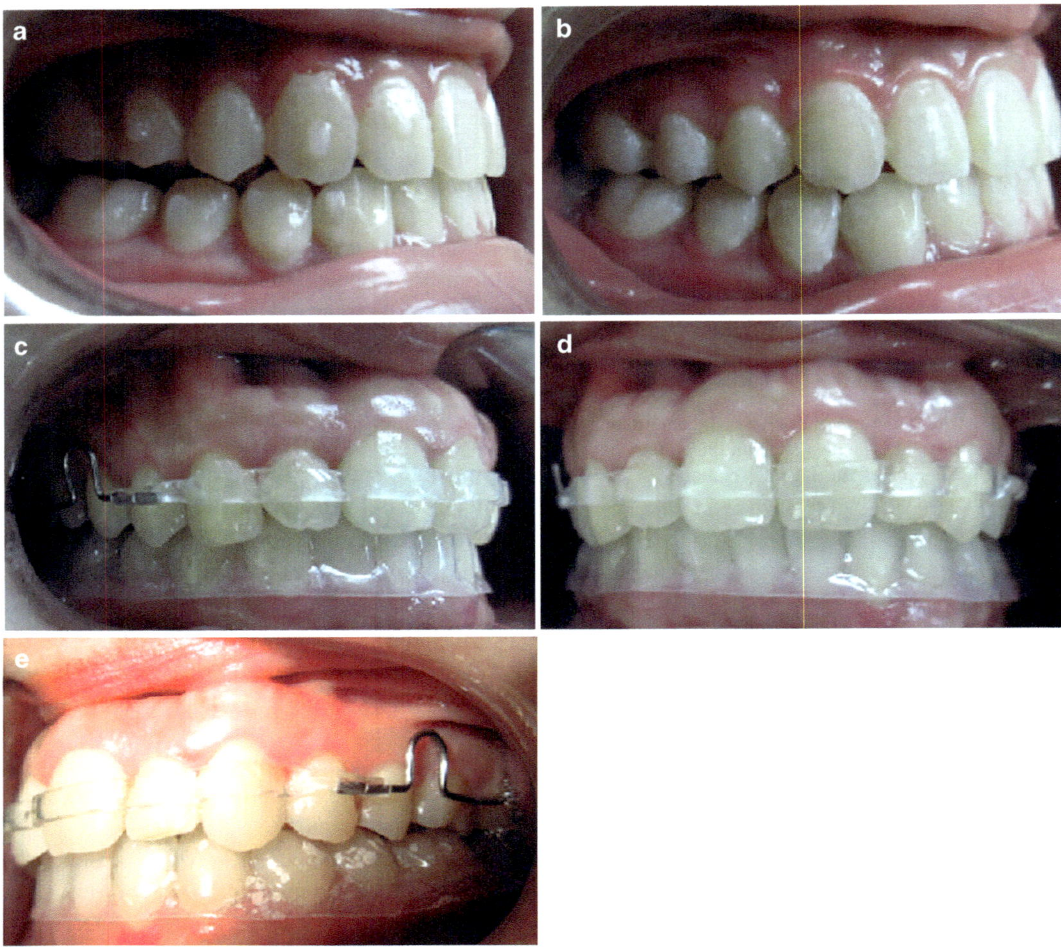

Fig. 11.16 (**a, b**) For this patient who completed a single refinement course but still showed a lateral open bite, the upper aligner was sectioned distal to both maxillary canines for settling of the posterior teeth. After 2 months of patient wear with the sectioned upper aligner, the maxillary posterior teeth extruded into ideal interdigitation. (**c–e**) During retention, a wraparound maxillary Hawley retainer can allow for occlusal settling and proper interdigitation if a mild posterior open bite persists following clear aligner treatment

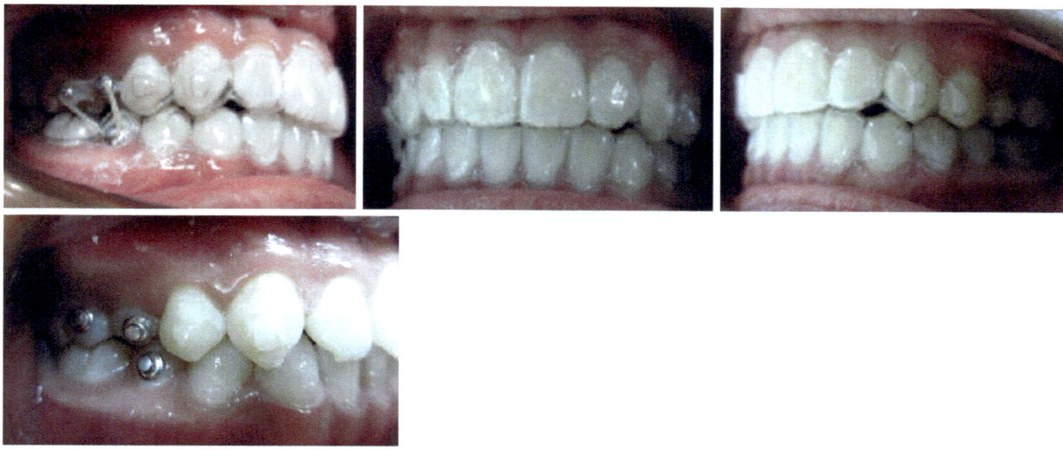

Fig. 11.17 For local posterior open bites caused by the infraeruption of 3–4 teeth, metal buttons can be bonded on the problematic teeth for a short course of vertical elastics to achieve lateral open bite closure

nician can either bond buttons and run vertical elastics between the infraerupted teeth or develop an additional refinement course to extrude the posterior segments.

Severe posterior open bites (greater than 2 mm) often result from residual heavy anterior interferences, overly tipped posterior teeth, or a combination of both. In extraction therapy, undesired tipping of premolars and molars often occurs resulting in severe lateral open bites. If the posterior open bite is local and caused by 3–4 posterior teeth, the clinician might consider vertical elastics between the improperly tipped teeth to close the open bite (Fig. 11.17). We have successfully demonstrated this method of posterior open bite closure in complex cases involving extraction therapy [11]. In other cases, when the posterior open bite is severe or widely distributed, the most effective means of closure is most likely an additional course of refinement.

In certain cases, a patient may develop a combination of an anterior open bite and lateral open bites, often due to a heavy posterior interference. This scenario is commonly seen in adolescent patients whose second maxillary or mandibular molars were not completely covered with aligner material due to complete lack of eruption or partial eruption. During treatment, the eruption of the second molars leads to a posterior premature contact and significant bite opening in both the anterior and posterior segments. The most prudent resolution would be for the clinician to rescan the arches and to develop a refinement course of aligners for coverage and intrusion of the erupting second molars for open bite closure.

Finishing for Treatment Efficacy

A number of intraocclusal and interocclusal discrepancies can arise during the finishing stages largely due to the limitations of the clear aligner appliance. A variety of methods including hand instruments and other adjunctive means can be employed for both finishing and correcting more global discrepancies during the course of treatment in order to reduce treatment time and increase effectiveness of therapy. The clinicians should exercise clinical judgment when deciding when to intervene with adjunctive measures as opposed to immediately continuing toward an additional course of refinement. There are situations when discrepancies are too significant, such as significant rotations and residual deep overbites, for hand instruments and adjunctive strategies and require more extensive intervention. Nevertheless, the appropriate use of auxiliaries can alleviate minor discrepancies as well as enhance aligner biomechanics.

References

1. Rossini, et al. Efficacy of clear aligners in controlling orthodontic tooth movement: a systematic review. Angle Orthod. 2015;85(5):881–9.
2. Izhar A, Singh G, Goyal V, Singh R, Gupta N, Pahuja P. Comparative assessment of clinical and predicted treatment outcomes of clear aligner treatment: an in vivo study. Turk J Orthod. 2019;32(4):229–35.
3. Kravitz ND, Kusnoto B, Agran B, Viana G. How well does Invisalign work? A prospective clinical study evaluating the efficacy of tooth movement with Invisalign. Am J Orthod Dentofac Orthop. 2009;35:27–35.
4. Kravitz ND, Kusnoto B, Agran B, Viana G. Influence of attachments and interproximal reduction on the accuracy of canine rotation with Invisalign: a prospective clinical study. Angle Orthod. 2008;78(4):682–7.
5. Simon M, Keilig L, Schwarze J, Jung BA, Bourauel C. Treatment outcome and efficacy of an aligner technique—regarding incisor torque, premolar derotation and molar distalization. BMC Oral Health. 2014;14:68.
6. Djeu G, Shelton C, Maganzini A. Outcome assessment of Invisalign and traditional orthodontic treatment compared with ABO objective grading system. Am J Ortho Dentofac Orthop. 2005;128:292–8.
7. Dasy H, Dasy A, Asatrian G, Rózsa N, Lee H-F, Kwak JH. Effects of variable attachment shapes and aligner material on aligner retention. Angle Orthod. 2015;85(6):934–40.
8. Ikeda Y, Kokai S, Ono T. A patient with mandibular deviation and 3 mandibular incisors treated with asymmetrically bent improved superelastic NiTi alloy wires. Am J Ortho Dentofac Orthop. 2017;153(1):131–43.
9. Papadimitriou A, Mousoulea S, Gkantidis N, Kloukos D. Clinical effectiveness of Invisalign® orthodontic treatment: a systematic review. Prog Orthod. 2018;19(1):37.
10. Garnett BS, Mahood K, Nguygen M, Al-Khateeb A, Liu S, Boyd R, Oh H. Cephalometric comparison of adult anterior open bite treatment using clear aligners and fixed appliances. Angle Orthod. 2019;89(1):3–9.
11. Cisneros G, Huang AT, Huang D. Situational extraction therapy with clear aligner therapy in complex malocclusions. Orthod Pract US. 2019;10(2):14–20.

When and How to Overcorrect? 12

Contents

The Various Roles of Overcorrection

One of the most controversial aspects of clear aligner therapy is the role of overcorrection during treatment planning and the design of virtual setups. Frequently, overcorrection serves as a measure to counteract the inaccuracy of unpredictable tooth movements. Various studies have recommended overcorrection to achieve planned movements considered difficult for clear aligners, including anterior tooth extrusion and intrusion, posterior tooth expansion, and canine and premolar derotation [1, 2]. Overcorrection should also be considered for tooth movements involved in the treatment of Class II malocclusions, especially those involving posterior teeth distalization. Studies have shown effective maxillary molar distalization within the range of 2–3 mm, but overcorrection should be considered for movements at the upper end or beyond this range to achieve desired outcomes [3].

The method of overcorrection also plays a vital role in the treatment planning of extensive jaw movements, such as mandibular autorotation for open bite closure, the simulation of jaw growth, and mandibular forward repositioning with the MA appliance (Chap. 3).

A less commonly discussed application of overcorrection is for residual space closure, especially following extractions or IPR. The planning for precise space closure can pose a dilemma, as underprescribing virtual C-chains can result in unclosed spaces, while overprescribing can cause adverse effects, such as an excessive overjet. These considerations are especially important for extraction cases, as extraction space closure has been shown to be highly unpredictable [4].

One of the most controversial uses of overcorrection has been for the proper finishing of the occlusion. Specifically, the correction of deep bites and posterior open bite closure can benefit from overcorrection [5]. However, excessive overcorrection can introduce another element of

A. T. Huang, D. Huang, *Controversies in Clear Aligner Therapy*,
https://doi.org/10.1007/978-3-030-92810-0_12

unpredictability to treatment and result in adverse effects, especially in the vertical dimension. There remains uncertainty regarding the most judicious methods of overcorrection for achieving a proper final occlusion.

Overcorrection has emerged as a viable approach for enhancing the predictability of both dental and jaw movements, as well as an essential tool for achieving a harmonious final occlusion. However, although overcorrection has been frequently referenced in the literature, its exact use has not been thoroughly discussed. To address the ambiguities surrounding overcorrection, this chapter details its indications and methods for clinical applications ranging from treatment planning challenging movements to occlusal finishing.

Indications and Methods for Overcorrection

Unpredictable Tooth Movements

Unpredictable Tooth Movements: Anterior Teeth Intrusion

One of the most common indications for overcorrection is the intrusion of maxillary and mandibular anterior teeth for the correction of deep overbites (Table 12.1). Recent studies have shown low predictability in the clinical expression of overbite reduction programmed in the Clincheck software [6]. This result is likely associated with the low accuracy of incisor intrusion, even following technological advancements, such as the G5 protocol [7]. Various studies have recommended the incorporation of auxiliary appliances, such as TADs, or the modification of the software projection, in the form of overcorrection, to improve overbite control with clear aligners [5]. The clinician should seriously consider overcorrection for severe overbites, as the deeper the initial overbite, the more difficult it will be to achieve overbite reduction [6].

Table 12.1 Indications for overcorrection among challenging tooth movements

Indications for overcorrection	Guidelines for overcorrection
Intrusion	Overcorrect 1–1.5 mm/arch
Extrusion	0.5–1 mm for extensive extrusive movements
Derotation	Overcorrect canine and premolar rotations by 5°
Expansion	Overcorrection of an additional 1 mm of expansion
Root uprighting	Overcorrection of root tip by approximately 5°
Relative extrusion/ relative intrusion	1–2 mm intrusion/1–2 mm extrusion
Lingually displaced maxillary lateral incisors	Overcorrect labial root torque by approximately 5°

Because of these limitations in the predictability of overbite control with clear aligners, it is recommended in the treatment of deep bite cases that the clinician overcorrect the amount of intrusion of maxillary incisors and mandibular incisors by 1–1.5 mm for each arch so that the programmed final occlusion shows 0 mm overbite. This is in accordance with the findings of previous studies, which have shown significant overbite reduction through the G5 protocol, adequate leveling of curves of Spee, and overcorrecting overbites to 0 mm [5]. A similar overcorrection approach can be employed in programming maxillary incisor intrusion supplemented with TADs: 2 mm of additional intrusion can be incorporated for the maxillary incisors (Fig. 12.1).

Unpredictable Tooth Movements: Anterior Teeth Extrusion

Recent studies suggest the accuracy of incisor extrusion has significantly improved from earlier generations of clear aligners [7]. These improvements are likely due to multiple factors, including the introduction of SmartTrack material in 2013, the use of optimized extrusion attachments, and variations in study designs. Studies have also observed efficacy in clear aligners for open bite closure through incisor extrusion, molar intrusion, and autorotation of the mandible. However, despite these improvements, extrusion accuracy remains low, relative to other movements such as rotation or crown tip [1]. As discussed in Chap. 7, the predictability of anterior teeth extrusion, especially in

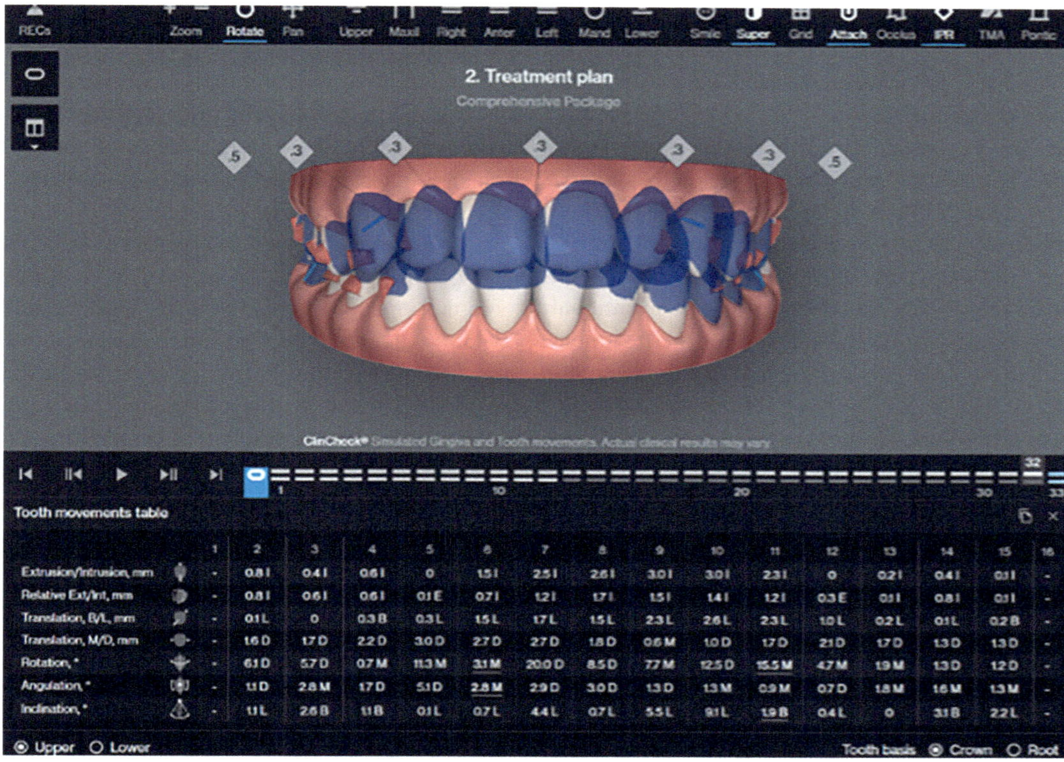

Fig. 12.1 For maxillary incisor intrusion assisted with TADs, an additional 2 mm of intrusion can be programmed to simulate the supplementary intrusive force

treatments of open bite closure where a significant amount of incisor extrusion is required, can be enhanced by combining pure extrusion with retraction for relative extrusion and through overcorrection of the movement.

Specifically, the clinician should consider an overcorrection of approximately 0.5–1 mm for extensive extrusive movements, such as those >3.5 mm, which Align Technology classifies as an advanced amount of extrusion (<2.5 mm is considered mild extrusion, while 2.5–3.5 mm is classified as moderate extrusion). Recent studies have similarly advocated for overcorrection by 0.5 ± 0.1 mm, based on a difference between predicted and achieved values for extrusion, whether with optimized or conventional attachments [1]. For open bite cases, the amount of extrusion for the maxillary and mandibular incisors can be overcorrected by 1 mm per arch to enhance the predictability of open bite closure.

Unpredictable Tooth Movements: Derotation

The rotation of canines and premolars has been shown to be imprecise when compared to planned movements on virtual setups, even in aligner systems alternative to Invisalign [8]. Various studies have shown mandibular canine rotation is one of the least accurate movements and its accuracy falls significantly in rotations exceeding 15° [9]. Because of the low accuracy in both canine and premolar rotation, since early generations of clear aligners, clinicians have recommended measures such as IPR adjacent to the tooth to be rotated, slowing down the velocity of rotation per aligner, and overcorrection [10]. Recent studies have suggested overcorrection for canines and premolars, even with the incorporation of optimized attachments [1].

Various strategies have been proposed for overcorrection in the derotation of canines and premolars, including overcorrecting by an additional 10% of the programmed amount of rotation [11]. It is recommended that the clinician overcorrect the rotations of canines and premolars by 5°, especially for rotations greater than 15°. This method was also suggested by a recent study which found the mean difference between predicted and achieved amounts of rotation ranging from 4.01° to 6.01° (with the use of optimized attachments for the former and conventional attachments for the latter) [1]. For the treatment of extremely rotated teeth, such as those requiring greater than 45° rotation, the clinician should consider adjunctive fixed appliances [12].

Unpredictable Tooth Movements: Expansion

Studies that have investigated the predictability of expansion with clear aligners have observed discrepancies between planned and achieved movements in both arches. One of the most inaccurate sites for expansion has been bodily expansion for the maxillary molars, while the canine region has been demonstrated to show greater accuracy for expansion [13]. Therefore, the clinician should consider overcorrection for significant expansion of the posterior region of the maxilla, especially for the first and second maxillary molars.

Studies have observed in the treatments of patients with transverse malocclusions, a discrepancy between predicted and achieved values of expansion of 0.69 mm at the first molar, 0.81 mm at the second premolar, and 0.77 mm at the first premolar [2]. To correct for this inaccuracy, in cases that require significant maxillary expansion, such as patients with teeth in posterior crossbite, an overcorrection of an additional 1 mm of expansion can be incorporated for the posterior segment with the transverse discrepancy to achieve desired outcomes. In addition to overcorrecting the amount of expansion, the clinician should also consider presetting buccal root torque for posterior expansion due to the low accuracy of bodily expansion with clear aligners (although this efficacy may have improved since the incorporation of Invisalign's G8 modifications).

Unpredictable Tooth Movements: Complex Movements

We have discussed the significance of overcorrection for complex movements, such as molar uprighting and root torquing. Studies on the performance of clear aligners in extraction cases have suggested overcorrecting the distal tip by 6° on first molars adjacent to extraction spaces to maintain root angulation and to achieve more bodily tooth movement [4]. For significant space closure in both extraction and non-extraction cases, the amount of root tip may have to be overcorrected in the teeth adjacent to the edentulous space for bodily movement and proper root parallelism.

For extensive space closure, the virtual gable bend should be requested as a form of overcorrection to help ensure root parallelism. Similarly, for significant root tipping for uprighting teeth, such as in the preparation for implant restorations, the clinician should consider overcorrecting the amount of root tip by approximately 5° to achieve desired movements.

Controlling the Vertical Position of Incisors

Studies on efficacy of clear aligners in first premolar extractions have shown greater loss of torque than planned in incisors during retraction, resulting in relative extrusion of incisors and undesired deepening of overbite [4]. A loss of torque also occurs even with the application of attachments or power ridges [14]. To control the vertical position and angulation of incisors during significant retraction, it has been recommended to overcorrect lingual root torque for the maxillary incisors. Additionally, the clinician should consider overcorrection of the amount of intrusion prescribed for the maxillary incisors to counteract the relative extrusion associated with loss of torque. Similarly, in non-extraction cases with significant retraction of the maxillary or mandibular incisors, overcorrection should be considered for both torque and intrusion of the incisors to be retracted.

Conversely, for incisors planned for movements associated with relative intrusion, the clinician should consider overcorrection for the amount of extrusion to maintain the desired vertical position of the incisors. For example, for cases involving expansion or significant labialization of the incisors, such as the protraction of maxillary incisors for the treatment of Class III malocclusions, extrusive movements should be incorporated to counteract the relative intrusion associated with labialization (Fig. 12.2).

For incisors planned for significant retraction, the clinician can incorporate power ridges in addition to an overcorrection of 1–2 mm intrusion to counteract loss of torque and relative extrusion. Likewise, for incisors that will be labialized, an overcorrection of 1–2 mm extrusion can be employed to compensate for the effects of relative intrusion.

Irregularly Positioned Teeth

Severely displaced teeth, such as high maxillary canines or lingually displaced maxillary lateral incisors, will require difficult movements including extrusion and derotation. Overcorrection should be incorporated as high maxillary canines will require extensive extrusion, which as discussed, remains a weakness for clear aligner therapy. The clinician should consider an overcorrection of an additional 1 mm extrusion for high maxillary canines to counteract the unpredictability of the appliance in extrusive movements, as observed in previous studies. Often, even with overcorrection, high maxillary canines will need auxiliary measures, such as vertical elastics for a supplementary extrusive force, for ideal finishing.

Lingually displaced maxillary lateral incisors will typically require significant derotation, exceeding 15°, and therefore warrant overcorrection of approximately 5°. The roots of these lateral incisors also tend to be lingually inclined and often require labial root torque to achieve

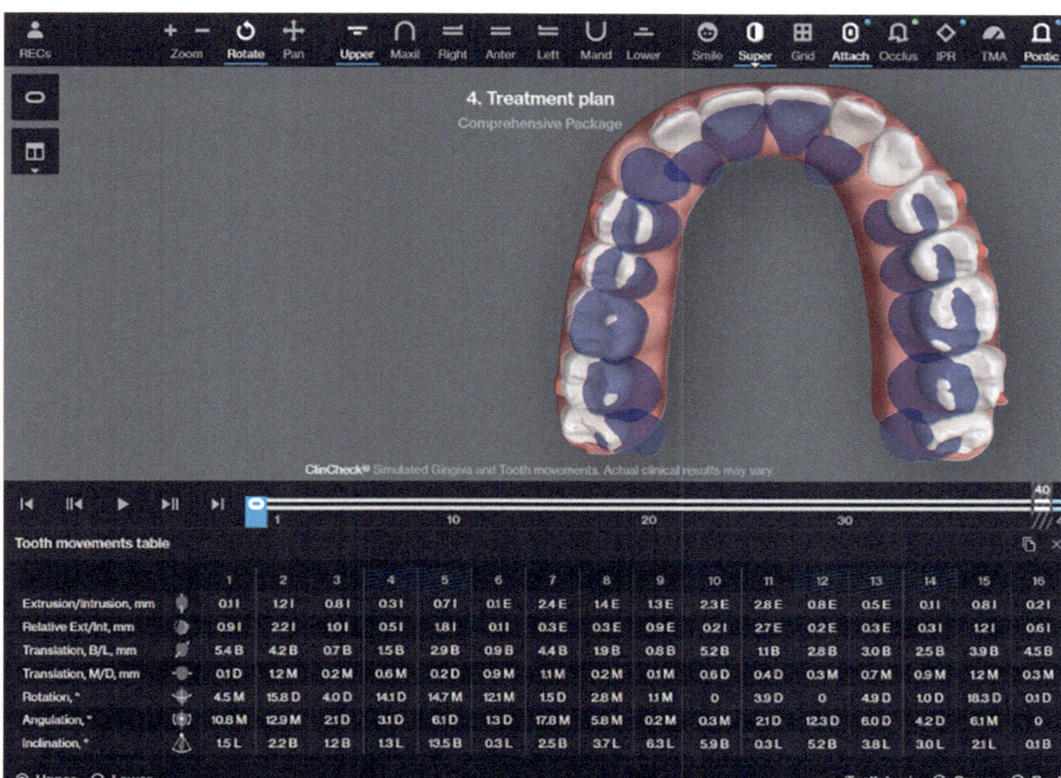

	1	2	3	4	5	6	7	8	9	10	11	12	13	14	15	16
Extrusion/Intrusion, mm	0.1 I	1.2 I	0.8 I	0.3 I	0.7 I	0.1 E	2.4 E	1.4 E	1.3 E	2.3 E	2.8 E	0.8 E	0.5 E	0.1 I	0.8 I	0.2 I
Relative Ext/Int, mm	0.9 I	2.2 I	1.0 I	0.5 I	1.8 I	0.1 I	0.3 E	0.3 E	0.9 E	0.2 I	2.7 E	0.2 E	0.3 E	0.3 I	1.2 I	0.6 I
Translation, B/L, mm	5.4 B	4.2 B	0.7 B	1.5 B	2.9 B	0.9 B	4.4 B	1.9 B	0.8 B	5.2 B	1.1 B	2.8 B	3.0 B	2.5 B	3.9 B	4.5 B
Translation, M/D, mm	0.1 D	1.2 M	0.2 M	0.6 M	0.2 D	0.9 M	1.1 M	0.2 M	0.1 M	0.6 D	0.4 D	0.3 M	0.7 M	0.9 M	1.2 M	0.3 M
Rotation, °	4.5 M	15.8 D	4.0 D	14.1 D	14.7 M	12.1 M	1.5 D	2.8 M	1.1 M	0	3.9 D	0	4.9 D	1.0 D	18.3 D	0.1 D
Angulation, °	10.8 M	12.9 M	2.1 D	3.1 D	6.1 D	1.3 D	17.8 M	5.8 M	0.2 M	0.3 M	2.1 D	12.3 D	6.0 D	4.2 D	6.1 M	0
Inclination, °	1.5 L	2.2 B	1.2 B	1.3 L	13.5 B	0.3 L	2.5 B	3.7 L	6.3 L	5.9 B	0.3 L	5.2 B	3.8 L	3.0 L	2.1 L	0.1 B

Fig. 12.2 For incisors to be labialized by significant amounts, the clinician should consider overcorrecting extrusion by 1–2 mm to compensate for relative intrusion

proper labiolingual inclination. As clear aligners tend to perform inaccurately with torque control, it would be prudent for the clinician to overcorrect for labial root torque by approximately 5° [14].

Unpredictable Jaw Movements

Mandibular Autorotation

We have discussed the significance of posterior intrusion for mandibular autorotation and successful open bite closure (Chap. 7). Though the intrusion of mandibular second molars has been shown to be more accurate than their extrusion, intrusion remains unpredictable at about 50% accuracy [7]. A study on the efficacy of open bite closure with clear aligners without auxiliaries demonstrated that even with intrusion programmed into the trays, a mean of only about 0.6 mm of intrusion of maxillary molars and 0.4 mm of intrusion of mandibular molars were achieved during treatment [15]. These data suggest in severe open bite cases, measures such as overcorrection and skeletal anchorage should be employed to enhance molar intrusion.

For severe open bite cases, the clinician should consider overcorrection by an additional 1 mm of intrusion for both the maxillary and mandibular molars (Table 12.2). This amount of overcorrection should also be incorporated for TAD-supported molar intrusion to realistically simulate the effects of supplementary intrusive force from the TADs.

Table 12.2 Indications for overcorrection among jaw movements

Indications for overcorrection	Guidelines for overcorrection
Molar intrusion for mandibular autorotation	Additional 1 mm for maxillary and (or) mandibular molars
MA appliance	Correction to 1–2 mm beyond edge-to-edge for severe discrepancies
Orthopedic treatment of growing Class III patient	Overcorrect positive overjet by 1–2 mm

Jaw Growth in Growing Patients

As discussed in Chap. 3, the MA appliance advances the mandible, typically in a stepwise fashion, for the treatment of Class II malocclusions. The position of the mandible should be overcorrected to an edge-to-edge incisor relationship with slightly overcorrected Class I canine and molar relationships, bilaterally (Fig. 12.3). This method accounts for relapse and simulates the protocol successfully employed in treatments with the Herbst appliance, which frequently advance the mandible to edge-to-edge incisor relationships [16]. For cases requiring significant advancement, such as an overjet >6 mm, the clinician should consider overcorrection of the mandible 1–2 mm forward of the edge-to-edge position so that the canines and molars will lie in Class III relationships, bilaterally.

Conversely, the virtual setups for the orthopedic treatment of a growing Class III patient, such as with the RPFM, should be overcorrected so that the final occlusion shows 1–2 mm of positive anterior overjet (Fig. 12.4). This setup will account for the supplementary orthopedic forces applied to the maxilla and maxillary teeth. Studies have also frequently recommended overcorrection in skeletal Class III correction for long-term stability [17].

Occlusal Finishing

Overjet

As discussed in Chap. 11, one of the most frequent challenges of clear aligner therapy is the development of a posterior open bite during treatment. Though some practitioners have claimed that posterior open bites can be attributed to intrusion of the molars from a bite block effect of the clear aligners, recent studies have shown posterior intrusion does not occur with clear aligners when not prescribed [18]. Therefore, it is likely that most posterior open bites are due to heavy anterior interferences. The primary method for avoiding heavy anterior interferences is to confirm light contacts in the maxillary and mandibular anterior teeth within the final occlusion of the

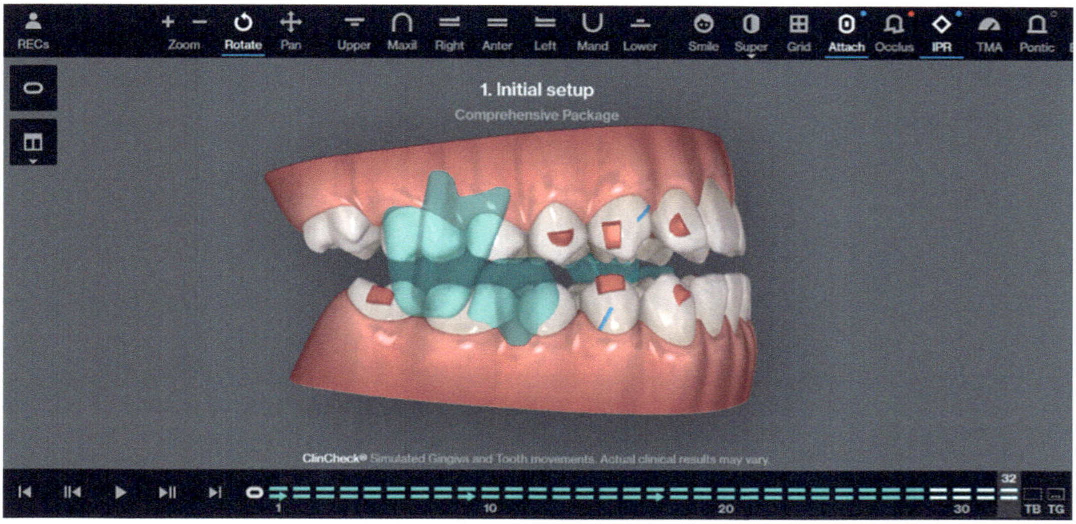

Fig. 12.3 For cases with severe overjets treated with the MA appliance, the clinician shoulder consider overcorrecting the final occlusion to Class III molar and canine relationships and 1 mm beyond the edge-to-edge position. This approach can more predictably achieve ideal sagittal relationships and overjet reduction

virtual setup. The clinician should also set a 0.5 mm more than normal overjet of 1–2 mm to reduce the likelihood of heavy anterior interferences (the G7 modifications may automatically trigger this default overcorrection in the Invisalign system, which the clinician should consider accepting during the development of the virtual setup).

Overbite

In programming the final overbite in the virtual setup for the treatment of deep bite cases, the clinician should consider overcorrection of 0.5–1 mm for both the maxillary and mandibular incisors to approximately 0 mm overbite, as suggested by studies on efficacy of incisor intrusion with clear aligners [19]. It is important to note that overcorrection to beyond 0 mm overbite is not recommended, as this method may result in an anterior open bite if the patient is not closely monitored.

Posterior Interdigitation

Often, the reduction or equilibration of heavy anterior interferences may not be adequate for the closure of a posterior open bite. Instead, the posterior teeth may have to be extruded for proper interdigitation. Because extrusion of posterior teeth remains inaccurate relative to movements like crown tipping and intrusion and the amount of extrusion necessary is typically extensive, exceeding 0.5 mm, it is recommended that the clinician overcorrect extrusion of posterior teeth within 0.5 mm to achieve posterior open bite closure (Fig. 12.5).

Residual Space Closure

Virtual C-Chain

The judicious use of virtual C-chains, the equivalent of the power chain in fixed appliances, is essential for proper closure of residual spaces in both extraction and non-extraction cases and the avoidance of adverse effects, such as excessive overjet or undesired tipping. In premolar extraction cases, the canine to canine C-chain should not be employed or employed sparingly, as its overuse will result in the reopening of extraction spaces distal to the canines. Instead, in these cases, a first molar to first molar or second molar to second molar C-chain should be requested for complete closure of all residual spaces. A canine to canine C-chain is suitable for cases with extractions of exclusively anterior teeth, such as a single mandibular incisor.

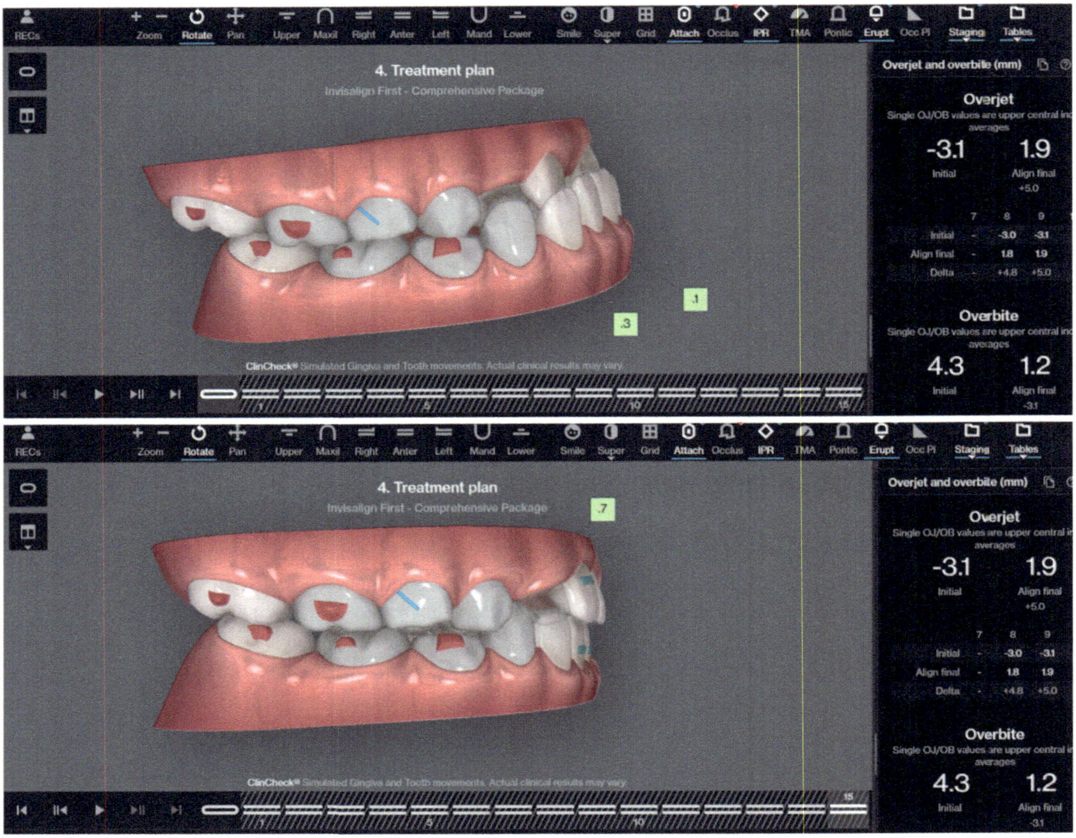

Fig. 12.4 Orthopedic treatment of growing patients with Class III patients should employ a bite jump with overcorrected amount of positive overjet. This method accounts for the supplementary forces supplied by orthopedic maxillary protraction

For non-extraction cases, a C-chain from canine to canine can be employed for cases involving anterior spacing or exclusively anterior IPR. Typically, a single C-chain should be adequate if the IPR prescribed were not excessive for the initial severity of crowding. However, for non-extraction cases with generalized spacing or requiring posterior IPR, a first molar to first molar or second molar to second molar C-chain, rather than a canine to canine chain, should be requested for complete closure of all residual spaces.

The overuse of C-chains can result in adverse effects, such as the skewing of the arches, the tipping of posterior teeth due to significant mesial movement without adequate root control, and posterior open bite due to the tipping of posterior teeth (Fig. 12.6). Excessive use of C-chains in the mandibular arch can result in over-retraction of the mandibular incisors and increased overjet. Therefore, C-chains should be used in a conservative fashion to prevent compromising proper occlusal outcomes. In most cases, a single C-chain for either arch should be adequate; if greater than one C-chain for a single arch is necessary, then the clinician should program passive aligners for the opposing arch to avoid excessive movements.

Distalization

Studies have shown that clear aligners in the absence of auxiliaries can distalize molars by approximately 2 mm without significant tipping

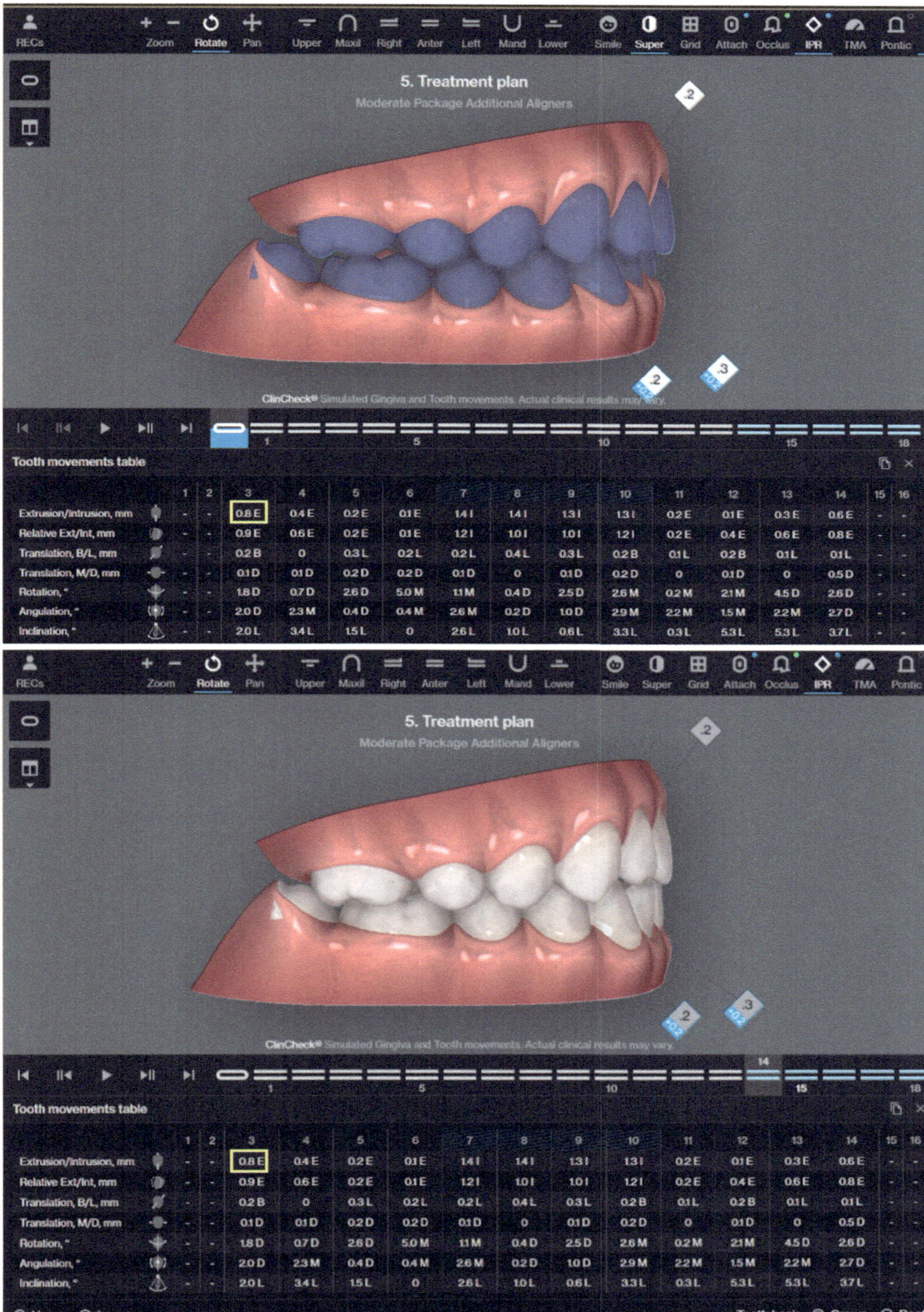

Fig. 12.5 It is recommended that the clinician overcorrect the extrusion of posterior teeth within 0.5 mm when seeking to achieve ideal interdigitation. In this case, the amount of extrusion for the right maxillary first molar has been overcorrected by about 0.3 mm

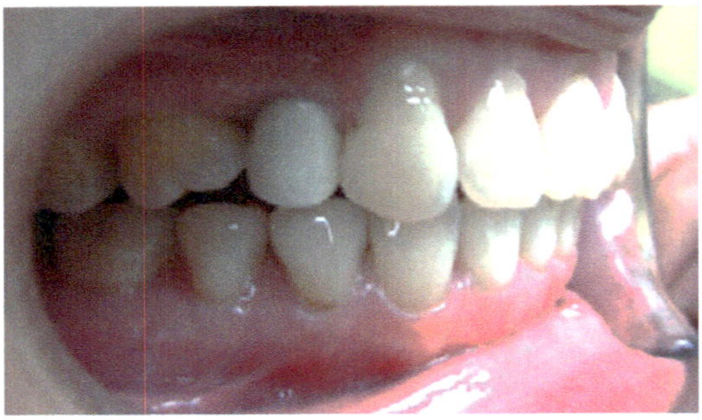

Fig. 12.6 The excessive application of VCCs can result in tipping of posterior teeth. In this patient, excessive VCCs for the maxillary arch resulted in tipping of the right maxillary first molar. This tipping was treated by bonding a metal button on the mesiobuccal cusp of the right maxillary first molar and short round of vertical elastics to the opposing arch

or extrusive movements [3]. Distal movements of molars significantly greater than 2 mm are likely to be more unpredictable than more minor movements. As a result, for extensive distalization of molars, such as movements exceeding 2 mm, the clinician should consider auxiliaries, such as a bonded molar distalizer, and overcorrect the amount of distalization by 0.5–1 mm to account for the supplementary distalizing force (Fig. 12.7).

A Conservative Approach for Overcorrection

Despite an abundance of conflicting perspectives on the proper use of overcorrection, there exist clear indications for its application in challenging

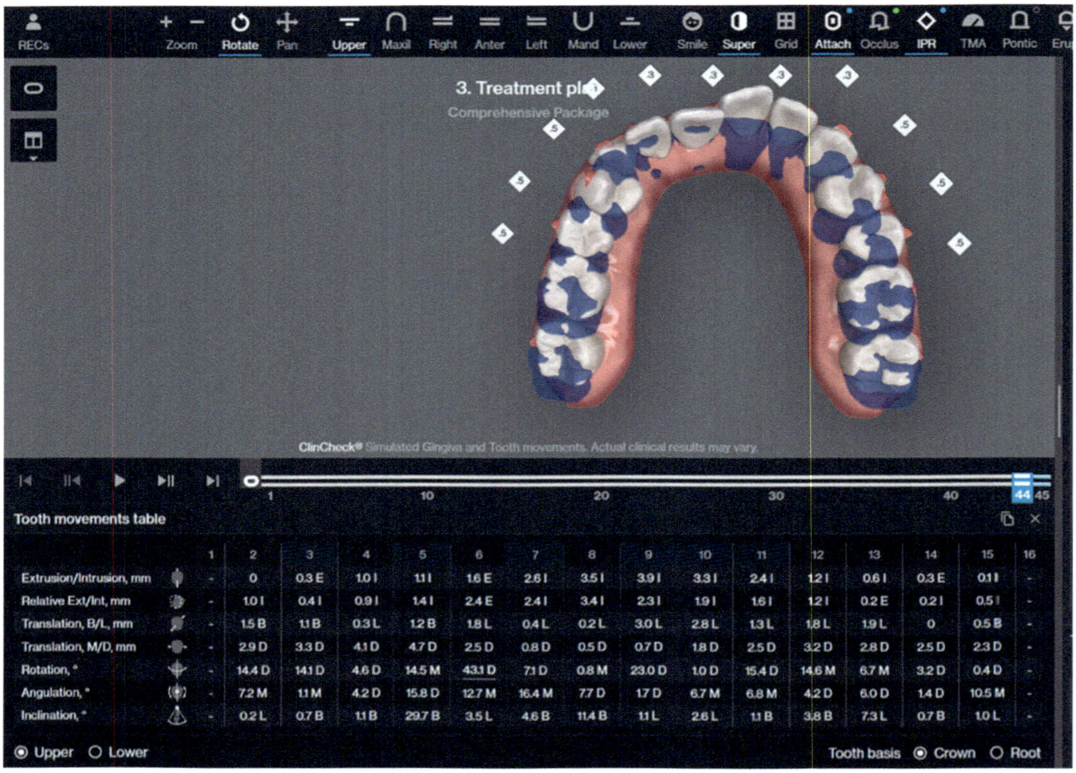

	1	2	3	4	5	6	7	8	9	10	11	12	13	14	15	16
Extrusion/Intrusion, mm	-	0	0.3 E	1.0 I	1.1 I	1.6 E	2.6 I	3.5 I	3.9 I	3.3 I	2.4 I	1.2 I	0.6 I	0.3 E	0.1 I	-
Relative Ext/Int, mm	-	1.0 I	0.4 I	0.9 I	1.4 I	2.4 E	2.4 I	3.4 I	2.3 I	1.9 I	1.6 I	1.2 I	0.2 E	0.2 I	0.5 I	-
Translation, B/L, mm	-	1.5 B	1.1 B	0.3 L	1.2 B	1.8 L	0.4 L	0.2 L	3.0 L	2.8 L	1.3 L	1.8 L	1.9 L	0	0.5 B	-
Translation, M/D, mm	-	2.9 D	3.3 D	4.1 D	4.7 D	2.5 D	0.8 D	0.5 D	0.7 D	1.8 D	2.5 D	3.2 D	2.8 D	2.5 D	2.3 D	-
Rotation, °	-	14.4 D	14.1 D	4.6 D	14.5 M	43.1 D	7.1 D	0.8 M	23.0 D	1.0 D	15.4 D	14.6 M	6.7 M	3.2 D	0.4 D	-
Angulation, °	-	7.2 M	1.1 M	4.2 D	15.8 D	12.7 M	16.4 M	7.7 D	1.7 D	6.7 M	6.8 M	4.2 D	6.0 D	1.4 D	10.5 M	-
Inclination, °	-	0.2 L	0.7 B	1.1 B	29.7 B	3.5 L	4.6 B	11.4 B	1.1 L	2.6 L	1.1 B	3.8 B	7.3 L	0.7 B	1.0 L	-

Fig. 12.7 Maxillary distalization supplemented with distalizing appliances should be represented by overcorrecting the amounts of distalization for the maxillary posterior teeth. For patient A.C., who received treatment with clear aligners and a Carriere distalizer, the amount of distalization programmed for the maxillary posterior teeth was overcorrected by about 0.5 mm

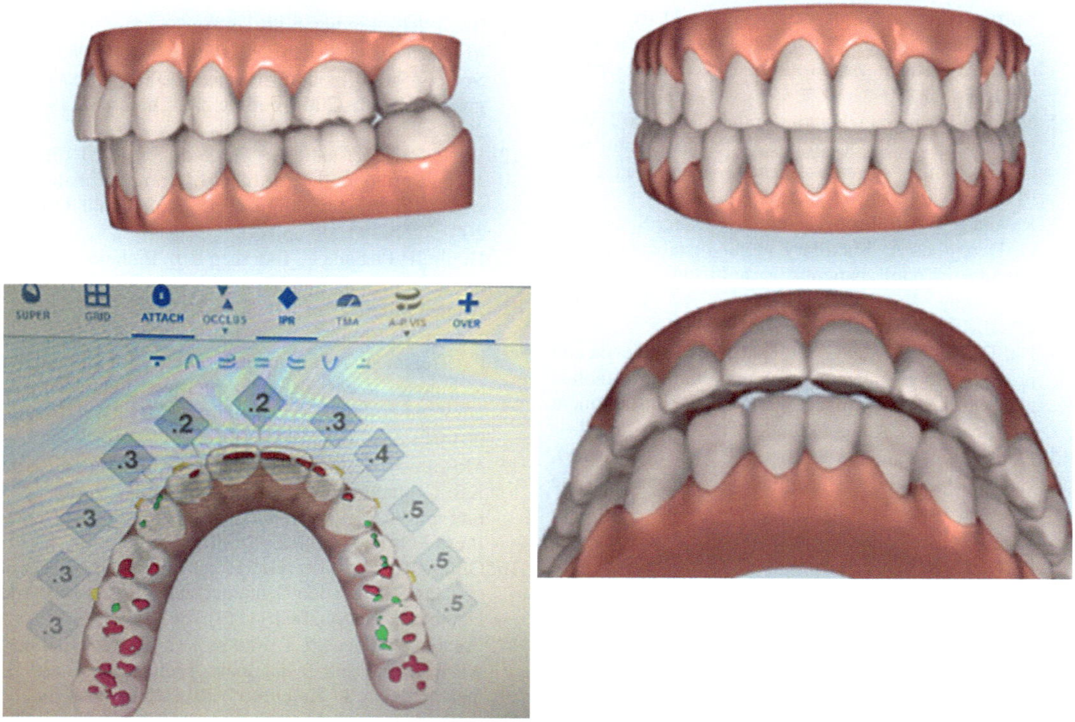

Fig. 12.8 Ideal overjet should not be deliberately compromised for the sake of preventing heavy anterior contacts. Above, the clinician has deliberately increased overjet and added excessively heavy posterior contacts to minimize anterior contacts. However, this maneuver results in an end-on Class II canine relationship, as well as a nonideal excessive overjet. Instead, the clinician should consider alternative measures, such as adjusting maxillary and mandibular incisor inclinations or incorporating intrusion to these incisors. The clinician can also accept Invisalign's G7 default adjustment for minimizing anterior interferences

movements, modeling jaw movements, and occlusal finishing. The method has been shown to be viable for improving the predictability of both teeth and jaw movements.

Nevertheless, overcorrection should be applied in a conservative, targeted manner, as its overuse can adversely affect occlusal outcomes. Notably, the overuse of virtual C-chains can result in excessive overjet, molar tipping, posterior open bites, and crowding. Similarly, overcorrection should not be employed in a manner that compromises another aspect of the occlusion. For example, the overjet should not be significantly increased for the prevention of heavy anterior interferences and posterior open bites (Fig. 12.8). Instead, the clinician should find alternative therapeutic means to maintain an acceptable overjet while minimizing heavy anterior interferences, such as adjusting the maxillary and mandibular incisor inclinations or intruding the maxillary or mandibular incisors.

The rapidly evolving nature of clear aligner therapy suggests that improvements will occur in the accuracy of tooth movement. For example, studies have shown a significant increase in the accuracy of incisor extrusion between generations of Invisalign. Therefore, the methods of overcorrection will also have to evolve to remain abreast of these improvements for the appliance.

References

1. Karras T, Singh M, Karkazis E, Liu D, Nimeri G, Ahuja B. Efficacy of Invisalign attachments: a retrospective study. Am J Orthod Dentofac Orthop. 2021;160(2):250–8.
2. Morales-Burruezo I, Gandía-Franco JL, Cobo J, Vela-Hernández A, Bellot-Arcís C. Arch expansion with the Invisalign system: efficacy and predictability. PLoS One. 2020;15(12):e0242979.
3. Ravera S, Castroflorio T, Garino F, Daher S, Cugliari G, Deregibus A. Maxillary molar distalization with aligners in adult patients: a multicenter retrospective study. Prog Orthod. 2016;17:12. https://doi.org/10.1186/s40510-016-0126-0.
4. Dai FF, Xu TM, Shu G. Comparison of achieved and predicted tooth movement of maxillary first molars and central incisors: first premolar extraction treatment with Invisalign. Angle Orthod. 2019;89(5):679–87.
5. Khosravi R, Cohanim B, Hujoel P, Daher S, Neal M, Liu W, Huang G. Management of overbite with the Invisalign appliance. Am J Orthod Dentofac Orthop. 2017;151(4):691–699.e2.
6. Blundell HL, Weir T, Kerr B, Freer E. Predictability of overbite control with the Invisalign appliance. Am J Orthod Dentofac Orthop. 2021;160:725–31:S0889–5406(21)00441–8.
7. Haouili N, Kravitz ND, Vaid NR, Ferguson DJ, Makki L. Has Invisalign improved? A prospective follow-up study on the efficacy of tooth movement with Invisalign. Am J Orthod Dentofac Orthop. 2020;158(3):420–5.
8. Lombardo L, Arreghini A, Ramina F, Huanca Ghislanzoni LT, Siciliani G. Predictability of orthodontic movement with orthodontic aligners: a retrospective study. Prog Orthod. 2017;18(1):35.
9. Kravitz ND, Kusnoto B, Agran B, Viana G. Influence of attachments and interproximal reduction on the accuracy of canine rotation with Invisalign. A prospective clinical study. Angle Orthod. 2008;78(4):682–7.
10. Boyd RL. Predictability of successful orthodontic treatment using Invisalign. The Greater Philadelphia Society of Orthodontists page. 2002. http://www.gpso.org/events/2003_outline.pdf. Accessed 12 Sep 2021.
11. Boyd RL. Predictability of successful orthodontic treatment using Invisalign. The Greater Philadelphia Society of Orthodontists page. 2002. http://www.gpso.org/events/2003_outline.pdf. Accessed 19 Sep 2021.
12. Boyd RL, Vlaskalic V. Three-dimensional diagnosis and orthodontic treatment of complex malocclusion with the Invisalign appliance. Semin Orthod. 2001;7:274–93.
13. Houle JP, Piedade L, Todescan R Jr, Pinheiro FH. The predictability of transverse changes with Invisalign. Angle Orthod. 2017;87(1):19–24.
14. Simon M, Keilig L, Schwarze J, Jung BA, Bourauel C. Treatment outcome and efficacy of an aligner technique—regarding incisor torque, premolar derotation and molar distalization. BMC Oral Health. 2014;14:68–74.
15. Moshiri S, Araújo EA, McCray JF, Thiesen G, Kim KB. Cephalometric evaluation of adult anterior open bite non-extraction treatment with Invisalign. Dental Press J Orthod. 2017;22(5):30–8.
16. Obijou C, Pancherz H. Herbst appliance treatment of Class II, division 2 malocclusions. Am J Orthod Dentofac Orthop. 2002;112(3):287–91.
17. Franchi L, Baccetti T, Masucci C, Defraia E. Early Alt-RAMEC and facial mask protocol in Class III malocclusion. J Clin Orthod. 2011;45(11):601–9.
18. Rask H, English JD, Colville C, Kasper FK, Gallerano R, Jacob HB. Cephalometric evaluation of changes in vertical dimension and molar position in adult non-extraction treatment with clear aligners and traditional fixed appliances. Dental Press J Orthod. 2021;26(4):e2119360.
19. Al-Balaa M, Li H, Ma Mohamed A, Xia L, Liu W, Chen Y, Omran T, Li S, Hua X. Predicted and actual outcome of anterior intrusion with Invisalign assessed with cone-beam computed tomography. Am J Orthod Dentofac Orthop. 2021;159(3):e275–80.

Index

A. T. Huang, D. Huang, *Controversies in Clear Aligner Therapy*,
https://doi.org/10.1007/978-3-030-92810-0

GPSR Compliance

The European Union's (EU) General Product Safety Regulation (GPSR) is a set of rules that requires consumer products to be safe and our obligations to ensure this.

If you have any concerns about our products, you can contact us on ProductSafety@springernature.com

In case Publisher is established outside the EU, the EU authorized representative is:

Springer Nature Customer Service Center GmbH
Europaplatz 3
69115 Heidelberg, Germany

Batch number: 10732801

Printed by Printforce, the Netherlands